Neonatal Infections

To Carmel and Marianne for their constant support.

Neonatal Infections

David Isaacs, MD, MRCP, FRACP
Wellcome Trust Senior Lecturer and Honorary Consultant, Department of
Paediatrics, John Radcliffe Hospital, Oxford, UK
Currently Head, Department of Immunology and Infectious Diseases, Royal
Alexandra Hospital for Children, Sydney, Australia

and

E. Richard Moxon, MA, FRCP
Professor and Head of Paediatrics, University of Oxford Department of
Paediatrics, John Radcliffe Hospital, Oxford, UK

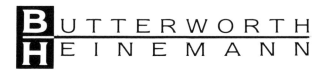

Butterworth-Heinemann Ltd
Linacre House, Jordan Hill, Oxford OX2 8DP

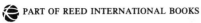 PART OF REED INTERNATIONAL BOOKS

OXFORD   LONDON   BOSTON
MUNICH   NEW DELHI   SINGAPORE   SYDNEY
TOKYO   TORONTO   WELLINGTON

First published 1991

British Library Cataloguing in Publication Data
Isaacs, David
    Neonatal infections.
    I. Title   II. Moxon, E. Richard
    618.92

Library of Congress Cataloguing in Publication Data
A catalogue record for this book is available from the Library of Congress

ISBN 0 7506 1319 X

Photoset, printed and bound in Great Britain by
Redwood Press Limited, Melksham, Wiltshire

Contents

Appendices

Preface

The signs of neonatal sepsis are often subtle: they may be poorly localized and not specifically indicative of infection, so may therefore be mimicked by many non-infectious conditions. Untreated sepsis results in rapid deterioration which is often irreversible. When sepsis is suspected, therefore, the rule in neonatal medicine is to treat early, with or without the benefits of ancillary laboratory tests, and before the results of cultures are available. This appropriate but empirical approach to the management of suspected sepsis generates many problems. The neonatologist has to decide whether invasive investigations, such as lumbar puncture and suprapubic aspiration of urine, should be performed on all babies before starting antibiotics; which babies should be treated, and the relative importance of laboratory and clinical criteria in deciding who to treat; whether to prescribe antibiotics according to a general antibiotic policy or based on the circumstantial evidence provided by surveillance cultures; and how long to continue antibiotics if subsequent cultures are negative.

Because antibiotics are frequently prescribed in neonatal units, often for long periods, selection of organisms resistant to one or many antibiotics is a perennial problem. The incidence of fungal infections is increasing, particularly in infants of very low birth-weight. The intensive care environment and the extreme susceptibility of the babies who are relatively immunocompromised and justifiably subjected to invasive procedures make hospital-acquired infections a major consideration.

The neonatologist may be consulted by obstetric colleagues about the timing of preterm delivery, the relative importance of infection and prematurity in preterm prolonged rupture of the membranes and the possible benefits of giving antibiotics to the mother to prevent neonatal infection.

This book is not intended as a comprehensive reference work on neonatal infections. There are medical textbooks in which specific problems with infection are dealt with in a learned and exhaustive manner. Our intention is to offer a personal view of the principles and thinking behind the management of neonatal infections, caused by bacteria, viruses and fungi, both in terms of individual babies and in the wider context of all babies in the newborn nursery.

We would like to thank Andrew Wilkinson, Peter Hope, David Lindsell, Simon Dobson, and our other colleagues for frequent discussions on aspects of neonatal infection; Jonathan Austyn and Katharine Wood for their excellent lectures which formed the basis for the chapter on immunity in this book; the Department of Medical Illustration for their fine art-work; and Gail Davies, Claire Deeley and Betty Nicholson for secretarial assistance. The radiographs are predominantly courtesy of Dr Lindsell and the X-ray Department at the John Radcliffe Hospital, Oxford. The following colleagues and friends kindly provided constructive comments on different chapters in the book: Carole Baker, John Bennett, Simon Dobson, David Dorman, Morven Edwards, Maureen Gapes, Peter Hope, Jerome Klein, Bob Leggiadro, John Modlin, John Nelson, Francisco Noya, Tim Townsend and Andrew Wilkinson. We would also like to thank all the junior doctors, nursing and other staff on the neonatal unit whose energy and enthusiasm has helped us to study newborn babies and to formulate our ideas about neonatal infections.

David Isaacs
E. Richard Moxon

Abbreviations

ADCC	antibody-dependent cellular toxicity
ADH	antidiuretic hormone
AZT	zidovudine
BCG	bacille Calmette-Guérin
CIE	countercurrent immuno-electrophoresis
CMV	cytomegalovirus
CNS	central nervous system
CPAP	constant positive airway pressure
CRP	C-reactive protein
CSF	cerebrospinal fluid
CT	computed tomography
CTL	cytotoxic T lymphocyte
DHSS	Department of Health and Social Security
DIC	disseminated intravascular coagulation/coagulopathy
DMSO	dimethylsulphoxide
DNA	deoxyribonucleic acid
DPT	diphtheria, pertussis, tetanus
DTPA	diethylenetriamine penta-acetate
EEG	electroencephalogram
ECG	electrocardiogram
ELISA	enzyme-linked immunosorbent assay
EPEC	enteropathogenic *E. coli*
ESR	erythrocyte sedimentation rate
ETA	endotracheal (tube) aspirate
ETEC	enterotoxigenic *E. coli*
FTA	fluorescent treponemal antibody
GBS	group B streptococcus
GFR	glomerular filtration rate
GI	gastrointestinal
G6PD	glucose-6-phosphate dehydrogenase
HBcAg	hepatitis B core antigen
HBeAg	hepatitis B e antigen
HBIg	hepatitis B immunoglobulin
HBsAg	hepatitis B surface antigen
HIV	human immunodeficiency virus
HSV	herpes simplex virus
ICP	intracranial pressure
IDU	idoxuridine
IgA	immunoglobulin A

IgG	immunoglobulin G
IgM	immunoglobulin M
i.m.	intramuscular
IMV	intermittent mandatory ventilation
IPPV	intermittent positive pressure ventilation
i.v.	intravenous
IVP	intravenous pyelography
LP	lumbar puncture
LPA	latex particle agglutination
MBC	minimum bactericidal concentration
MCU	micturating cysto-urethrography
MIC	minimum inhibitory concentration
MRSA	methicillin-resistant *Staphylococcus aureus*
NBT	nitro-blue tetrazolium
NEC	necrotizing enterocolitis
NK	natural killer
NPA	nasopharyngeal aspirate
PCP	*Pneumocystis carinii* pneumonia
PUJ	pelvi-ureteric junction
RDS	respiratory distress syndrome
RNA	ribonucleic acid
RSV	respiratory syncytial virus
SCBU	special care baby unit
SPA	suprapubic aspirate
TB	tuberculosis
THAM	tris-hydroxymethyl aminomethane
TORCH	*Toxoplasma gondii*, rubella, cytomegalovirus, herpes simplex virus
TPHA	*Treponema pallidum* haemagglutinating antibody
TTN	transient tachypnoea of the newborn
UAC	umbilical arterial catheter
UTI	urinary tract infection
VA	ventriculoatrial
VDRL	Venereal Disease Research Laboratory
VDRT	Venereal Disease Research Test
VP	ventriculoperitoneal
VUJ	vesico-ureteric junction
VUR	vesico-ureteric reflux
VZV	varicella–zoster virus
WBC	white blood cell
ZIG	zoster immune globulin

Chapter 1

Pathogenesis and epidemiology

PATHOGENESIS

The incidence of infection is higher in the neonatal period than at any other time in life, even if preterm babies are excluded. Some of the factors that determine this increased susceptibility to infection are summarized in Table 1.1. In addition to immaturity of the immune system, which is discussed in detail in Chapter 2, there are several reasons why preterm babies are more susceptible to infection than term babies (Table 1.2). Many studies have shown that the incidence of infection increases with falling birth-weight or gestation and that *low birth-weight is the single most important independent variable in predisposing to sepsis*.

Table 1.1 Reasons for increased susceptibility to infection in the neonatal period (term infants)

1 Immaturity of the immune system
    (a) Poor humoral response to organisms (IgG, IgM and IgA)
    (b) Relatively poor neutrophil response
    (c) Relatively poor complement activity
    (d) Possibly impaired macrophage function
    (e) Relatively poor T-cell function

2 Exposure to micro-organisms from the maternal genital tract
    (a) Ascending infection via amniotic fluid
    (b) Transplacental haematogenous spread

3 Exposure to viruses from mother without antibody
    (a) Antenatal, e.g. rubella, CMV, HIV
    (b) Viraemic spread, e.g. chickenpox
    (c) Perinatal, e.g. herpes simplex virus, hepatitis B

4 Peripartum factors
    (a) Trauma to skin, vessels, etc. during parturition
    (b) Scalp electrodes and other invasive obstetric procedures

5 Portals of colonization and subsequent invasion
    (a) Umbilicus
    (b) Mucosal surfaces
    (c) Eye
    (d) Skin

6 Exposure to organisms postnatally
    Exposure in neonatal unit or lying-in wards to organisms from other babies
    (a) Overcrowding
    (b) Understaffing

Table 1.2 Reasons for greater susceptibility to infection of preterm infants

1 Immunological
  (a) Reduced transplacental transfer of maternal IgG
  (b) Relative immaturity of all immune mechanisms

2 Exposure to micro-organisms from maternal genital tract
  Preterm labour may be precipitated by infection (chorioamnionitis)

3 Invasive procedures
  (a) Endotracheal tubes
  (b) Intravascular catheters
  (c) Chest drains
  (d) Cerebrospinal fluid shunts

4 Increased postnatal exposure
  Organisms from other babies on neonatal unit
  Overcrowding and understaffing

5 Poor surface defences
  Skin thin, easily traumatized

6 Increased risk of conditions predisposing to sepsis
  (a) Prolonged artificial ventilation
  (b) Intravenous feeding
  (c) Necrotizing enterocolitis

7 Antibiotic pressures
  (a) Resistant organisms
  (b) Fungal infection

Early-onset sepsis

The fetus and newborn infant are exposed to infection in unique ways. The amniotic fluid is bacteriostatic or bactericidal for many organisms with the exception of group B streptococci. Thus, despite the fact that the maternal genital tract and rectum are frequently colonized with potential pathogens, amnionitis is rare and most babies are not born infected. Nevertheless, amnionitis can occur. Sometimes this produces maternal symptoms or signs of frank chorioamnionitis with fever, a tender uterus and purulent, foul-smelling amniotic fluid. More commonly, however, amnionitis is asymptomatic and the amniotic fluid is not frankly purulent or even cloudy. There is good evidence that infection of the amniotic fluid can actually initiate preterm labour, possibly through the formation of bacterial products with prostaglandin-like activity.

The amniotic fluid is in continual contact with the fetal lungs *in utero* and although the latter are collapsed, ascending infection causing pneumonia and secondary septicaemia is probably the most important route of early-onset sepsis. Certainly, most babies with sepsis in the first 48 h postnatally present with pneumonia as well as septicaemia.

Babies with group B streptococcal pneumonia are frequently septicaemic at delivery. This might suggest transplacental haematogenous spread from a maternal septicaemia, but there is little evidence to support this mechanism in most instances of early-onset sepsis. It is more likely that the bacteraemia occurs secondary to multiplication of organisms within the fetal lung.

Benirschke (1960) proposed ascending infection as the major cause of early-onset sepsis. To examine this hypothesis he looked at infections occurring in twin pregnancies. He argued that twins *in utero* could lie either horizontally or vertically. If the twins were horizontal (the commonest position), twin one would be affected by ascending infection before twin two, whereas if they were vertical, simultaneous infection was likely (see Figure 1.1). In the former case, twin one alone or both twins would be infected; in the latter case, both twins were likely to be infected. Of the 23 infected twin pregnancies that he studied, both twins were infected in 7 cases, twin one alone in 16, but in no case was twin two alone infected.

In infection with *Listeria monocytogenes*, transplacental haematogenous spread is probably the most important mechanism. A history of maternal flu-like illness with fever, often two or more weeks before delivery, is usual. Signs of neonatal infection are often present at birth, and the placenta often shows granulomata and inflammatory changes suggestive of placental infection. In other infections the precise contribution of transplacental spread is less clear.

Occasionally, early-onset sepsis occurs in babies delivered by caesarean section through intact membranes. Although rare, these infections suggest either that transplacental spread has occurred, or that bacteria can cross intact membranes to set up an amnionitis, or that colonization has occurred at operation and led to rapid spread of infection.

Skin trauma during delivery may provide a portal of entry for micro-organisms. Instrumentation of the baby before delivery, for example with scalp electrodes, vacuum extraction or forceps, is particularly likely to damage the skin, and skin sepsis, osteomyelitis and disseminated sepsis may occur.

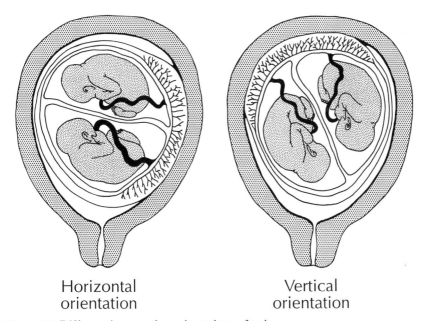

Horizontal
orientation

Vertical
orientation

Figure 1.1 Different intrauterine orientations of twins

Table 1.3 Early-onset sepsis: cases of septicaemia or meningitis in the first 48 h after birth; Neonatal Unit, Oxford 1984–1989

Organism	Cases	Deaths
Group B streptococcus	19 (4)[a]	7 (2)
Listeria monocytogenes	8 (1)	1
Gram-negative bacilli (mainly E. coli)	6 (1)	1
Streptococcus pneumoniae	4	2
Haemophilus influenzae	3	1
Anaerobes	2	0
Staphylococcus epidermidis	1	0
Total	43	12 (28%)

[a] Numbers in parentheses are cases of bacterial meningitis

We have used the term 'early-onset sepsis' and implied that such sepsis is distinct from sepsis occurring later. The micro-organisms causing early-onset sepsis, which we have defined as sepsis within 48 h of birth, and those causing late-onset sepsis in babies on the neonatal unit in Oxford over a 5-year period are shown in Tables 1.3 and 1.4, respectively. It is clear that early-onset sepsis in Oxford is predominantly due to group B streptococci, whereas *Staphylococcus epidermidis*, Gram-negative bacilli and faecal streptococci are the main causes of late-onset sepsis. Some organisms, such as group B streptococci and *Listeria*, can cause both early- and late-onset sepsis but in these cases the clinical picture and pathogenesis are different.

The well-documented maternal risk factors for early-onset sepsis are spontaneous preterm onset of labour (with or without membrane rupture), prolonged rupture of the membranes, and maternal fever (Boyer *et al.*, 1983). Approximately 75% of all cases of early-onset sepsis are associated with one or more such risk factors; the remaining 25% of cases occur in term babies without recognized predisposing factors. Perinatal asphyxia has also

Table 1.4 Late-onset sepsis: organisms isolated from 77 cases of septicaemia or meningitis after 48 h of age; Neonatal Unit, Oxford 1984–1989[a]

Organism	Cases
Staphylococcus epidermidis	23
Enterococci	16 (7)[b]
Klebsiella oxytoca	16 (5)
Pseudomonas aeruginosa	12 (4)
Escherichia coli	8 (3)
Other Gram-negative bacilli	8 (2)
Staphylococcus aureus	3
Anaerobes	2
Total	88

[a] These figures include 4 cases of meningitis caused by *Pseudomonas aeruginosa* (1), *Klebsiella oxytoca* (1), *Achromobacter xylosoxidans* (1) and both *Klebsiella oxytoca* and *Escherichia coli* (1).
[b] Polymicrobial episodes indicated in parentheses.

been described as a risk factor for sepsis but it is not clear whether this causes sepsis or is a sign of pre-existing sepsis. Gluck and colleagues (1966) noted that 20% of babies with sepsis had severe respiratory depression at birth requiring artificial intubation. Risk factors for early-onset sepsis are further considered in Chapter 4.

Late-onset sepsis

Early- and late-onset infections have a different pathogenesis. In early-onset infections (whether ascending or transplacental), sepsis occurs rapidly and babies are often systemically infected at delivery. In late-onset infections, in contrast, the organism first colonizes the baby and only later invades to cause sepsis. The most important sites colonized are the upper respiratory tract, conjunctivae, other mucosal surfaces, umbilicus and skin. Because the time interval between colonization and invasion will vary, it is clear that the distinction between early- and late-onset sepsis is an artificial one, based on the timing of onset of signs and symptoms of infection. Many authors use 7 days as the cut-off point between early- and late-onset sepsis; we favour 48 h because many of our cases of infection with hospital-acquired organisms present between 2 and 7 days of age. Nevertheless, some infections with hospital-acquired organisms, such as *Staphylococcus epidermidis*, still occur in the first 48 h after birth and are called early-onset sepsis (see Table 1.3), suggesting rapid colonization and invasion.

Factors predisposing to sepsis

The organisms causing late-onset sepsis on a neonatal unit are evidently very different from those causing sepsis in term babies at home. The organisms causing sepsis in a neonatal intensive care unit are very similar to those in an adult intensive care unit: Gram-negative enteric bacilli and staphylococci predominate. Neonates may become colonized with these organisms, as well as enterococci, group B streptococci and other organisms, at the time of delivery (sometimes called 'auto-infection'), but may also become colonized from other babies (hospital-acquired or nosocomial infection, from the Greek: *nosocomos* = hospital).

Neonatal units and, indeed, postnatal wards are often *overcrowded* and *understaffed*. Crowded wards (Goldmann *et al.*, 1978, 1981) and increases in workload (Isaacs *et al.*, 1988a) have been shown to lead to increased spread of colonizing organisms and to an increase in the incidence of nosocomial infections.

Babies receiving intensive care are subjected to other invasive procedures. *Intravascular cannulas*, particularly if they remain in place for some time, are a potent source of infection. As might be expected, skin organisms such as *Staphylococcus epidermidis* and *Staphylococcus aureus* are a common source of infection of these cannulas. *Staphylococcus epidermidis*, an organism of relatively low virulence, adapts well to colonization of foreign bodies such as indwelling cannulas. It has the capacity to erode into, and gain sustenance from, the plastic cannulas and to secrete a protective 'slime' layer resulting in the formation of microcolonies on the cannula.

Intravenous feeding is another risk factor for developing sepsis. Not only can the cannulas used for such feeding become infected, but the intravenous fluids themselves can provide a culture medium for micro-organisms. If quality control is lax, i.v. fluids can readily become contaminated with organisms such as *Staphylococcus epidermidis* and Enterobacteriacae. Fat emulsions are also excellent growth media for fungi such as *Malassezia furfur*, and intravenous feeding is associated with an increased risk of systemic candidiasis.

One of the most important risk factors for late sepsis is prolonged *endotracheal intubation* for ventilatory support (Goldmann *et al.*, 1981; Isaacs *et al.*, 1987a). Humidified air provides an excellent growth medium for hydrophilic organisms such as Gram-negative bacilli, and the mucociliary clearance mechanisms are bypassed by the endotracheal tube. Routine suctioning of the endotracheal tube has been shown to cause a transient bacteraemia (Storm, 1980) and, especially in the presence of vascular endothelial damage or an indwelling cannula, this may lead to sustained bacteraemia.

Necrotizing enterocolitis or lesser degrees of necrosis of the gut mucosa can provide a ready portal of entry for gut organisms such as Gram-negative bacilli and anaerobes. This subject is dealt with in detail in Chapter 12.

Because sepsis can be rapidly fatal and the signs of sepsis are non-specific, antibiotics are used liberally in neonatal units. This *antibiotic pressure* may select for antibiotic-resistant organisms. Resistant organisms are not necessarily more virulent than other organisms: there is some evidence that aminoglycoside-resistant Gram-negative bacilli may be less virulent than sensitive ones (White *et al.*, 1981; Isaacs *et al.*, 1987a). Nevertheless, some methicillin-resistant *Staphylococcus aureus* (MRSA) seem to exhibit enhanced virulence and can cause serious outbreaks of systemic infection. The indiscriminate use of antibiotics also selects for colonization by, and infection with, fungi: *the duration of prior antibiotic therapy for a baby is one of the most important risk factors for the development of systemic candidiasis.*

Portals of entry

The umbilical cord is an important potential portal of entry of bacteria. In the 1950s *Staphylococcus aureus* sepsis was widespread in the USA and UK. It was almost certainly not coincidence that these outbreaks resolved at the time that umbilical cord care (antisepsis), i.e. cleaning the umbilical stump with powerful antiseptics, became universal. Whenever this lesson has been forgotten and umbilical cord care relaxed, outbreaks of impetigo and systemic staphylococcal sepsis tend to occur and remind us of the predilection of *Staphylococcus aureus* for the umbilical stump, and of its ability to spread to the skin and thence to cause disseminated sepsis.

The skin of the newborn, and particularly that of preterm infants, is thin and susceptible to trauma both during delivery and subsequently. Skin sepsis is common in the neonatal period, usually with *Staphylococcus aureus*; skin abscesses in babies receiving intensive care may also be caused by Gram-negative bacilli, *Staphylococcus epidermidis* and fungi. Organisms may be inoculated directly into areas of traumatized skin or may be blood borne and seed embolically.

Neonatal conjunctivitis is common, possibly because IgA production in tears is poor. Conjunctivitis may be caused by organisms acquired in hospital, such as *Staphylococcus aureus* and *Pseudomonas aeruginosa*, or during passage through an infected vaginal canal, such as *Chlamydia trachomatis* or *Neisseria gonorrhoeae*.

Urinary tract infections are rare and when they do occur are often associated with structural abnormalities causing urinary stasis.

Ischaemic lesions of the gastrointestinal tract secondary to necrotizing enterocolitis, Hirschsprung's disease or other diseases causing bowel obstruction and/or vascular damage can lead to septicaemia due to the passage of organisms from the bowel flora (enteric bacilli, anaerobes) through the necrotic bowel wall.

Virus infections

Virus infections are often more severe in the neonatal period than at any other time in life, including infections occurring in severely immunocompromised patients. Infections caused by enteroviruses, herpes simplex virus and varicella–zoster virus can be devastating and rapidly fatal. In all these examples previous maternal infection tends to protect the baby, probably because of the transplacental passage of maternal antibody; in contrast, peripartum primary maternal infection is associated with a poor outcome, as there is often a large inoculum of virus and little or no passively acquired antibody to protect the baby.

Virulence

Thus far we have concentrated on host factors in the pathogenesis of neonatal infection and little attention has been given to the organisms and their virulence. It is clear that the different patterns of sepsis seen with different organisms are, in part, attributable to the different propensity with which they colonize epithelial surfaces and invade the bloodstream and meninges to cause severe sepsis. Some organisms cause meningitis in a high proportion of cases (e.g. group B streptococci and *Listeria*); others do so much more rarely (e.g. *Staphylococcus epidermidis*). Meningitis results from high-level bacteraemia and the causative organisms must multiply efficiently in the vascular spaces or seed the blood from extravascular sites, in order to cause a sufficient bacteraemia to lead to meningitis.

There may also be variation in virulence within strains. For example group B streptococci can be subdivided into subtypes I, II and III. These are found with approximately equal frequency in the maternal vaginal tract and also causing early-onset sepsis, suggesting that, for early sepsis, environmental factors are as important as any particular interstrain variation in virulence. Late-onset group B streptococcal septicaemia and meningitis, however, is largely caused by subtype III organisms, implying that these are more pathogenic than the other subtypes.

Clones of group B streptococcus of high virulence have been identified in the United States and may explain the relatively high incidence of neonatal group B streptococcal infection in the USA, despite levels of maternal colonization comparable to those in other countries.

Because newborns, particularly preterm infants, are immunologically immature they may become infected with organisms of low virulence that normally only cause opportunist infections. A number of organisms that rarely cause serious disease in older children may cause neonatal septicaemia and even meningitis; examples are alpha-haemolytic streptococci, anaerobes and fungi.

Inoculum effect

Severity of disease is determined in part by the size of the inoculum of potentially pathogenic organisms. The inoculum size may help to explain the observation that 'vertical' infections caused by bacteria or viruses are generally far more severe than postnatally acquired infections with the same organisms. For example early-onset group B streptococcal infection has a much worse prognosis than the late-onset infection. Similarly, in infections with enteroviruses and chickenpox, perinatal vertical infection is often fatal whereas postnatal infection is generally benign.

EPIDEMIOLOGY

Incidence

The incidence of neonatal sepsis varies with a number of different factors, which are considered below. In the United States the incidence of neonatal infection has varied from 1 to 8.1 per 1000 live births (Klein and Marcy, 1990), although in one region the rate has remained fairly constant over many years at 2–4 cases per 1000 live births (Freedman et al., 1981).

Organisms

The organisms causing early-onset sepsis reflect the vaginal flora of pregnant women. The prevalent organisms may vary rapidly over time, and may be altered by external factors. In the United Kingdom all pregnant women are screened for syphilis and gonorrhoea and treated if positive. As a consequence, neonatal infection with these organisms is very rare, but this is not the case in many other parts of the world. There may be marked geographical variations: maternal carriage of group B streptococci has approximately the same prevalence in the United Kingdom and United States of America, but neonatal group B streptococcal infection is 3 to 10 times more common in the USA than in the UK. There is evidence that particularly virulent clones of group B streptococci may circulate in the USA and be responsible for the increased rate of neonatal sepsis. There are also annual fluctuations in the incidence of neonatal group B streptococcal infection in the same institution that are not easily explicable.

Late-onset infections, as already emphasized, can result from invasion of organisms colonizing the maternal genital tract or from the environment. The organisms colonizing babies and causing sepsis on a neonatal unit may change with time, for no apparent reason. Although we have not made deliberate attempts to eliminate any particular organisms nor altered our antibiotic policy significantly in the last 5 years, there have none the less been marked fluctuations in the organisms causing sepsis from year to year (see Table 1.5). In 1984–1985 *Pseudomonas aeruginosa* predominated, to be succeeded by enterococci and *Klebsiella oxytoca* in 1985–1987. We have not detected any babies colonized with *Pseudomonas* for 2 years. Over the years 1986–1989 *Staphylococcus epidermidis* became the major pathogen causing septicaemia; less than one-half of these cases were associated with infected intravascular cannulas. Despite these variations, the annual total number of cases of late-onset sepsis has remained constant.

Geographical

In many developing countries infections with *Salmonella* species are common, whereas they are rare in most developed countries. Neonatal tetanus is one of the major killers of babies world wide: in developing countries this is commonly caused by applying mud, ghee or other contaminated materials to the umbilical stump and compounded by the low level of tetanus immunization of mothers.

There are also regional differences within countries and sometimes between hospitals which are geographically close. Such differences may be due to identifiable environmental factors such as hygiene or antibiotic pressures, but often the cause remains obscure.

Age

As already stated, gestational age is one of the most important factors in determining the incidence of sepsis. There is an inverse correlation between gestational age or birth-weight and the incidence of group B streptococcal sepsis (Boyer *et al.*, 1983) suggesting this is an important determinant in early-onset sepsis. In late-onset sepsis we, among others, have shown a similar relationship (see Table 1.6). The risk of both early- and late-onset sepsis increases markedly in very preterm babies, particularly those weighing < 1000 g at birth. We found no difference in rates of late sepsis between term babies on our unit and those weighing between 1500 and 2499 g (Table 1.6) but a > 20-fold increase in babies < 1000 g at birth. Systemic candidiasis occurs virtually only in babies of very low birth-weight (< 1500 g).

Table 1.5 Late-onset septicaemia (occurring after 48 h of age) in babies on the Neonatal Unit, John Radcliffe Hospital, Oxford, 1984–1989

Year	Pseudomonas sp.	Klebsiella sp.	Other Gram-negative enteric bacilli	Enterococci	Staphylococcus epidermidis	Staphylococcus aureus	Other	Total episodes of sepsis[a]	No. of babies on Neonatal Unit	Late sepsis % of admissions
1984	7	1	6	2	1	0	0	15	497	3.0
1985	4	5	3	8	3	0	1	19	523	3.6
1986	0	4	4	5	5	1	1	16	482	3.3
1987	0	4	4	1	5	0	2	14	507	2.8
1988	0	1	1	0	13	2	0	17	472	3.6
1989	2	0	5	1	8	2	2	19	589	3.2

[a] Number of organisms sometimes exceeds episodes of sepsis because occasional cases were polymicrobial but felt to be genuine episodes of sepsis.

Table 1.6 Incidence of late-onset sepsis (bacteraemia or meningitis) in babies on newborn intensive care unit by birth-weight; Oxford, 1 May 1984–31 October 1985

Birth-weight (g)	Number with sepsis	Number on unit	Proportion infected (%)
> 2500	3	371	0.8
1500–2499	2	266	0.8
1000–1499	11	95	11.6
< 1000	11	54	20.4
Total	27	786	3.4

The effects of postnatal age are less clear-cut, but in general the incidence of infection decreases with increasing postnatal age. This is because early-onset infections relate to the special conditions of exposure already outlined, and because of increasing immunological maturity with age. Nevertheless, the risk of sepsis remains high for very preterm infants, particularly those requiring long-term respiratory support and intravenous feeding.

Sex

Early-onset sepsis affects both sexes equally, implying that overwhelming exposure is a more important determinant than host factors in the pathogenesis of early-onset sepsis. In late-onset sepsis, when host factors might be expected to be more important, boys are more susceptible in almost all studies, and may have more than twice the incidence.

Multiple pregnancies

Preterm twins are at greater risk (nearly five times) of group B streptococcal infection than preterm singletons (Pass *et al.*, 1980). As already stated, the first-born twin is at greater risk of early-onset infection than the second (Benirschke, 1960).

Mortality and morbidity

Many factors influence mortality and morbidity from bacterial infections. One of the most important is whether infection is due to early-onset (ascending or transplacental) or late-onset (hospital-acquired) infection. Although there has been a general improvement in mortality from early-onset sepsis, this nevertheless remains as high as 25–50% in many centres. In Oxford over the 5 years from 1984 to 1989 the mortality from early sepsis was 28% (see Table 1.3). In contrast, the mortality from late bacterial sepsis was considerably lower: in Oxford only 3 of 77 episodes (4%) were responsible for babies' deaths over the same period. However, late-onset infection can be an important cause of death in babies < 1000 g (La Gamma *et al.*, 1983).

Naeye (1977) estimated that amniotic fluid infection was responsible for 17% of perinatal deaths, of which about two-thirds were neonatal deaths. A far more conservative definition of perinatal infection led Edouard and

Alberman (1980) to attribute only 1.3–1.8% of perinatal deaths to infection in the United Kingdom, from 1966 to 1978.

There may be considerable morbidity, not just from bacterial meningitis, but from pneumonia which may contribute to chronic lung disease, and from other infections. Furthermore, viral and parasitic infections may be severe, particularly congenital infections acquired early in gestation and those acquired around delivery.

Chapter 2

Immunity

Introduction

Infection is more common in the neonatal period than at any other time in life. This is partly attributable to exposure to large numbers of organisms, but is also due to a relative failure of the neonatal host defences to clear micro-organisms from blood and tissues. The 'immune deficiency' of the newborn infant is relative rather than absolute: babies rarely become infected with opportunistic organisms such as *Pneumocystis carinii* unless their immunity is further compromised. Most neonatal infections are caused by organisms that are also capable of causing infection in older children and adults, but neonatal infection is usually more severe and more likely to disseminate and be fatal.

The basis of the defective immunity in the newborn period can be illustrated by considering the mechanisms involved in protection against infection. Invading micro-organisms may be thought of as predominantly extracellular or intracellular (Table 2.1). This convenient oversimplification allows us to examine adult host defence mechanisms and the ways in which the newborn is relatively poor in overcoming infection.

Extracellular organisms are mainly bacteria, both Gram-positive bacteria such as group B streptococci and staphylococci, and Gram-negative organisms such as *E. coli*. These organisms are predominantly cleared by phagocytosis by polymorphonuclear leucocytes (neutrophils or granulocytes). Phagocytosis is enhanced if the surface of the organism is altered by being coated with antibody and complement (opsonization).

Once infection is established within cells, *intracellular organisms* such as *Listeria, Salmonella, M. tuberculosis*, viruses and parasites are protected from antibodies, complement and neutrophil phagocytosis. In these circumstances other host defence mechanisms, which rely on recognition of

Table 2.1 Different host defence mechanisms predominantly employed in response to extracellular and intracellular micro-organisms

Mechanism	Extracellular organisms	Intracellular organisms
Non-immune	Neutrophils Complement	Natural killer cells Macrophage/monocyte
Immune	B lymphocytes Antibody	T lymphocytes Cytotoxicity Delayed-type hypersensitivity Memory

infected cells as well as of infecting organisms, are required. Cells of the macrophage/monocyte lineage are the most important phagocytic cells in combating intracellular infection. Natural killer cells recognize and destroy infected cells non-specifically, whereas recognition of infected cells by thymus-derived (T) lymphocytes is an antigen-specific, immune mechanism. Macrophages/monocytes interact with T lymphocytes, which themselves produce soluble proteins (lymphokines) that enhance the activity of macrophages/monocytes and natural killer cells. Thus there is interaction between cells, resulting in amplification of the immune response to intracellular organisms.

In this chapter we deal first with immune (antigen-specific) and non-immune host cellular defences against invading micro-organisms and the extent to which such cellular defences are immature or defective in the neonatal period. We then illustrate the neonatal response to infection with different groups of organisms.

Antigen-specific immune response

Antibody production

Antibody molecules share certain structural features (see Figure 2.1). Their main role is to coat the surface of micro-organisms and alter the surface structure (opsonize them), rendering the organisms more susceptible to

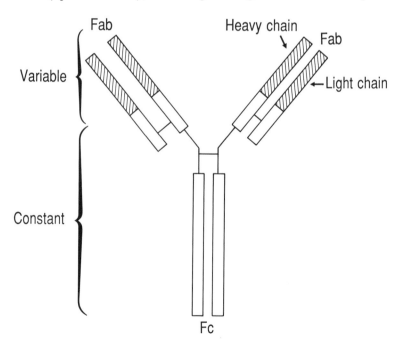

Figure 2.1 Antibody molecule. There are two antigen-binding sites (Fab) with variable regions (shaded) allowing different specificities of antigen recognition. The F_c region is constant, allowing recognition by cell receptors

phagocytosis. This process is particularly important in recovery from infections with extracellular organisms. In contrast, antibody may be important in preventing infection and reinfection with intracellular organisms but is less important in recovery from acute infection.

Antibodies are produced by *B lymphocytes* or B cells, lymphocytes which have immunoglobulins on their surface. The 'B' stands for the bursa of Fabricius, the organ in birds in which such cells develop. The equivalent human fetal organ is the liver, and B cells bearing surface immunoglobulin appear in the fetal liver from about 8 weeks' gestation.

B cells do not secrete antibodies into the serum until they have differentiated into 'plasma cells', and this requires assistance from cells called helper T lymphocytes or T helper (T_H) cells; in general these T cells express the CD4 antigen (formerly called OKT4) on their surface. B cells will respond to unaltered or 'native' antigens and do not require antigens to be 'processed' by other cells (see below) in order to recognize them. B cells secrete different classes of immunoglobulin (G, A, M, D or E), according to which heavy chain (see Figure 2.1) is incorporated into the immunoglobulin (Ig) molecule.

IgG

The human newborn produces relatively little IgG compared with older children and adults, and IgG production remains low until 4–6 months postnatally. This is frequently forgotten when interpreting serological responses to viral infections: it is not useful to look for a rise in IgG titre in the neonatal period.

Fetal and neonatal IgG are acquired transplacentally from the mother. Placental transfer occurs in two ways, passive and active. Passive transfer of IgG increases progressively from about 17 weeks' gestation. The active, enzymatic transfer is primarily a regulatory mechanism allowing

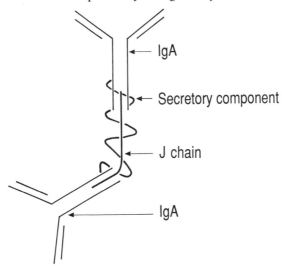

Figure 2.2 Secretory IgA molecule. Two molecules of IgA are held together by a joining (J) chain and secretory component to form a dimer

compensation for abnormally high or low levels of maternal IgG levels (Gitlin *et al.*, 1964). Levels of IgG subclasses in the newborn are the same as in the mother (IgG1, 70%; IgG2, 20%; IgG3, 7%; IgG4, 3%). IgG2, produced primarily in response to polysaccharides, has the shortest half-life and newborns and infants mount a poor antibody response to polysaccharide antigens.

IgA

The newborn is also relatively poor at producing IgA, the antibody present on mucosal surfaces which is important in protection against respiratory and gastrointestinal pathogens. Furthermore, IgA does not cross the placenta. Secretory IgA (see Figure 2.2), is a dimeric molecule composed of two IgA molecules joined by a J (joining) chain and a secretory component. It is produced in exocrine gland secretions. Plasma cells in the gland produce IgA and J chain, whereas epithelial cells contribute the secretory component. Secretory IgA is not found in tears until 10–20 days after birth, which may partly explain the propensity of neonates to conjunctivitis. Secretory cells do not appear in the intestinal mucosa until about 4 weeks postnatally, but colostrum and breast milk do contain secretory IgA, so that the incidence of respiratory and gastrointestinal infections is lower in breast-fed infants. The role of IgA is an important reason for early introduction of enteral feeds with breast milk for preterm babies.

IgM

IgM is a single molecule at the cell surface, but when secreted it can form a pentameric structure in the serum in conjunction with the same joining J chain as appears in secretory IgA (see Figure 2.3). Because each IgM

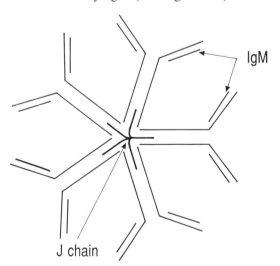

Figure 2.3 IgM molecule. Pentameric structure of IgM in serum with five antibody molecules joined by J chain

molecule has two binding sites (Fab), each pentamer has 10 binding sites. IgM does not interact with complement in the way that IgG does.

The fetus can produce IgM from about 30 weeks' gestation. As this immunoglobulin does not cross the placenta, the detection of IgM specific to a given organism, e.g. rubella, in cord blood indicates congenital infection. Babies born before 30 weeks' gestation are at increased risk of infection because transplacental passage of maternal IgG is relatively poor and IgM production occurs at only a low level.

IgM, unlike IgG, does not activate the classic pathway of complement (see below). Recent work suggests that IgM may have a major role in recovery from Gram-negative infections.

IgD

The role of IgD is uncertain and it is found in only low levels in serum. There is evidence that IgD can cross the placenta and can activate the classical pathway of complement.

IgE

IgE does not cross the placenta and very little is produced in the neonatal period. It has been suggested that IgE specific to respiratory syncytial virus (RSV) may appear in the nasopharynx of infected babies and its persistence may contribute to recurrent wheezing (Welliver *et al.*, 1981).

Antigen presentation

T lymphocytes do not recognize antigens unless they are first 'processed' and presented on the surface of *antigen-presenting cells*. The latter are phago-cytic cells which ingest the micro-organism and process it by degrading its proteins to small peptides which are transported to, and presented on, the

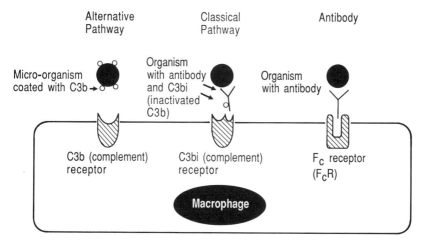

Figure 2.4 Mechanisms by which macrophages recognize micro-organisms using surface receptors. (Courtesy of Dr Jonathan Austyn, Nuffield Department of Surgery, Oxford)

cell surface. Almost any cell can be an antigen-presenting cell but the most important of these are probably macrophages and monocytes. *Macrophages possess receptors to the Fc portion of the antibody molecule which allow them to associate with organisms coated with antibody* (see Figure 2.4). Macrophage complement receptors bind to two different C3 breakdown products, C3b and its further degradation product, inactivated C3b (C3bi). The macrophage therefore can recognize organisms through three distinct immune mechanisms (Figure 2.4), and although macrophages can ingest organisms without previous exposure to the organism they can also use immune recognition. Activated macrophages can kill organisms using the same respiratory burst as neutrophils (see below). Macrophage and monocyte function has been studied in newborn infants: interleukin-1 production is normal but chemotaxis, phagocytosis and antigen processing are all variably diminished. Furthermore neonatal macrophages are less readily activated by lymphokines, such as interferon-gamma. As lymphokines are relatively poorly produced by neonatal T lymphocytes there is a cumulative defect in response to intracellular organisms.

T lymphocytes (cellular immunity)

T lymphocytes (thymus-derived lymphocytes) are responsible for cellular or cell-mediated immunity. They recognize, through specific T-cell receptors, antigens that have been processed (degraded to peptides) and presented on the surface of antigen-presenting cells. The antigen-presenting cell presents degraded antigen in association with its own major histocompatibility complex (MHC) or HLA molecule on the cell surface (see Figure 2.5). T cells recognize processed antigen through a receptor which has constant and variable regions analogous to immunoglobulin. Once the T cell has

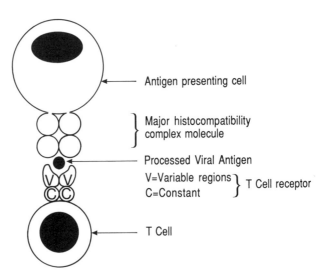

Figure 2.5 T cell uses T-cell receptor to recognize 'processed viral antigen' (degraded to a peptide) presented on the surface of an antigen-presenting cell in association with a molecule of its major histocompatibility complex

recognized processed antigen it starts to proliferate. It may then either mature into a *memory cell*, which becomes quiescent but can recognize the same antigen if re-exposed, or into an *effector cell* responsible either for destroying infected cells (*cytotoxic T cell*) or for helping B cells to produce antibody (*T-helper cell*). Cytotoxic T cells are important in recovery from infection with intracellular pathogens, particularly viruses. T cells are also responsible for delayed-type hypersensitivity, important in recovery from tuberculosis.

T cells produce soluble proteins or lymphokines, such as the interleukins and immune interferon (interferon-gamma). The lymphokines can act on B cells, natural killer cells (see below), macrophages and activated T cells themselves to recruit these cells to the site of infection and amplify the immune response.

T-cell function is only marginally poorer in preterm and term neonates than in adults. Immunization with BCG is protective in most term infants (although this is somewhat controversial), suggesting near-normal delayed-type hypersensitivity. Neonatal T cells can proliferate and produce lympho-kines in response to appropriate stimuli, although some workers have found lower levels of lymphokine production (e.g. interferon gamma) in newborns than in adults. Some babies as young as 3 weeks old have been shown to mount a cytotoxic T-lymphocyte response to infection with respiratory syncytial virus (Isaacs *et al.*, 1987c). Newborns and infants will not mount an antibody response to polysaccharide antigens such as the capsules of *Haemophilus influenzae* type b or pneumococcus but if the capsular polysaccharide is linked to a T cell-dependent antigen such as diphtheria toxoid, babies as young as 2 months may make an antibody response to both the diphtheria toxoid and the capsular polysaccharide.

Antibody-dependent cellular cytotoxicity (ADCC)

ADCC, the importance of which in most infections is unknown, depends on cytotoxic (killer) cells recognizing organisms coated with antibody, presumably via Fc receptors, and effecting cell lysis. Various cell types including killer cells, macrophages and granulocytes are capable of ADCC. ADCC is augmented by interferon.

Non-immune responses

Neutrophils

Polymorphonuclear leucocytes or neutrophils are important in phagocytos-ing extracellular organisms such as *Staphylococcus aureus*. To kill these organisms, neutrophils need to be able to detect them and move towards them (*chemotaxis*), ingest them (*phagocytosis*) and kill them by intracellular generation of toxic oxygen metabolites such as superoxide ions (*respiratory burst*). Studies of neutrophil function in the neonatal period have given conflicting results, but no gross defects have been shown. The main problem appears to be that there is a diminished bone marrow reserve of immature neutrophils. If infection leads to peripheral destruction of neutrophils, the neutrophil reserve rapidly becomes depleted, resulting in neutropenia. Neutropenia is relatively common in neonatal bacterial infections and carries a poor prognosis.

Complement

The complement system consists of a series of proteins which interact in a sequence or cascade to generate other proteins responsible for important defences to micro-organisms (chemotaxis, opsonization and cell lysis). The complement system also regenerates its component proteins so that complement activation continues in the presence of infecting organisms. The central event in the complement cascade is the conversion of C3 to the activated molecule C3b (or C̄3). This can be achieved either by the classic pathway or the alternative pathway (see Figure 2.6). *The classic pathway requires the presence of antibody and is best activated by immune complexes. The alternative pathway can be activated by bacterial cell-wall products, such as endotoxin or polysaccharide, in the absence of antibody.* However, antibody may augment alternative pathway-mediated killing. Both pathways catalyse the conversion of C3 to C3b by an enzyme, C3 convertase. This then leads to a series of reactions, the common pathway, which generates chemotactic factors which attract inflammatory cells, anaphylotoxins which increase vascular permeability and hence access of inflammatory cells, opsonins which coat micro-organisms, and the terminal attack complex which punches holes in cell walls and lyses them. An important feature is that *the complement cascade occurs on the cell surface of the infecting organism.*

Complement levels in the term newborn are approximately one-half those of normal adults, and preterm babies have even lower levels (Miller, 1978).

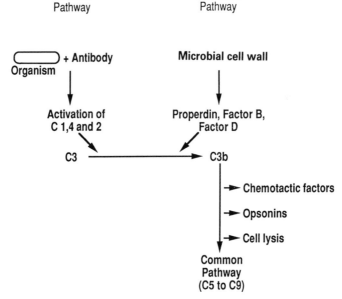

Figure 2.6 Simplified representation of complement cascade

Natural killer cells

Natural killer (NK) cells resemble large granular lymphocytes morphologi-
cally but probably derive from a lineage distinct from B and T cells. They kill
virus-infected cells, some micro-organisms, and tumour cells spontaneously
and do not require antigen processing or MHC recognition. NK activity is
stimulated by interferon and is generally somewhat lower in neonates than
in adults. NK cells are particularly important in recovery from infections
with herpesviruses (Biron *et al.*, 1989). In neonates there are fewer NK cells
and they respond less well to interferons (Kohl, 1989).

Interferon production

There are three types of interferon, alpha, beta and gamma. Interferon-
alpha can be produced by almost any nucleated cell in the body and inter-
feron-beta by fibroblasts and epithelial cells in response to various stimuli,
particularly virus infections. The interferons act on neighbouring cells,
stimulating them to produce various antiviral proteins that render the cell
resistant to viral infection. The production of interferons alpha and beta is
not a specific immune mechanism: they can be produced in response to a
wide range of viruses and can protect against a number of different viruses.

Interferon-alpha is produced locally in most respiratory virus infections
before antibody can be detected and is probably one of the most important
mechanisms of recovery from such infections. Production of interferons
alpha and beta appears to be quantitatively normal in the neonatal period,
even by preterm neonates.

Interferon-gamma, or immune interferon, in contrast to interferon-alpha,
is produced by T cells on re-exposure to an antigen to which they have
already been sensitized and is thus an immune mechanism. Although interferon-gamma has antiviral properties, its major role is as a modulator of the
immune response. Macrophages and monocytes are activated by interferon-
gamma, thus improving their ability to process and present antigen, whereas
NK cells and the cells responsible for ADCC are activated to increase lysis of
virus-infected cells. In the newborn period less interferon-gamma is produced and macrophages, NK cells and ADCC cells are less sensitive to its
action.

The various interactions between immune and non-immune responses to
infection are summarized in Figure 2.7.

Immunological response to infection

Pyogenic bacteria

Pyogenic bacteria are extracellular organisms. They generally colonize a
mucocutaneous surface before invasion. In the neonate, production of
secretory IgA and fibronectin, which would normally decrease bacterial
adherence, is relatively poor.

Once the organism is locally established, the most important defence
mechanism is *phagocytosis and killing by neutrophils, enhanced by opsonization by specific antibody and complement* (see Figure 2.8). The relative

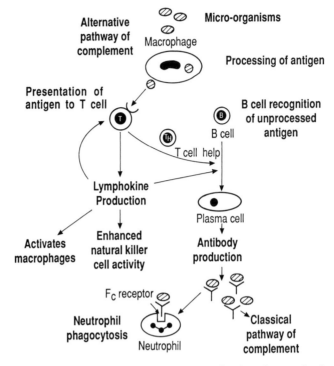

Figure 2.7 Immune (specific) and non-immune mechanisms interacting in response to infection. T, T cell; T_H, T-helper cell; B, B cell

importance of these factors may vary depending on the organism, e.g. defects in the terminal components of the complement pathway are peculiarly associated with *Neisseria* infections. In general, however, invasive disease with pyogenic organisms such as group B streptococci is more likely in the absence of type-specific antibody. The ready depletion of the

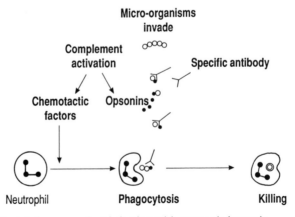

Figure 2.8 Host defences against infection with pyogenic bacteria

pool of neutrophil precursors means that neutropenia, an unusual occurrence in older children, readily occurs in neonatal infections with pyogenic organisms.

Viruses

A critical factor determining the severity of most neonatal virus infections is the timing of infection. The fetus is poorly protected against viruses so that intrauterine infection readily occurs. Infections in the first trimester, the time of maximum organogenesis, are most likely to be teratogenic. Infections acquired just before or at delivery are often severe because there is a large amount of virus and little or no maternal antibody. Enterovirus and varicella zoster virus infections due to postnatal acquisition of the same virus, even in the absence of maternal antibody, are generally relatively mild. On the other hand, postnatal herpes simplex virus infection in the absence of maternally acquired antibody may be devastating. This suggests that the newborn may be able to mount an immune response to slow-growing or less virulent viruses but not to rapidly multiplying, virulent viruses like herpes simplex.

Apart from antibody, important early mechanisms in limiting viral replication are probably interferons, NK cells and ADCC, which act in the presence of maternal IgG (Figure 2.9). IgM directed against viruses can be produced by neonates but is less efficient at neutralizing virus than IgG and

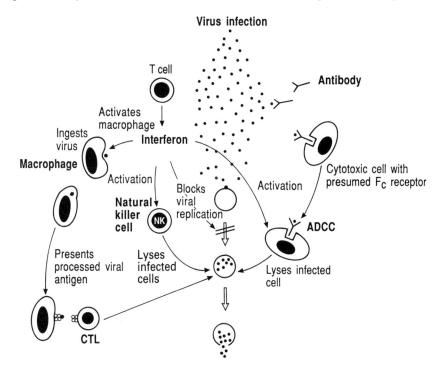

Figure 2.9 Host defences against virus infection. ADCC, antibody-dependent cellular cytotoxicity; CTL, cytotoxic T lymphocytes; NK, natural killer cells

will not sensitize virus-infected cells to lysis by effector cells. Neonatal IgG production is poor so the newborn without specific maternal IgG is disadvantaged in combating virus infections. ADCC cannot operate in the absence of IgG, NK-cell activity is generally lower in newborns, and gamma (but not alpha) interferon production is diminished. The role of cytotoxic T lymphocytes (CTL) in clearing infection has not been well established in newborns.

Intracellular pathogens

The immunological response to intracellular pathogens other than viruses is predominantly mediated by cellular immunity. *Listeria, Salmonella* and *Mycobacterium tuberculosis* are facultative intracellular pathogens whereas *Chlamydia trachomatis* and *Toxoplasma gondii* are obligate intracellular pathogens. In animals, macrophage depletion increases susceptibility to *Listeria*, whereas T-cell depletion increases susceptibility to all intracellular pathogens, and immunity to intracellular pathogens can be restored by passive transfer of sensitized T cells.

Monocytes and macrophages produce interleukins, messenger proteins which activate T cells, whereas T cells produce lymphokines, including interferon-gamma which activates macrophages and interleukin-2 which activates T cells. Thus there is amplification of the cellular response to infections (see Figure 2.10). *The cytokine-dependent interaction between T lymphocytes and macrophages is poor in neonates* (Wilson, 1986) and largely explains the increased susceptibility to intracellular pathogens.

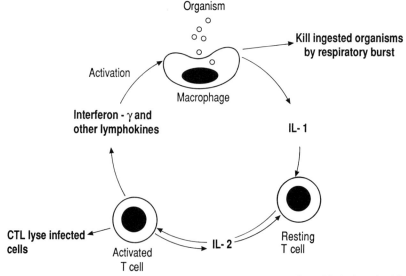

Figure 2.10 Host defences against intracellular pathogens, IL-1, IL-2, interleukins 1 and 2; CTL, cytotoxic T lymphocytes

Chapter 3

Clinical manifestations

Introduction

It is well known that the signs of neonatal bacterial sepsis are often non-specific and may be clinically indistinguishable from those occurring in non-infectious conditions. Furthermore, rapid deterioration is usual if the appropriate antibiotics are not given, so that antibiotics must be prescribed early if sepsis is suspected.

Septicaemia

The signs of septicaemia vary somewhat according to whether the sepsis is acquired by vertical infection (early onset) or following colonization and later invasion (late onset). In general, early-onset sepsis is far more likely to be associated with respiratory distress and babies are more likely to be shocked, whereas the onset is often, but by no means always, more insidious in late-onset sepsis.

Fever

Only about one-half of the babies with proven sepsis are febrile; about 15% have hypothermia or temperature instability, while the remaining babies, about one-third, are normothermic. Thus, although fever should suggest infection, the absence of fever certainly does not exclude it. Fever is an important defence mechanism against infection and failure to mount a febrile response may contribute to the poor outlook in neonatal infections.

Tachycardia

In one study of babies < 72 h old, almost half of the babies with sustained tachycardia > 160 beats per minute were septic with positive blood cultures, giving a specificity of nearly 50%. Furthermore, tachycardia was a sensitive index of sepsis, being present in 12 out of 13 babies with proven sepsis (Graves and Rhodes, 1984).

No similar evaluation has been made of tachycardia in late-onset sepsis.

Respiratory distress

In early-onset sepsis the clinical picture may be identical to that of hyaline membrane disease (idiopathic respiratory distress syndrome), with tachypnoea, recession, cyanosis, grunting and flaring of the alar nasae. Furthermore, the chest radiograph may show a generalized fine granularity, focal pneumonic changes or even be completely normal.

In late-onset sepsis, with or without pneumonia, respiratory distress is less common. Tachypnoea may occur in bacterial meningitis due to central stimulation of the respiratory centres with or without acidosis.

Apnoea

Apnoea is common in septic babies, but apnoea of prematurity occurs in a large proportion of preterm babies. The two types of apnoea ('septic' and apnoea of prematurity) cannot be readily distinguished by the duration, frequency or severity of the episodes, nor by the response to aminophylline derivatives, because apnoea may temporarily respond to aminophylline in babies with sepsis.

Jaundice

Jaundice occurs in about one-third of babies with sepsis. For unknown reasons it is particularly associated with Gram-negative infections, particularly of the urinary tract, but may also occur in Group B streptococcal and other Gram-positive infections. The hyperbilirubinaemia is characteristically unconjugated, although it may occasionally be conjugated.

Hepatomegaly

Hepatomegaly occurs in about one-third of cases of sepsis, often in association with jaundice.

Splenomegaly

This is rarely described in reported series of septic babies, but this may be because of difficulty in eliciting the sign. If present, it suggests bacterial sepsis or intrauterine infection.

Skin lesions

Petechial rash is a feature of congenital infections but also occurs in immune thrombocytopenia and can result from disseminated intravascular coagulopathy (DIC) in severe sepsis. A raised papular rash is often present in early-onset listeriosis. A fine macular rash is fairly common in enteroviral infections and also occurs in congenital syphilis. Vesicular lesions as well as purpura or erythema may occur in herpes simplex virus infection. Ecthyma gangrenosum, necrotic skin lesions, may occur in *Pseudomonas* sepsis or

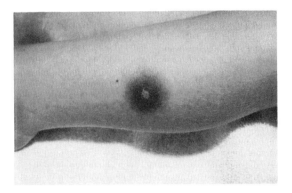

Figure 3.1 Ecthyma gangrenosum associated with *Pseudomonas* sepsis

sepsis due to fungi (Figure 3.1), while sclerema can occur in babies with advanced sepsis from any cause.

Omphalitis may range from a slightly red skin around the umbilicus to a purulent discharge with spreading necrosis of surrounding tissues (necrotizing fasciitis) which can be caused by *Staphylococcus aureus* but also by Gram-negative bacteria and anaerobes (Mason *et al.*, 1989).

Lethargy, irritability, anorexia

Non-specific symptoms of lethargy or irritability and, in term infants, poor feeding are present in less than one-half of all babies with sepsis. The baby who 'handles well' may, nevertheless, be infected.

Vomiting, abdominal distension

Failure to tolerate enteral feeds, causing abdominal distension or vomiting due to ileus, is a common and important early sign of sepsis.

Meningitis

The signs of meningitis do not differ markedly from those of systemic sepsis without meningeal involvement. Neck rigidity is rare in neonatal meningitis and a full or bulging fontanelle is seen in less than one-third of these babies (Klein and Marcy, 1990). Convulsions occur in < 50%. Irritability is common, as is lethargy. Fever only occurs in about 60%. The cry may be high-pitched, suggesting cerebral irritation.

The clinical diagnosis of meningitis, particularly in preterm babies, is difficult and, unless there are good reasons for not performing a lumbar puncture, a sample of CSF should be examined and cultured in all cases of suspected neonatal sepsis (see Chapter 4).

Urinary tract infection

The signs of urinary tract infection (UTI) are no more specific than those of septicaemia or meningitis. Although there is a well-recognized association

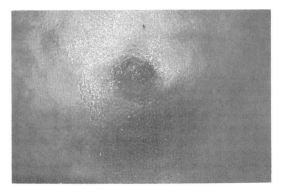

Figure 3.2 Omphalitis and early necrotizing fasciitis

between UTI and jaundice, jaundice is actually present in < 20% of babies with UTI (Klein, 1990a). Other signs of UTI, such as gastrointestinal manifestations (vomiting, abdominal distension, diarrhoea), irritability, lethargy and fever, are variably present and do not distinguish babies with UTI, which is frequently associated with bacteraemia in the newborn period, from those with sepsis without UTI.

Osteomyelitis or septic arthritis

The clinical features are described in detail in Chapter 9. Osteomyelitis or septic arthritis (or both) may present insidiously with the baby afebrile and feeding well but with progressive enlargement of a bone or joint, or alternatively with pseudoparesis of a limb mimicking Erb's palsy (osteomyelitis of the humerus or clavicle) or foot drop. Alternatively, the onset may be abrupt, with signs indistinguishable from systemic sepsis until multiple areas of bony involvement become apparent.

Viral infections

Systemic viral infections may present with a clinical picture similar to that of bacterial sepsis, whereas respiratory viruses tend to cause milder, but often equally non-specific, signs.

Enterovirus infections

Most vertically (maternally) acquired enterovirus infections are associated with a history of peripartum maternal illness. This may be fever, gastroenteritis, upper respiratory tract infection or severe abdominal pain mimicking appendicitis. Babies classically present at 3–5 days, although occasionally at birth and as late as 7 days, with fever, irritability or lethargy, rash, abdominal distension, vomiting and poor feeding. Most develop hepatomegaly with a severe bleeding diathesis. Tachycardia or heart failure due to myocarditis is most likely with coxsackievirus infections but can also occur with echovirus infections. Meningitis with or without typical signs may occur. The timing of the onset of illness, the severe bleeding and the maternal history all help to suggest a diagnosis of enteroviral infection.

Hospital-acquired enteroviral infection may cause diarrhoea, respiratory signs (apnoea, tachypnoea, recession, increased oxygen requirements), rash, signs of meningitis or myocarditis, or may be completely asymptomatic.

Herpes simplex virus infection

Herpes simplex virus (HSV) infection may be localized to the skin (usually causing vesicular lesions), eye (keratitis, conjunctivitis, cataracts, chorioretinitis), oral cavity (ulcers) or central nervous system. Alternatively it may be disseminated, involving the liver, the above organs plus the lungs, GI tract and other organs. Disseminated infection presents with a sepsis-like picture; a bleeding diathesis is common. CNS involvement often results in intractable convulsions. Fever, jaundice, apnoeic episodes, lethargy or irritability, poor feeding, abdominal distension or vomiting, and respiratory distress may all occur. The onset of signs is variable. Occasionally babies are born with skin or eye lesions, but usually these present in the first week after birth. Disseminated infection usually presents in the first week. Isolated CNS infection, presenting with lethargy, irritability, poor feeding and convulsions, tends to be later, usually between 7 and 30 days.

Respiratory viruses

Infections with several respiratory viruses, notably respiratory syncytial virus (RSV), influenza virus, parainfluenza viruses and rhinoviruses can present a similar non-specific clinical picture. Apnoeic episodes, respiratory distress with or without added pulmonary shadowing and increased oxygen requirements, lethargy and irritability are all common. Rhinitis is by no means common in neonatal respiratory viral infection.

Fungal infections

Fungal infections affect preterm infants with birth-weights < 1000 g almost exclusively, particularly those babies who have received a great deal of antibiotics or are receiving total parenteral nutrition. The clinical picture closely mimics bacterial sepsis. The only clinical distinguishing features may be oropharyngeal candidiasis (often not present despite systemic fungal infections), fungal skin abscesses or endophthalmitis, which sometimes accompanies fungaemia.

In certain tribes in New Guinea there is a cultural response to illness of any kind, which is to groan, clutch the abdomen and complain of abdominal pain. The newborn infant presents a similar problem in that the signs of sepsis, whether attributable to different bacteria, viruses or fungi, are non-specific. Not only is it difficult to predict clinically what sort of organism is causing sepsis, but non-infectious conditions, such as patent ductus arteriosus, may cause an almost identical clinical picture. It is clear that the paediatrician will treat many babies with antibiotics and must rely heavily on the laboratory to confirm or refute his suspicion of sepsis and to identify the causative organisms.

Chapter 4

Investigations for suspected sepsis

Microbiological investigations

Blood cultures

Antibiotics should not be started without taking at least one blood culture. Preferably, blood should be taken from a peripheral vein or artery, after cleaning the overlying skin with an alcohol or iodine-based solution which is first allowed to dry. Blood drawn through umbilical catheters that have just been inserted is unlikely to be contaminated; blood cultures taken through umbilical arterial or venous or peripheral arterial catheters that have been present for some time are less reliable, as growth of organisms not found in simultaneous peripheral venous blood cultures is a frequent finding. On the other hand, Pourcyrous *et al.* (1988) found that, of 318 paired simultaneous umbilical arterial catheter (UAC) and peripheral venous cultures, the same organism was grown in 13 episodes of sepsis. Six UAC and five peripheral cultures grew organisms not found in the other blood culture pair. In the authors' opinion most of these were true episodes of sepsis and contamination rates for UAC cultures were actually marginally lower than those for peripheral blood cultures. Capillary blood cultures are easily contaminated by skin bacteria and should not be used.

Quantitative blood cultures may distinguish true sepsis from contamination when organisms, such as *Staphylococcus epidermidis*, which may be pathogens or contaminants are grown in blood cultures, but quantitative cultures are not usually routinely available.

Because of the large numbers of organisms generally present, only small volumes of blood may be needed to detect neonatal bacteraemia. As little as 0.2 ml of blood will detect *E. coli* bacteraemia (Dietzman *et al.*, 1974). It is, therefore, worth culturing blood even if only a small volume is obtained.

Because it is sometimes difficult to decide later about the validity of blood culture results, we record in the case notes the indications for blood culture, the site from which blood is taken and the quantity put in the bottles. Paired aerobic and anaerobic bottles are usually inoculated with blood. These are under vacuum and tend to suck in the whole specimen if the doctor is not careful.

Buffy coat microscopy

Because of the number of organisms present in neonatal septicaemia, organisms may be seen in neutrophils. These can be obtained by centrifuging a small volume of heparinized blood and aspirating the 'buffy coat' layer just above the red cells, or breaking a spun heparinized capillary tube full of blood at the buffy coat layer. The neutrophils are smeared on a slide and stained with Gram's iodine, methylene blue or acridine orange stains.

In expert hands the sensitivity can be up to 80–90% (Faden, 1976; Boyle *et al.*, 1978; Kleiman *et al.*, 1984) and some false negatives are due to neutropenia, itself strongly suggestive of sepsis. However, Rodwell *et al.* (1989) found a sensitivity of only 17%. Buffy coat examination may occasionally reveal intracellular budding yeasts (Cattermole and Rivers, 1987) and allow a rapid diagnosis of fungaemia.

Examination of cerebrospinal fluid

Lumbar puncture (LP) may interfere with respiration and cause a fall in neonatal oxygenation. This can be minimized by flexing the hips and knees but not the neck during the procedure. Approximately 20–30% of cases of neonatal septicaemia have simultaneous bacterial meningitis, which is thus not a rare occurrence. It has been suggested that LP is not immediately necessary in all cases of suspected early sepsis because LP can lead to severe deterioration in the baby's respiratory status (particularly if the baby has pulmonary hypertension), because meningitis is relatively rare and because the antibiotics used are often the same for septicaemia with or without meningitis. However, we believe that there are risks if LP is omitted for babies with suspected early sepsis.

Visser and Hall (1980) retrospectively reviewed 39 cases of neonatal bacterial meningitis and found that six (15%) had sterile blood cultures at the time of diagnosis. Nine babies with meningitis were aged < 24 h and three of these had negative blood cultures. Thus, negative blood cultures do occur in babies with both early- and late-onset bacterial meningitis and, therefore, if a lumbar puncture is not performed at the time of starting antibiotics there needs to be some safeguard so that babies with meningitis are not missed. The data from Visser and Hall suggest that it is insufficient to do an LP only in babies with positive blood cultures, because approximately one-third of cases of early-onset meningitis and one-tenth of cases of late-onset meningitis are associated with sterile blood cultures.

In early-onset bacterial meningitis the antibiotic treatment for early-onset sepsis would usually be the same whether or not meningitis was present. *E. coli* meningitis can be treated adequately with ampicillin and an aminoglycoside, so if an LP is not done for early-onset sepsis this combination might be better than penicillin and an aminoglycoside. For this reason, and because LP in early-onset sepsis can be deleterious, it could be argued that LP can be omitted from the 'sepsis screen' for early-onset infection and performed later when the baby's respiratory status is more stable. One problem with this approach is that it can be difficult to interpret the later CSF findings. For example, if there has been an intraventricular haemorrhage there is often lysis of red cells leaving a falsely raised CSF white cell count. Occasionally, meningitis (growth of a pathogen from CSF) occurs with normal CSF microscopy, Gram stain and biochemistry; although the initial LP is then negative it is uncertain what would be found in a delayed LP after the baby has been given antibiotics.

Our policy is that a lumbar puncture is performed before starting antibiotics on all babies with suspected sepsis, with the exception of babies with severe early-onset respiratory distress with a high risk of pulmonary hypertension in whom the deleterious effects of LP are felt to outweigh the advantages. We would then perform an LP as soon as the baby's condition was stable. Our reasoning is that, in addition to the prognostic and supportive treatment implications of making a diagnosis of bacterial meningitis, the later interpretation of CSF findings can often be difficult. Furthermore, the examination of CSF is equivalent to a biopsy in that organisms are usually seen immediately on Gram stain if there is meningitis. Because our antibiotic policy for treating late-onset sepsis (flucloxacillin and an aminoglycoside) provides very poor cover for late-onset meningitis, we are obliged to perform an LP on all babies with suspected late-onset sepsis. Nevertheless, even where the antibiotic policy provides good cover (as when it includes a third-generation cephalosporin), surprises may occur: fungal infections are increasing in infants of very low birth-weight, and *Candida* meningitis, for example, may mimic bacterial sepsis.

The interpretation of the CSF microscopy is considered in Chapter 7.

Examination of the urine

Urinary tract infection may present acutely as a septicaemic illness or more insidiously with vomiting and/or jaundice. Urine collected in a sterile plastic bag ('bag urine') is easily contaminated by faeces, whereas a suprapubic aspirate of urine (SPA) is rarely contaminated unless the bowel is accidentally perforated. A catheter specimen of urine is occasionally used as an alternative. In investigating babies with prolonged jaundice or vomiting, a bag urine is appropriate initially because antibiotics need not be prescribed immediately and further urines can be obtained if necessary. In apparently septic babies, when antibiotics must be started immediately, consideration should be given to performing an SPA before starting treatment. Visser and Hall (1979) have questioned the need for SPA urines, at least in early-onset sepsis. They analysed urine culture results in early ($< 72\,h$) and late-onset sepsis. In early sepsis a positive urine culture was rare: they only had 3 in a year; one baby also had positive blood cultures, while one of the urines was probably contaminated. In late-onset sepsis they had more positive urine cultures (14) but details of the organisms and the presence or absence of white cells in the urine were not reported and it is difficult to assess the likelihood of contamination.

Urinary tract infection is associated with pyuria (> 10 WBC per high-power field) in about 70–75% of cases (Ginsburg and McCracken, 1982). Suprapubic aspiration can lead to complications, is traumatic (to babies, parents and medical staff) and may lead to hypoxaemia. We have seen no cases of early-onset UTI over 5 years ($> 25\,000$ live births) except in association with disseminated sepsis in which blood cultures were also positive. Late-onset UTI is more common but we still diagnose only one or two cases annually in our newborn nursery, which serves 5000 live births. This incidence is lower than that usually quoted for neonatal UTI. Our policy is to perform urine microscopy on a bag urine obtained from all babies with suspected late-onset sepsis, but we have elected not to culture routinely the urine of babies with suspected early-onset sepsis. We would obtain urine by SPA if there were one or more of the following: a strong clinical suspicion of UTI; persistent pyuria (> 10 WBC per high-power field); organisms seen on urine microscopy, or growth of organisms from two or more bag urines. The main problem with this approach is that a 'positive' urine culture (as defined by growth of $\geq 10^5$ organisms per ml of a single bacterial strain) does not necessarily indicate a true UTI, because bag specimens can be contaminated. In practice we find that this is rarely a problem, as bag specimens are usually either sterile or yield multiple organisms on culture, indicating probable contamination. In the occasional equivocal case, when antibiotics have already been started and there is a 'pure growth' of $> 10^5$ organisms per ml, with or without pyuria, from a bag urine specimen, we would treat and investigate as for UTI. We have seen only four such cases in > 5 years of a policy in which bag urine specimens were used to investigate possible UTI. As our initial radiological investigations of neonatal UTI are now relatively non-invasive (see Chapter 10), we think that the possibility of failing to detect a few children with possible UTI is offset by avoiding several hundred SPA procedures per year.

Gastric aspirate

Gram's stains of gastric aspirates taken in the first few hours of life are frequently used to assess babies with respiratory distress for possible infection, particularly with group B streptococcus. However, the presence of polymorphonuclear leucocytes, which are maternal in origin, only indicates exposure to infection: <6% of babies born to mothers with clinical chorioamnionitis develop sepsis (Siegel and McCracken, 1981). Ingram *et al.* (1980) performed Gram's stains on gastric aspirates from 109 newborns with respiratory distress or suspected sepsis. Of 13 babies with early-onset group B streptococcal sepsis, 10 had positive Gram's stains but three (23%) had false-negative smears. This means that too much reliance should not be placed on a negative gastric-aspirate Gram's stain. Furthermore, there is a high rate of false positives, with bacteria and leucocytes identified in gastric aspirates from babies who are shown subsequently not to be septic. We no longer obtain gastric aspirates in suspected sepsis because our impression has been that too much reliance may be placed on a negative result, whereas the presence of pus cells and/or a scanty number of organisms is often over-interpreted as indicating probable sepsis.

Tracheal aspirate

In early-onset neonatal sepsis, ascending infection is the commonest mode of infection, with the respiratory tract an important early site of bacterial replication, and early pneumonia is usual. Sherman and colleagues (1980) evaluated the use of Gram's stains on smears of early tracheal aspirates in detecting congenital pneumonia. They obtained tracheal aspirates, during or immediately following laryngoscopy, from 320 newborns with respiratory distress. Twenty-five babies had bacteria seen on the Gram's stain; 14 of the 25 grew a compatible organism from blood cultures. The authors compared these babies with 25 of the babies with no organisms seen on tracheal aspirate smear: three of these 25 'controls' had positive blood cultures. The authors do not state how many of the remaining 270 babies with negative tracheal aspirate smears had positive blood cultures but, extrapolating from the 25 'control' babies, one might suppose that > 30 had bacteraemia. Thus, for the total population of 320 babies, the sensitivity of early tracheal aspirate in detecting early sepsis may have been < 30%. In a second study they found that, of those babies who had organisms seen on Gram's stain of the tracheal aspirates, 47% had early-onset bacteraemia, and 74% of all babies with early-onset bacteraemia had positive tracheal aspirate microscopy (Sherman *et al.*, 1984). This is a much-improved sensitivity, although one-quarter of the babies with early-onset sepsis had negative tracheal aspirate microscopy.

Endotracheal aspirate cultures are frequently performed on babies requiring long-term artificial ventilation for surveillance purposes and to identify likely pathogens should sepsis be suspected. It is known that endotracheal suction frequently causes transient bacteraemia, and it seems likely that the upper respiratory tract is a common site of entry of invading pathogens in late sepsis, occurring as frequently as it does in artificially ventilated babies. We have, nevertheless, found that endotracheal cultures are relatively insensitive in predicting the organisms causing late-onset septicaemia: either no organism is grown from the endotracheal aspirate when a baby is septicaemic (50–62% of cases) or the cultures yield many different organisms (Isaacs *et al.*, 1987a; Evans *et al.*, 1988). Furthermore, clinicians rarely pay any attention to the culture results, even when these are available (Evans *et al.*, 1988). Slagle *et al.* (1989) found that endotracheal cultures were insensitive in predicting the organisms causing late sepsis in ventilated babies and that, in 42% of cases, an antibiotic regimen based on the endotracheal culture would have resulted in inappropriate antibiotic therapy for the septicaemia.

The proportion of endotracheal tubes colonized with potential pathogens increases with time and is almost inevitable in babies on long-term artificial ventilation (Webber *et al.*, 1990). Antibiotics should not be given merely because of growth of a potential pathogen, e.g. *Pseudomonas*, from the endotracheal aspirate.

Surface cultures

Surface cultures and cultures from deep sites are commonly obtained when early- or late-onset sepsis is suspected. Evans and colleagues (1988) examined the sensitivity and specificity of cultures from the nasopharynx, external ear canal, axilla, rectum, umbilical cord, skin and eye. They found the sensitivity of each of these tests to be < 50% in predicting the organisms causing sepsis.

In our opinion it is important to know if a newborn with suspected early-onset sepsis is colonized, as blood cultures may be negative despite a strong clinical suspicion of sepsis. Thus we would treat a baby with heavy group B streptococcal (GBS) colonization and a clinical picture suggestive of early GBS sepsis for a full 7–10 days of antibiotics despite negative blood cultures. Similarly, we have seen babies with a clinical diagnosis of congenital listeriosis (rash, hepatosplenomegaly and respiratory distress) who are colonized with *Listeria monocytogenes* but have a negative blood culture; again, we treat such babies as infected.

In view of the low yield of surface cultures for late-onset sepsis and the fact that cultures from multiple sites scarcely improve the sensitivity of these tests, we have been able to reduce greatly the number of surface cultures performed in cases of suspected sepsis (see Chapter 17). For sepsis in the first 48 h of life we now culture an external ear swab and a nasopharyngeal or endotracheal aspirate, whereas for later sepsis we obtain only a naso-pharyngeal culture or endotracheal aspirate. We do, of course, culture from other sites if there is a clinical indication, such as an umbilical swab for omphalitis or eye swab for conjunctivitis.

It has been estimated by our microbiology department that the annual saving from our reduction in the number of surface swabs is > £20,000. Our monitoring has not suggested that this reduction in the number of swabs has impaired our ability to detect sepsis, nor to anticipate problems with resistant organisms.

Antigen detection

Rapid tests to detect bacterial antigens have been developed to identify infected babies before culture results are available. Countercurrent immuno-electrophoresis (CIE) involves placing the test specimen (usually serum or concentrated urine) in one well cut in an agar plate opposite a well containing antibody to the antigen being tested. When a current is placed across the agar, the antigen and antibody move towards each other, forming a precipitin line. Latex particle agglutination (LPA) employs latex particles coated with specific antibody which agglutinate in the presence of antigen. Enzyme-linked immunosorbent assays (ELISAs) are performed in plastic microtitre plates (solid phase). They depend on detecting antigen, using antibodies to the test antigen which have been linked to an enzyme which then catalyses a colour change in an indicator, detected spectrophoto-metrically.

Other techniques include immunofluorescent staining using a fluorescent substance attached to an antibody, and co-agglutination by specific antisera conjugated with protein A-containing staphylococci.

Rapid antigen detection is most sensitive on concentrated urine but has also been used to detect antigen in serum and CSF and, occasionally, other body fluids. The tests are, of course, specific for a single organism, which limits their usefulness: thus, in early-onset sepsis, group B streptococcal antigen tests will miss those babies with sepsis caused by other organisms, such as pneumococcus or *Haemophilus influenzae*, who may have an identical clinical presentation. The sensitivity of CIE and LPA for group B streptococcus on concentrated urine is 88–96% but for serum it is < 50% and for CSF it is 67–88% (Baker and Edwards, 1990). Most babies with clinically suspected GBS sepsis who have heavy colonization but negative blood cultures, have GBS antigen in urine detectable by LPA (H. Jeffrey, personal communication). Antigen-detection tests are thus useful in early sepsis, particularly when group B streptococcus is the commonest pathogen, but not in late sepsis.

Serum IgM

Total serum IgM rises in about one-half of all babies with bacterial sepsis but often as much as one week after the onset of sepsis. It is, therefore, of little value in diagnosis of sepsis.

Haematological investigations

Total white cell count

The total white cell count is of limited value in evaluating a baby for suspected sepsis: about one-third of all babies with sepsis have normal white cell counts, and about one-half of all those babies evaluated for sepsis who have abnormal white cell counts are not, in fact, infected. White cell counts may be $> 50\,000 \times 10^9/l$ in healthy newborns in the first 24 h of life. A white count should always be performed in suspected sepsis. A low total white cell count is an ominous finding in such a baby and, although it may be caused by other factors such as birth asphyxia, indicates a worse prognosis if the baby is, indeed, infected.

Morphology of white cells

Although there may be morphological changes, such as vacuoles, toxic granules and Dohle bodies, in the white cells in bacterial infections, these changes are non-specific and may be seen in white cells from normal babies.

Neutrophil count

Because the total white cell count is an unreliable indicator of sepsis, the total neutrophil count has been used as an alternative measure. It is important to relate this to the age of the baby, as the normal range of neutrophil counts varies with age, being far higher in the first 24 h after birth (Manroe *et al.*, 1979). At presentation, up to about one-third of babies with proven sepsis have normal neutrophil counts, the rest being either high or low. Neutropenia is particularly suggestive of severe sepsis and, as this finding suggests depletion of the granulocyte pool in the bone marrow, is a poor prognostic sign.

Immature neutrophils

Immature neutrophils are seen in the peripheral blood of even healthy preterm babies. Most are non-segmented neutrophils, also known as band or stab forms. In sepsis an increased number of immature neutrophils enter the circulation from the bone marrow, causing a so-called shift to the left in the blood film. Because the bone marrow granulocyte pool is quickly exhausted in neonatal sepsis, there is rarely an increase in the total immature neutrophil count in septic babies and this value alone is an unreliable indicator. As the total white count also tends to drop, the ratio of immature to total white cells is more reliable (see below).

Neutrophil ratios

Various methods of describing the ratio of immature to mature neutrophils have been examined to quantify the 'left shift'. These include the ratio of band to segmented forms, the ratio of immature to segmented neutrophils and the ratio of all immature or just band forms to the total neutrophil count. In studies of many different variables that might indicate sepsis, the immature to total white cell count (I:T) ratio has proved the single most sensitive indicator of sepsis (Manroe *et al.*, 1979; Philip and Hewitt, 1980). The I:T ratio has a sensitivity of about 90% and a specificity of 80–90%, so a number of cases will still be missed if this is used as the only indicator of sepsis. Rozycki *et al.* (1987) found that 13 (21%) of 61 babies with early sepsis had a normal white cell profile (total neutrophil count, total immune neutrophil count and I:T ratio) early in their illness, so that if sepsis was strongly suspected but the white cell profile was normal it was important to repeat the profile within a few hours.

Platelet count

Thrombocytopenia may be caused by bacterial endotoxin acting directly on platelets or damaging endothelium and causing mild thrombosis, or by cytokines. It is present in about 50% of cases of sepsis. Established disseminated intravascular coagulation (DIC) is rare in neonatal sepsis. Platelet counts fall late in disease and thrombocytopenia may also be caused by birth asphyxia, among other conditions. Thus, although thrombocytopenia may indicate sepsis, it is a finding of relatively low sensitivity and specificity. We have found the progressive development of thrombocytopenia to be a useful indicator of continuing sepsis when managing babies with *Staphylococcus epidermidis* septicaemia.

Haematological profile

Rodwell *et al.* (1989) used a scoring system based on various white cell parameters (totals and ratios) and platelet count to assess babies with suspected sepsis. They found that if three or more parameters were abnormal, this identified 96% of septic babies with a specificity of 86%.

Erythrocyte sedimentation rate (ESR)

The ESR test usually requires too much blood, but can be modified to use very small samples (Philip and Hewitt, 1980). The ESR tends to rise too late in most infections (not until 24–48 h after onset) to be of great diagnostic value.

Nitro-blue tetrazolium (NBT) test

Phagocytosing but not resting neutrophils will generate free oxygen radicals that will reduce the dye NBT to a purple colour due to formazan. This colour change can be detected using spectrophotometric techniques. The NBT test may be abnormal in normal preterm neonates and is less sensitive and harder to standardize than many of the other tests described.

Acute-phase reactants

Acute-phase reactants are serum proteins produced primarily in the liver but also, in the case of orosomucoid, in the intestine in response to various stimuli. These stimuli include bacterial infection but also other forms of stress, such as necrotizing enterocolitis or surgery. The proteins can be produced by the fifth week of gestation and are probably of primitive origin; their role in limiting infection is unknown.

Of the various serum acute-phase reactants that have been measured, C-reactive protein (CRP, named after the C-carbohydrate of *Pneumococcus* with which it combines) has proved the most useful in suspected sepsis. It starts to rise within 12–24 h of the onset of sepsis, earlier than the other acute phase reactants. Tests for measuring CRP include qualitative latex tests and quantitative tests such as laser nephelometry; they are cheap and rapid. Serum CRP is elevated in 50–90% of cases of sepsis and necrotizing entero-colitis but, as with all tests for sepsis, may be normal in some cases of true sepsis. It returns to normal within 2–7 days of successful treatment, and persistent elevation of the serum CRP may indicate persistent bacterial meningitis (Sabel and Hanson, 1974) or abscess formation in necrotizing enterocolitis (Isaacs *et al.*, 1987d). Serial CRP levels may also be useful in monitoring the response to treatment for osteomyelitis or septic arthritis.

Other acute-phase reactants such as orosomucoid (alpha-1-acid glycopro-tein), fibrinogen and haptoglobin increase more slowly than CRP during infection and their measurement has generally been far less useful.

Sepsis screens

Various research workers have described the combined use of several differ-ent techniques for identifying sepsis in order to improve the sensitivity for detecting infected babies. The haematological screen of Rodwell *et al.* (1989) has already been described. Philip and Hewitt (1980) showed that a panel of screening tests (white cell count, band/total neutrophil ratio, CRP, micro-ESR and haptoglobin) available within an hour identified 93% of babies with sepsis. Nevertheless, their criterion of two or more positive tests indicating sepsis missed two of 30 cases of sepsis, and the authors stressed the importance of accurate clinical evaluation of each baby and stated that, if sepsis was strongly suspected, antibiotics should be started, regardless of test results. These screens are expensive and none has 100% sensitivity. They can certainly reduce antibiotic use (Philip & Hewitt, 1980) but this must not be at the expense of delayed treatment of sepsis. We prefer to use an individual clinical decision on each baby as to whether or not antibiotics should be prescribed, in conjunction with the guidelines on risk factors which are described in Chapter 5.

Antibiotic policies

Which babies to treat

We have already discussed the risk factors for the development of early and late sepsis, and possible adjuncts to the diagnosis of sepsis. Some babies will develop sepsis, either early or late, with no known risk factors. Furthermore, no ancillary laboratory tests for sepsis have 100% sensitivity. If cases of sepsis are not to be missed, therefore, treatment should always be initiated if there is strong clinical suspicion of neonatal sepsis, regardless of whether there are risk factors or laboratory tests supporting sepsis. This inevitably means that far more babies receive antibiotics than ever have documented sepsis: approximately one baby has proven sepsis of every 10 babies treated for suspected sepsis. We go on to argue that the effects of such widespread use of antibiotics can be minimized by using antibiotics for as short a duration as possible.

Certain clinical situations, in which the use of antibiotics on a routine basis is often considered, recur regularly in the newborn intensive care nursery. We attempt to discuss these situations and describe our policy and reasonable alternatives below.

Preterm baby with respiratory distress from birth and one or more risk factors for sepsis

It is our policy that, for any preterm baby with early respiratory distress, an abnormal chest radiograph and one or more risk factors for sepsis, cultures are taken and antibiotics given. The risk factors in these babies are prolonged rupture of the membranes, smelly liquor, maternal fever, and spontaneous preterm onset of labour with or without rupture of the membranes. These risk factors are known to be associated with sepsis attributable to group B streptococci (Boyer *et al.*, 1983), pneumococci (Bortolussi *et al.*, 1977) and enterococci (Dobson and Baker, 1990), and probably apply to other organisms. Prolonged rupture of membranes is a continuum of increased risk: the greatest risk is after 18 h but the risk of sepsis increases when membranes are ruptured for > 12 h (Boyer *et al.*, 1983).

In our experience, the admitting doctor is highly likely to consider sepsis in the differential diagnosis of a baby with early respiratory distress and any of the first three risk factors. In contrast, respiratory distress in association with spontaneous preterm onset of labour is almost always called hyaline membrane disease and early pneumonia is rarely considered (Webber *et al.*,

1990). In our series of babies with early-onset pneumonia, however, spontaneous preterm onset of labour was by far the commonest risk factor (Webber *et al.*, 1990). In practice, this means that the only preterm babies with respiratory distress who do not receive at least 48 h of antibiotics are the small group in which caesarean section is performed or labour is induced early for maternal reasons.

We have specifically mentioned an abnormal chest radiograph in this context, usually a fine, generalized granularity but sometimes showing focal areas of consolidation. Where the radiograph is normal but there is respiratory distress, clinical suspicion of sepsis and one or more risk factors, we would nevertheless start antibiotics, because we have occasionally seen a normal chest radiograph early in severe GBS sepsis.

Some authors have suggested that it is possible to distinguish babies with early-onset bacterial pneumonia from those with hyaline membrane disease by the use of Gram's stains of surface swabs, total neutrophil counts and immature-to-total neutrophil count ratios (Leslie *et al.*, 1981). However, up to 21% of babies with early-onset sepsis have completely normal haematological profiles (Rozycki *et al.*, 1987) and there may be difficulties in obtaining these tests rapidly. Our view is that the decrease in the proportion of babies given antibiotics resulting from the use of sepsis screens (e.g. Philip and Hewitt, 1980) is outweighed by the danger of delay in administering antibiotics and the risk of placing too much reliance on a negative test.

Preterm baby with one or more risk factors for sepsis but no immediate symptoms after birth

The more risk factors present at birth, the more likely is the baby to be infected. Thus, if a baby is born with two or more risk factors for sepsis, e.g. a baby with spontaneous preterm onset of labour and prolonged rupture of membranes, we would perform a full septic screen and start antibiotics. We would do this even if the baby was asymptomatic and there was no information on maternal vaginal cultures. On the other hand, if only one risk factor was present, e.g. preterm onset of labour, but the baby was clinically well we would not necessarily start antibiotics.

Full-term baby with respiratory distress

Hyaline membrane disease is rare in full-term babies, and respiratory distress at term should suggest the possibility of sepsis. Most full-term babies with respiratory distress will have a final diagnosis of transient tachypnoea of the newborn (TTN). In this condition the initial chest radiograph shows a 'wet lung' appearance with increased vascular markings and often fluid in the horizontal fissure. Unfortunately, an identical radiographic appearance has been described in about 10% of cases of early-onset GBS pneumonia (Baker and Edwards, 1990). Thus, although most cases of early pneumonia at term will have a generalized granularity mimicking hyaline membrane disease or areas of focal consolidation, a chest radiograph that is normal or shows 'wet lung' does not exclude pneumonia. Mifsud and colleagues (1988) have described tachypnoea, as monitored routinely in newborn babies at their hospital, as a useful early indicator of sepsis. Early detection of infected babies in their study may have contributed to a fall in mortality from early sepsis.

Examination of Gram's stains performed on gastric aspirates (Ingram *et al.*, 1980) and tracheal aspirates (Sherman *et al.*, 1980, 1984) have shown these tests to be only moderately reliable, with sensitivities of 77% and 74% respectively, in predicting babies with early sepsis. Thus they may be used to aid diagnosis, but only in the knowledge that they will not identify all cases of early sepsis. For example, in the study by Ingram *et al.* (1980) the gastric aspirate was negative in three of 16 (23%) babies with early-onset GBS pneumonia. We do not use gastric aspirates because our junior staff are falsely reassured by a negative Gram's stain and have great difficulty in interpreting the results if the Gram's stain reveals a number of different organisms.

In term babies with respiratory distress, additional laboratory tests such as total neutrophil count, ratio of immature-to-total neutrophil counts and serum CRP level may help to decide whether to treat or observe, but the clinical picture should always be the final arbiter.

Severe perinatal asphyxia

Severe perinatal asphyxia may occasionally result from sepsis: up to 20% of babies with perinatal sepsis have respiratory depression requiring intubation (Gluck *et al.*, 1966). On the other hand, most babies with perinatal asphyxia are not septic. If the baby is severely obtunded, then clinical signs of sepsis may be masked. Additionally, the haematological picture is often abnormal in severe asphyxia and neutropenia may occur (Manroe *et al.*, 1979). As sepsis is a rare cause of asphyxia, the use of antibiotics should be determined on an individual basis for severely asphyxiated babies. Both asphyxia and infection may cause pulmonary hypertension ('persistent transitional circulation') and if this should supervene, full septic screen should be carried out and antibiotics started.

Meconium aspiration syndrome

Meconium aspiration may result from severe perinatal asphyxia. In addition, it has been argued that, although meconium is sterile, the plugging of airways resulting from meconium aspiration may predispose to secondary pneumonia. As is the case for severe perinatal asphyxia, it is not logical to prescribe antibiotics in case secondary pneumonia develops. We, therefore, do not routinely prescribe antibiotics in meconium aspiration syndrome but assess each baby for the likelihood of sepsis.

Dirty procedures around delivery

In some babies, usually those with perinatal asphyxia or acute blood loss, intravascular catheters are inserted hurriedly, often in the delivery suite and under less than optimally sterile conditions. Antibiotics are often prescribed to cover such 'dirty' procedures. There is extremely little evidence that sepsis occurs as a result of dirty procedures, nor that it can be prevented by giving antibiotics. Nevertheless, the practice of giving antibiotics under these conditions is likely to continue, whatever is argued, and is probably relatively harmless if antibiotics are stopped early when cultures are negative.

Prophylactic antibiotics

Some neonatologists routinely prescribe antibiotics to babies with venous and arterial cannulas and to those requiring endotracheal intubation, as prophylaxis against infection. There is evidence that prophylactic antibiotics do not prevent sepsis from umbilical venous or arterial catheters, peripheral artery catheters (where the risk of sepsis is low) and indwelling peripheral or central venous catheters (summarized in Nelson, 1983). Harris and colleagues (1976) found that antibiotics that were started at the time of endotracheal intubation and continued for a mean of 3–4 days protected against subsequent systemic infection, which invariably followed colonization of the endotracheal tube. However, they also found that colonization was almost invariable after 72 h of intubation. It may be that antibiotics decrease the number of colonizing organisms and hence the risk of sepsis. We and others have not found such a clear correlation between the organisms causing endotracheal colonization and subsequent sepsis (Slagle *et al.*, 1989; Webber *et al.*, 1990) and feel that the nature of late-onset sepsis may be changing since the time of Harris' study. We do not give prophylactic antibiotics to cover endotracheal intubation *per se* although, as stated previously, most artificially ventilated babies are given antibiotics in case they are already infected. The use of antibiotics in preterm babies with respiratory distress is often described as giving 'prophylactic' antibiotics. This is a misconception: antibiotics are being given to these babies to *treat* possible sepsis until culture results are obtained; a corollary of this is that antibiotics can be stopped when cultures are negative.

There are very few situations in which antibiotic prophylaxis has been shown to be effective in the neonatal period. Babies with structural abnormalities of the urinary tract are at high risk for UTI. Although antibiotic prophylaxis is often useful in preventing UTI in older children, we have found it less effective in neonates, although we continue to prescribe prophylactic antibiotics for babies with proven UTI. We are unaware of any formal studies on their efficacy in the newborn with urinary tract abnormalities. Intrapartum administration of intravenous ampicillin to women who are colonized with group B streptococcus and in a high-risk category (maternal fever, prolonged rupture of the membranes, spontaneous preterm onset of labour) been shown to reduce neonatal GBS sepsis (Boyer and Gotoff, 1986); this is discussed in more detail in Chapters 13 and 18. There are conflicting data on whether oral aminoglycosides prevent necrotizing enterocolitis and they are rarely used because of selection of resistant organisms. There is no evidence that antibiotics given at the time of insertion of cerebrospinal fluid shunts prevent shunt infections (Editorial, 1989). There is evidence that intravenous cefuroxime at induction for anaesthesia reduces the risk of subsequent sepsis in adult patients undergoing bowel surgery, but no such evidence exists for newborn infants. Prophylactic oral nystatin is frequently used for infants and babies of low birth-weight on antibiotics, but there is no firm evidence of its efficacy.

Which antibiotics to use

The antibiotics to use are those that most narrowly cover the spectrum of organisms causing sepsis in the nursery and that have been shown to be effective in treating cases of sepsis. However, there is great variation in the organisms causing sepsis, not only between but also in one region and even within any one hospital over time. It is important to keep up-to-date records, therefore, on the organisms causing systemic sepsis in the newborn nursery and the outcome of episodes of sepsis, and to review these regularly. No antibiotic policy can be deemed wrong unless it patently fails to cover organisms causing significant sepsis, and infection with these organisms causes significant morbidity or mortality (see Chapter 17).

Early-onset sepsis

Penicillin or ampicillin is generally used, together with an aminoglycoside (gentamicin, netilmicin or amikacin), as the empirical treatment of early sepsis. This is logical because in most countries in the developed world the group B streptococcus is currently the organism that most often causes early-onset sepsis and also causes the highest morbidity and mortality. Group B streptococcus has rarely been reported as causing sepsis in developing countries, although a recent report from Kingston, Jamaica showed it to be the commonest organism causing both early and late-onset sepsis (Macfarlane, 1987). Aminoglycosides are used with a penicillin because Gram-negative organisms, particularly *E. coli*, are a common cause of early sepsis. On the other hand *Listeria monocytogenes* is increasingly described as causing early sepsis, and in some European countries such as France it is one of the most common organisms. Ampicillin is preferred to penicillin for *Listeria* sepsis (with an aminoglycoside), although penicillin and an aminoglycoside is generally effective (see Chapter 13). The third-generation cephalosporins, which have sometimes been advocated for monotherapy of neonatal sepsis, are ineffective against *Listeria*.

We have tended to prefer penicillin G to ampicillin because widespread use of ampicillin is more likely to select for multiple drug resistance (Tullus and Burman, 1989) and colonization with *Candida*. On the other hand, there are theoretical but unproven advantages of ampicillin over penicillin in treating infections with *Haemophilus influenzae*, enterococci and *Listeria monocytogenes*, all of which are increasing in the UK. The aminoglycoside of choice is again a moot point. Gentamicin is cheaper, there is more experience with its use and, consequently, potentially toxic drug levels are less common. On the other hand, netilmicin causes less ototoxicity in adults (Davey, 1985) and is less likely to select for the emergence of resistant Gram-negative organisms (Isaacs *et al.*, 1988a). Amikacin may be the most ototoxic of these three aminoglycosides, although because of confounding causes of deafness it has been difficult to show this in small studies (Davey, 1985; Finitzo-Heiber *et al.*, 1985).

In most cases of suspected early-onset sepsis, little additional information is available on which to base antibiotic treatment. If the culture results of a high vaginal swab from the mother before delivery are known, the antibiotics used should cover these organisms effectively. The results from

Gram's stains of surface swabs, gastric and tracheal aspirates are insufficiently reliable to form the basis for changing a tried and tested antibiotic regimen.

The mortality from early-onset sepsis is high and it is important that there is the minimum possible delay in giving the first doses of antibiotics. In our unit, the admitting doctor takes blood cultures and gives intravenous antibiotics as soon as the decision is made to start treatment, usually within an hour of birth. Surface swabs and CSF can then be collected immediately after treatment has been started.

We are sceptical of the wisdom of attempts to introduce monotherapy with a ureidopenicillin or third-generation cephalosporin for early- and late-onset sepsis (Isaacs and Wilkinson, 1987). Such policies ignore the difference between the organisms causing early- and late-onset sepsis and do not sufficiently cover relatively common or increasing causes of sepsis such as *Listeria*.

Regardless of the antibiotic regimen used for early-onset sepsis, the mortality and morbidity of proven sepsis are extremely high. It seems unlikely that delayed therapy or ineffective antibiotics are responsible for the poor outcome; rather, the dissemination of a large microbial load, often in a compromised fetus without maternal antibody, has occurred before delivery. Our efforts should probably be centred on prevention of severe early-onset sepsis, perhaps by identifying and treating with intrapartum antibiotics those women at risk for delivering a baby with early sepsis (Boyer and Gotoff, 1986).

Late-onset sepsis

Three possible approaches can be taken to the choice of antibiotics for late-onset sepsis, as outlined below.

Treat the baby according to a standard antibiotic policy

This is probably the best way of limiting the emergence of resistant organisms. If a large range of antibiotics is used simultaneously, multiple drug resistance may become a significant problem. Use of a standard regimen will usually result only in selection of organisms resistant to a single antibiotic. Furthermore, colonization with resistant organisms does not necessarily lead to sepsis with resistant organisms, which are sometimes less virulent than sensitive ones (White *et al.*, 1981; Isaacs *et al.*, 1987a). If episodes of systemic sepsis with resistant organisms occur, and particularly when those babies most at risk for sepsis (artificially ventilated, low birth-weight) are also colonized with the resistant organisms, this can be used as an indication to change the antibiotic policy in order to withdraw the 'antibiotic pressure' (Isaacs *et al.*, 1988a).

There is no 'ideal' antibiotic regimen for treating suspected late-onset sepsis. When we surveyed neonatal units in the United Kingdom, a very wide range of antibiotic regimens was being used. Such regimens must cover the organisms most likely to cause systemic sepsis, and this information is best obtained by reviewing the recent cases of sepsis, rather than from surface cultures (Evans *et al.*, 1988). Nevertheless, there may be rapid changes in the organisms causing sepsis in a single unit (Table 1.5). At present, in most developed countries, late-onset sepsis is most commonly caused by Gram-negative enteric bacilli, enterococci (faecal streptococci), coagulase-negative staphylococci such as *Staphylococcus epidermidis* and sometimes *Staphylococcus aureus*.

The most commonly used regimens are (i) a penicillin and an aminoglycoside (the penicillin may be a semi-synthetic penicillinase-resistant penicillin such as cloxacillin or methicillin if staphylococcal infection is a particular problem); (ii) a third-generation cephalosporin with or without an aminoglycoside; (iii) a third-generation cephalosporin plus ampicillin; (iv) vancomycin plus an aminoglycoside or third-generation cephalosporin if methicillin-resistant *S. aureus* is a problem. The disadvantages of using aminoglycosides is their potential to cause oto- and nephrotoxicity and the consequent need to monitor drug levels. The third-generation cephalosporins do not need to be monitored and penetrate CSF well, but their use often leads to widespread colonization and sometimes sepsis with enterococci, while they provide relatively poor cover against staphylococci. Furthermore, widespread use of cephalosporins may lead rapidly to resistance (Modi *et al.*, 1987), although this is not always the case (Spritzer *et al.*, 1990). In general, different antibiotics will be needed for treating babies with meningitis (see Chapter 7).

The deciding factor on antibiotic policy must be the outcome of episodes of sepsis. Morbidity from sepsis is difficult to evaluate because of confounding factors such as extreme prematurity. In the John Radcliffe Hospital, Oxford, flucloxacillin and an aminoglycoside are used for late-onset sepsis and the third-generation cephalosporins are held in reserve for babies failing to respond to conventional treatment and those with Gram-negative enteric bacillary meningitis. An analysis of the organisms causing sepsis in Oxford (Table 1.5) might suggest that alternative antibiotic regimens could be envisaged; we have continued to use the same regimen, however, because the mortality from late-onset sepsis of babies in our Neonatal Unit is < 5% and the deaths would not have been avoided by an alternative antibiotic policy.

Treat according to the organisms colonizing that baby

Sprunt and colleagues (1973) found that nasopharyngeal colonization preceded the onset of systemic sepsis and that sepsis was almost always due to the colonizing organism. This has been used as one of the rationales for widespread and expensive surveillance of the organisms colonizing babies in the nursery. Recently, however, the value of surveillance cultures in this context has been questioned (Isaacs *et al.*, 1987a; Evans *et al.*, 1988). We did not find any false-positive surface cultures in 26 babies with late-onset septicaemia (i.e. no babies were colonized *only* with organisms other than the invading one) but only 10 of the septic babies had positive surface cultures, giving a sensitivity of 39% for such cultures in predicting the organism causing sepsis, and five of the 10 were colonized with multiple organisms (Isaacs *et al.*, 1987a). Evans and colleagues (1988) showed that surface cultures taken on the day of sepsis had a sensitivity of 56% and that this fell to 50% for cultures taken 1 day before sepsis, 32% 2 days before and < 30% for cultures taken earlier than this. Furthermore, they found a number of false-positive or misleading surveillance cultures.

Surveillance cultures are poor predictors of which babies will become infected, poor predictors of which organisms will cause systemic sepsis and not infrequently will wrongly identify the organism causing sepsis.

Treat according to the organisms prevalent colonizing babies in the neonatal unit

It would be suspected that rationalizing the choice of antibiotics for treating one baby on the basis of organisms found to be colonizing other babies in the nursery would be even less sensitive and specific than if the decision were based on the baby's colonizing organisms. Nevertheless, when there is widespread colonization with one organism, for example a gentamicin-resistant Gram-negative rod, it might seem rational to treat all babies as if they were infected with this organism. White and colleagues (1981), however, found substantial fluctuations in colonization rates of ampicillin- and gentamicin-resistant organisms and no correlation of patterns of colonization with episodes of sepsis. We have reported similar fluctuations in the rates of colonization with gentamicin-resistant organisms. As these bacteria rarely caused systemic sepsis, we continued to use gentamicin (Isaacs *et al.*, 1987a). Subsequently, all babies requiring artificial ventilation were found to be colonized with a gentamicin-resistant *Klebsiella oxytoca*; two babies developed sepsis due to this organism, although both survived. Under the circumstances we felt compelled to change from gentamicin to netilmicin as our aminoglycoside of choice for the treatment of suspected late-onset sepsis (Isaacs *et al.*, 1988a).

Our antibiotic management of suspected late-onset sepsis (with normal CSF and urine microscopy) is to prescribe antibiotics according to a standard regimen, currently flucloxacillin and netilmicin. We change the antibiotics for a given baby, as already described, if the blood culture results and deteriorating clinical picture suggest that this is necessary. We regularly review the results of blood cultures and limited surveillance cultures (an endotracheal aspirate taken once weekly from each ventilated baby only) and change our antibiotic policy if widespread colonization with resistant organisms is accompanied by episodes of systemic sepsis with the resistant organism.

Duration of antibiotics

An important corollary of the liberal use of antibiotics for suspected sepsis is that they should be stopped as early as possible if cultures prove negative. It used to be argued that stopping antibiotics before completing a 'full course' would select for antibiotic-resistant organisms; on the contrary, there is evidence that resistant organisms are selected by long courses of antibiotics (Lacey, 1984). Furthermore, babies who receive antibiotics for > 72 h are more likely to become colonized with Gram-negative enteric organisms

(Goldmann *et al.*, 1978). As 96% of positive blood cultures have grown within 48 h and 98% within 72 h (Pichichero and Todd, 1979), we stop antibiotics after 2–3 days' treatment if cultures are sterile. This policy has proved to be practical and reasonable (Isaacs *et al.*, 1987b).

The advantages of this approach are that antibiotics are used for a short duration, thereby reducing selection of resistant organisms, colonization with abnormal oropharyngeal and bowel flora (Goldmann *et al.*, 1978) and the risks of systemic candidiasis and aminoglycoside toxicity. In addition, there are cost savings (Isaacs *et al.*, 1987b) both from using less antibiotics and from rarely having to measure drug levels, because we do not usually measure aminoglycoside levels unless antibiotics are continued beyond 72 h. This approach has led to a 25–40% reduction in the average duration of antibiotic therapy (see Figure 17.1).

Some problems that we have encountered frequently regarding the use of antibiotics in different situations are discussed below.

Baby looked septic but cultures were negative

In general it is probably rare to get false-negative blood cultures, i.e. no growth from blood cultures despite bacteraemia, in the neonatal period. Neonatal bacteraemia is characterized by relatively large numbers of circulating organisms and therefore only small volumes of blood are needed to obtain a positive blood culture.

Nevertheless, negative blood cultures where the circumstantial evidence for sepsis is strong are common. In one study, blood cultures pre-mortem were negative in seven of 39 babies (18%) who died from infection (Squire *et al.*, 1979). In a study of babies with early-onset pneumonia we identified 11 who had blood cultures which grew group B streptococci, but also nine babies who were heavily colonized with group B streptococci but had sterile blood cultures (Webber *et al.*, 1990); in our opinion, this latter group almost certainly had pneumonia. Most of them would probably have had GBS antigen detected in concentrated urine (Baker and Edwards, 1990) but we did not perform this test. Thus the sensitivity of blood culture in GBS pneumonia is only 55%. We have also seen two babies with the clinical features of congenital listeriosis who were heavily colonized with *Listeria monocytogenes* but whose blood cultures were negative. Cases of neonatal meningitis, including cases in the first 24 h of life, with positive CSF microscopy and culture but negative (presumably false negative) blood cultures have been described (Visser and Hall, 1980).

Early-onset sepsis arises as a result of ascending or transplacental infection and heavy colonization almost invariably occurs concomitantly with septicaemia. If a baby with strongly suspected early-onset sepsis but negative systemic cultures (blood, urine, CSF) is heavily colonized with a probable pathogen such as group B streptococcus, it seems reasonable to continue a full course of antibiotics as if for proven sepsis. Conversely, if surface cultures as well as systemic cultures are negative, early-onset sepsis is unlikely and antibiotics can be stopped after 48–72 h (Isaacs *et al.*, 1987b).

In suspected late-onset sepsis, colonization with potential pathogens is a poor indicator of sepsis because colonization is extremely common in asymptomatic babies (Evans *et al.*, 1988). We have shown that stopping antibiotics after 48–72 h is safe in late-onset sepsis and in our experience babies did not subsequently need to be re-started on antibiotics (Isaacs *et al.*, 1987b). We did, however, perform lumbar punctures as part of our late-onset sepsis investigations. If these are not routinely performed before starting antibiotics it is advisable to do a LP before stopping, as ~ 10% of episodes of late meningitis have negative blood cultures (Visser and Hall, 1980).

Positive blood cultures, dubious organism or organisms

A common scenario is that the doctor has to decide whether or not a baby with a doubtful blood culture result requires a full course of antibiotics. Certain organisms are relatively common contaminants of blood cultures, contamination occurring either in taking blood from the baby or subsequently in the laboratory. Common, relatively common and rare contaminants are shown in Table 5.1 and, as might be expected, the commonest are organisms that colonize skin. Multiple organisms in blood cultures are usually, but not always, contaminants. As septicaemia is generally associated with large numbers of bacteria and contamination of blood cultures is generally associated with small numbers, rapid growth of an organism in both aerobic and anaerobic blood culture bottles is more likely to indicate true septicaemia whereas delayed growth in a single bottle is more likely to be due to contamination. Nevertheless, contaminants may grow in both bottles, and only one bottle may grow up in true sepsis. Some laboratories will perform quantitative or semi-quantitative blood cultures, which can

Table 5.1 Significance of blood culture isolates

Significance	Organisms
Almost always significant	Group B streptococcus
	Streptococcus pneumoniae
	Listeria monocytogenes
	Haemophilus influenzae
	Enterococci (*Streptococcus faecalis, S. faecium, S. bovis,* etc.)
	Group A streptococcus
	Group C/G streptococci
	Neisseria meningitidis
	Neisseria gonorrhoeae
	Gram-negative bacilli
	Candida and other fungi
Sometimes significant (about 50%)	*Staphylococcus aureus*
	Coagulase-negative staphylococci (*S. epidermidis* etc.)
	Streptococcus viridans group (including *S. mitis, S. mitior, S. milleri, S. sanguis,* etc.)[a]
	Clostridium species
	Multiple isolates (polymicrobial)
Almost always contaminants	Diphtheroids
	Propionibacterium
	Bacillus species

[a]In early-onset sepsis may be significant, in late-onset usually contaminants

help distinguish contamination from sepsis. It is always important to inter-pret blood culture results in the context of the clinical picture, and additional tests such as total and differential white cell count and serum CRP can be helpful. It should be noted that certain organisms are rare contaminants and should generally be taken seriously: for example, in disseminated candidia-sis it is common to find that there has been earlier growth of *Candida* from a blood culture, which has been dismissed as a probable contaminant (Weese-Mayer *et al.*, 1987).

It is always helpful to know, and preferably for the doctor taking the blood cultures to record in the notes, from whence the blood was drawn (vein, artery, through an umbilical or peripheral cannula) and the indications for taking blood. We have seen a baby whose blood culture taken one hour after birth grew *Staphylococcus aureus*, an unlikely early-onset pathogen. On questioning, the doctor admitted to having aspirated blood from the baby's skin after a difficult venepuncture. A menagerie of different organisms is suspicious of contamination: after one such example we discovered that junior doctors were using a 'broken needle' to collect blood which was dropped into specimen bottles. This useful technique for taking blood samples was also being used to take blood cultures by dropping the blood into the barrel of a syringe and needle from which the plunger had been removed. The plunger was then replaced to inject the blood into blood culture bottles. Sometimes a syringeful of blood is collected and some of the sample is injected into the porthole of a blood gas machine, which is often heavily contaminated, before filling blood culture bottles (which because of their vacuum tend to suck in the whole sample). Similarly, if blood is first injected into fluid-containing bottles such as ESR, clotting or urea and electrolyte bottles, even if the needle is changed before filling the blood culture bottles, water-loving organisms such as *Pseudomonas maltophilia* or *Acinetobacter* may grow. If this technique is repeated often, there can be an apparent outbreak of sepsis or 'pseudo-bacteraemia'.

If it is decided that the blood culture isolate is a contaminant we would stop antibiotics or, in the rare cases in which antibiotics had not been started, repeat the blood cultures. It is always wise to repeat the blood cultures, even if the baby seems well, because cases have been described of asymptomatic but persistent bacteraemia (Albers *et al.*, 1966). It should be remembered that neonates are extremely susceptible to infection and may become in-fected with organisms of low virulence. *Staphylococcus epidermidis*, which used to be considered only a contaminant, is increasingly recognized as a neonatal pathogen and babies may be infected with anaerobes secondary to chorioamnionitis. Thus, blood culture results must always be interpreted with care and in the appropriate clinical context.

Septicaemia

If the baby is clinically septic and has positive blood cultures, a full 'course' of antibiotics should be prescribed. There are no firm data on the correct duration of antibiotics for proven sepsis, as recurrence is rare. In the opinion of most authors, 7–10 days of antibiotics is appropriate, although we would continue longer if the baby remained ill. We treat *Listeria* septicaemia for

14 days because it is an intracellular pathogen. Meningitis requires longer antibiotic therapy (see Chapter 7).

Most antibiotic regimens incorporate a penicillin (penicillin G, ampicillin or a semi-synthetic penicillin such as flucloxacillin) and an aminoglycoside. Even if a baby is shown to have, say, GBS sepsis, the aminoglycoside is often continued because of the theoretical advantage, rather than any proven clinical benefit, of synergy between penicillin and aminoglycoside. The toxic effects of aminoglycosides are cumulative, particularly after 7 days of treatment, and in our opinion it is important to stop the aminoglycoside if a baby is infected with a penicillin-sensitive organism (group B streptococcus, *Listeria*, etc.) as soon as there is sustained clinical improvement.

In ~ 30% of episodes of neonatal septicaemia there is concurrent bacterial meningitis. If an LP was not performed in the initial investigations of sepsis because the baby's respiratory status was too unstable, or because that is the unit's policy, it is imperative to perform one as soon as possible. Even if this will not alter the antibiotics used, or the dose, it will affect the duration of antibiotics (see Chapter 7) and the earlier the LP can be done, the easier it will be to interpret the CSF findings.

Chapter 6

Supportive therapy for septic babies

Introduction

Despite the undoubted importance of specific antimicrobial therapy against pathogenic microbes, the role of other facets of the management of sepsis should not be underestimated: antimicrobials are only one aspect of the treatment of the septic baby. Because of real or perceived difficulties in recruiting sufficient babies and organizing controlled trials, many of the possible adjunctive therapies have not been critically evaluated and their use remains controversial.

Treatment of shock

It is necessary to assess whether a septic baby is shocked and, if so, to take immediate steps to reverse this. The diagnosis of shock is based on a clinical picture of pallor, paucity of movement, poor peripheral perfusion (as shown for example by slow return of colour when a digit is pressed) and tachycardia with poorly palpable pulses. Hypotension is not necessarily present, as peripheral vasoconstriction may maintain an adequate blood pressure despite hypovolaemia. There is oliguria or anuria. The rectal temperature is often low (< 35.5°C) (Messaritakis *et al.*, 1990). The peripheral core temperature gradient is a less useful indicator of shock in neonates than in older children (Messaritakis *et al.*, 1990).

The immediate use of fresh frozen plasma, 10–20 ml/kg given i.v. and repeated until shock is reversed, uses a physiological fluid that contains immunoglobulins and clotting factors. Plasma substitutes can be used until the fresh frozen plasma is thawed or if none is available. If there is significant bleeding, as for example in association with DIC, it is more appropriate to use fresh blood for volume replacement.

If the baby remains shocked despite adequate fluid replacement, or if cardiac output is profoundly depressed, it may be beneficial to use a continuous infusion of dopamine at 2–10 µg/kg per hour to improve myocardial function and renal perfusion. Infusion rates > 10 µg/kg per hour divert blood from the kidneys and are counterproductive. Central venous pressure monitoring is important in determining whether or not fluid replacement has been adequate, before using dopamine.

Echocardiography, if available, can be used to evaluate left ventricular function and, if myocardial contractility is depressed, can indicate the need for dopamine.

Artificial ventilatory support

Babies with severe sepsis, if not already shocked, are often in imminent danger of cardiovascular collapse, which may be prevented by initiating artificial ventilation. In our opinion, early elective intubation and ventilation of septic babies is an important supportive measure that is often neglected. Too often, severely ill babies are given antimicrobials and watched in the hope that they will not need artificial ventilation; some recover but others collapse and need emergency resuscitation for mixed metabolic and respiratory acidosis.

Correction of metabolic acidosis

Metabolic acidosis commonly accompanies systemic sepsis. The policy in the John Radcliffe Hospital, Oxford is to use the buffered alkali tris-hydroxymethyl aminomethane (THAM) as part of the management of metabolic acidosis if the base deficit exceeds 10, because $PaCO_2$ rises less with THAM than when sodium bicarbonate is used. If sodium bicarbonate is used it should be with caution because of its hypertonicity; we use it diluted 1:1 with 5% dextrose. Excessive use can cause hypernatraemia and hypercarbia. The latter may precipitate respiratory failure by depressing respiratory drive and lead to the need for urgent respiratory support.

Hypoglycaemia

Hypoglycaemia may accompany sepsis, particularly in babies who have also had perinatal asphyxia, and should be urgently corrected. We would give intravenous dextrose if the blood glucose concentration was below 2.6 mmol/l.

Thrombocytopenia

Significant thrombocytopenia may accompany sepsis. Thrombocytopenia may be caused by bone marrow suppression or by peripheral destruction due to the toxic effect of bacterial factors such as lipopolysaccharide (endotoxin), to peripheral immune platelet destruction or to DIC. Platelet transfusions are needed if significant bleeding accompanies thrombocytopenia or if thrombocytopenia is severe enough (usually $< 20 \times 10^9/l$) to threaten haemorrhage.

Convulsions

Convulsions accompany about one-half of all cases of meningitis, but may also occur in severe sepsis without meningitis. Convulsions are often subclinical or difficult to diagnose. Where these are a strong possibility, and particularly if the baby is receiving muscle relaxants, continuous EEG monitoring, if available, or serial EEGs may enable the diagnosis to be made and allow monitoring of the response to anticonvulsants.

Neutrophil transfusions

Christensen has been the keenest advocate of neutrophil transfusions for babies with severe sepsis who are neutropenic and have depleted bone-marrow neutrophil reserves, as shown by bone marrow examination. He has shown that transfusions of fresh neutrophils to septic neutropenic puppies can improve their survival rate. In a study in which neutropenic septic babies were randomly assigned to treatment with neutrophil transfusions or no neutrophil transfusions, all seven treated babies but only one of nine un-treated babies survived (Christensen *et al.*, 1982). Two other studies have shown improved survival of septic infants given neutrophil transfusions, even in the absence of neutropenia (Laurenti *et al.*, 1981; Cairo *et al.*, 1984). On the other hand, Baley and colleagues (1987) found no improvement in a small randomized controlled trial of buffy-coat neutrophil transfusions to neutropenic neonates, some of whom were septic.

The number of babies studied has been small and, although no adverse effects have been reported, there are a number of theoretical risks such as sensitization, graft-versus-host reactions and transmission of viruses such as CMV. In addition there are considerable logistic problems. Neutrophils for transfusion have to be obtained fresh by leucophoresis of one of an identified panel of donors who have to be regularly screened for CMV and HIV antibodies and who are available to be called at short notice. The process of leucophoresis is also time consuming, causing several hours' delay before neutrophils are available. In our experience, neutropenic sepsis is so rare (one or two cases a year) that the Blood Transfusion Service, who do not prepare neutrophil transfusions for other patients, are, quite reasonably, not prepared to offer such a service. In our opinion there is insufficient evidence to use neutrophil transfusions for all babies with suspected sepsis.

Exchange transfusion

Exchange transfusion is performed fairly frequently for severe sepsis but has never been subjected to a satisfactory controlled trial, so its efficacy is difficult to evaluate. In theory, there are many potential advantages: improvement of circulatory status; replacement of clotting factors and immunoglobulins (although these may be equally well served by plasma infusions); better oxygenation of the tissues by improving the oxygen-carrying capacity of the blood, and the removal of toxic bacterial products such as endotoxin. Exchange transfusion may cause untoward haemodynamic changes and we tend to use it only as a last resort. In one uncontrolled study, seven of ten babies with severe sepsis and sclerema improved immediately after exchange transfusion, and survived (Vain *et al.*, 1980).

Immunoglobulin therapy

The prophylactic use of intravenous immunoglobulin preparations is discussed in Chapter 18. The relatively low serum levels of IgG in the neonate, particularly before 32 weeks' gestational age, suggest that there might be a role for acute immunoglobulin therapy to improve serum opsonic capacity (Whitelaw, 1990). There have been two studies which have suggested that intravenous immunoglobulins may have a role in the *treatment* of systemic sepsis: Sidiropoulous *et al.* (1981) found that 500 mg/kg per day of Sandoglobulin reduced mortality from sepsis in preterm babies (four of nine in the control group died compared with one of 13 in the treatment group); similarly, Haque *et al.* (1988) found that six of 30 control babies with suspected sepsis died compared with one of 30 given Pentaglobin, an immunoglobulin preparation containing IgG, IgM and IgA. Larger studies are in progress and we await their results; at present we do not use intravenous immunoglobulins to treat septic babies.

Removal of indwelling cannulas

The incidence of sepsis with coagulase-negative staphylococci such as *Staphylococcus epidermidis* is rising in most neonatal units in the United Kingdom and elsewhere. In our unit, about one-half of the cases are associated with an indwelling UAC or a percutaneous intravenous silicone catheter ('central line'). A decision frequently must be made as to whether or not to remove an important line from a baby with suspected sepsis, who has poor vascular access. The two commonest scenarios are the *acute* presentation, in which the baby appears acutely septic with a UAC or silicone 'central line' *in situ*, and the *sub-acute* presentation in which the baby with such a line still in place has remained moderately unwell after 2 days on antibiotics and blood cultures are reported to be growing *Staphylococcus epidermidis*. An individual assessment of the baby must be made, with particular reference to the degree of illness, changes in the white cell and platelet counts, and the necessity for the UAC or silicone intravenous catheter.

If the baby is shocked, neutropenic and thrombocytopenic it is probably necessary to remove the vascular catheter and to treat the baby with antibiotics through peripheral venous cannulas. It should be remembered that, although *Staphylococcus epidermidis* is the commonest cause of catheter-associated sepsis and generally causes a relatively mild illness, *Staphylococcus aureus* can also infect catheters and tends to cause a much more fulminating illness (Decker and Edwards, 1988). Gram-negative organisms and fungi less commonly infect catheters but infections with fungi seldom resolve without catheter removal. As *Staphylococcus epidermidis* infection is rarely fulminant, we and others have tried to treat babies who are only moderately unwell, and whose catheter is particularly vital for feeding and vascular access, by using antibiotics and leaving the catheter in place. Sadiq *et al.* (1987) described the management of catheter-associated infections in neonates who predominantly were preterm and often were of very low birth-weight; their experience is summarized in Table 6.1. They were generally successful in managing *S. epidermidis* septicaemia without catheter

Table 6.1 Management of catheter-associated infections in neonates

Organism cultured from blood	No. of cases	No. managed without catheter removal	No. managed successfully without catheter removal
Staphylococcus epidermidis	8	6	5
Methicillin-resistant Staphylococcus aureus	8	6	3
Candida albicans	4	0	0
Escherichia coli	2	2	2
Miscellaneous streptococci	4	4	4
Total	26	18	14

After Sadiq et al. (1987)

removal, but only half the babies with methicillin-resistant *S. aureus* (MRSA) sepsis were successfully managed in this way.

Our current approach to suspected line-associated sepsis is as follows. If it is decided to treat a baby with antibiotics and to leave the catheter in place, the baby is constantly reviewed and if there is any clinical deterioration the catheter is removed. If, after 48–72 h, the blood cultures grow *Staphylococcus epidermidis*, the baby is reassessed; if the baby is well, the catheter is left in place, antibiotics are continued and repeat blood cultures performed. The further management depends on the clinical picture and repeat blood culture results. If there is anything to suggest continuing sepsis, either clinically or in the form of decreasing white cell or platelet counts (the latter is a particularly useful indicator of continuing sepsis with *S. epidermidis*), and the organism is sensitive to the antibiotics being used, the catheter is removed. Vancomycin is used for babies infected with methicillin-resistant staphylococci who have continuing clinical evidence of infection. The catheter is removed if fungi are cultured (Chapter 14).

Removal of CSF shunt

CSF shunt infections in older children and adults will not resolve unless the shunt is removed (Schoenbaum et al., 1975). Although this has not been formally confirmed in neonatal CSF shunt infections, it is generally accepted that the same principle applies, and that the infected shunt must be removed before the infection can be cured (see also Chapter 7).

Meningitis

Incidence

Meningitis is more common in the first month postnatally than at any other time and more common in the first week than later (Goldacre, 1976). About 20% of all cases of neonatal septicaemia, both early- and late-onset, are complicated by bacterial meningitis. In addition, viruses may cause meningitis or meningo-encephalitis, and fungal meningitis can occur in babies of very low birth-weight. The incidence of neonatal meningitis is higher in infants of low birth-weight; the reported incidence will therefore vary according to the population being studied. Nevertheless, whole population-based studies in the United States have consistently shown 0.2–0.5 cases of bacterial meningitis per 1000 live births. Reports to the Communicable Disease Surveillance Centre and a study by Goldacre (1976) suggest that the incidence in Britain is around 0.2 per 1000 live births, but this may well be an underestimate attributable to under-reporting. A recent study by J. de Louvois and D. Harvey (personal communication) suggests the true incidence is nearer 0.4 per 1000 live births. A study from Sweden suggests that, unlike other countries, their incidence of neonatal meningitis may be falling (Bennhagen *et al.*, 1987).

Certain groups of babies are at greatly increased risk of meningitis irrespective of birth-weight. Babies with open myelomeningoceles are particularly likely to develop bacterial meningitis, especially that attributable to Gram-negative enteric bacilli. CSF shunts are highly likely to become infected.

Dermal sinuses overlying the CSF anywhere from the bridge of the nose, over the skull and down the back to the sacrum may penetrate through to the dura and give rise to meningitis. If a dermal sinus is missed (and they can be very small and hidden under the hair), then recurrent meningitis can occur.

Organisms

In Britain, group B streptococcus is now the commonest cause of neonatal bacterial meningitis (about one-third of all cases), having overtaken *Escherichia coli*, which is easily the second commonest (~ 30%). *Listeria monocytogenes* is the third most prevalent, causing < 10% of cases but with the frequency rising. These are followed by various Gram-negative bacilli (*Pseudomonas, Proteus, Klebsiella, Enterobacter, Neisseria meningitidis* and *Haemophilus influenzae*) and Gram-positive cocci (*Streptococcus pneumoniae* and other streptococci). Anaerobic meningitis is rare. A list of

Table 7.1 Organisms causing neonatal bacterial meningitis, in approximate order of frequency for United Kingdom

Group B streptococcus
Escherichia coli
Listeria monocytogenes
Pseudomonas species
Streptococcus pneumoniae
Enterococci
Proteus species
Staphylococcus aureus
Klebsiella species
Neisseria meningitidis
Haemophilus influenzae
Citrobacter species
Enterobacter species
Serratia species
Salmonella species
Other Gram-negative bacilli
Other streptococci
Anaerobes
Mycobacterium tuberculosis
Campylobacter species
Coagulase-negative staphylococci (shunt infections)

organisms causing bacterial meningitis is given in Table 7.1, in the approximate order of frequency for the United Kingdom (approximate because bacterial meningitis is under-reported). In other parts of the world the frequency of the different organisms may be very different: *Salmonella* and *Mycobacterium tuberculosis* are common in developing countries and group B streptococcus is only occasionally reported from these countries. *Shigella* meningitis almost only ever occurs in the newborn period.

Shunt infections are most commonly due to coagulase-negative staphylococci. A specimen of CSF should always be obtained in suspected shunt infections because these may also be caused by *Staphylococcus aureus*, Gram-negative bacilli or fungi.

Meningitis due to myelomeningocele is usually caused by Gram-negative enteric bacilli.

The isolation of certain organisms should alert the physician to special problems. For example, *Citrobacter* meningitis is frequently associated with brain abscess, although abscess may occur with other organisms such as *Proteus*.

Pathogenesis

When infant rats are inoculated intranasally with *Haemophilus influenzae* type b, organisms colonize and invade the nasopharyngeal epithelium, resulting in bacteraemia (Moxon *et al.*, 1974). In this model infection, the magnitude of bacteraemia correlates strongly with the probability of meningitis; bacterial concentrations of 10^3/ml of blood were found to be necessary, but not always sufficient, to result in meningitis (Moxon and Ostrow, 1977).

These observations are consistent with observations in human neonates (Dietzman *et al.*, 1974), also showing an association between the magnitude of bacteraemia and the occurrence of Gram-negative meningitis.

Less commonly, meningitis can be due to direct spread either from an infected scalp lesion with spread through skull sutures and thrombosed veins (Morrison, 1970) or from otitis media (Ermocilla *et al.*, 1974).

Certain organisms are far more likely to cause bacterial meningitis than others, so that the virulence of the invading organism as well as host factors are important in determining whether or not meningitis occurs. The K1 capsular antigen of *Escherichia coli*, which is similar to the capsular poly-saccharide of Group B *Neisseria meningitidis*, is important in facilitating bloodstream survival. More than 80% of cases of neonatal *Escherichia coli* meningitis are caused by strains carrying the K1 antigen (Robbins *et al.*, 1974). The importance of the type III capsular polysaccharide of group B streptococcus as a virulence factor for late-onset meningitis has already been mentioned. Although neonatal septicaemia due to *Staphylococcus epidermidis* is increasingly being described, meningitis attributable to this organism virtually never occurs unless there is a CSF shunt *in situ*.

Despite earlier diagnosis and more effective antimicrobial therapy, the mortality and morbidity from neonatal meningitis remain extremely high. Various reasons can be advanced for this. Neonatal meningitis occurs at an age when host defences are poor and the brain is at its most susceptible to damage. The high bacterial load in neonatal meningitis means that toxic products of the bacterial cell wall, peptidoglycans and teichoic acid from Gram-positive and lipopolysaccharide (endotoxin) from Gram-negative organisms, cause substantial damage to the endothelial cells of the cerebral capillaries which form the so-called 'blood–brain barrier'. Disruption of the tight junctions between the endothelial cells increases the permeability and allows entry of bacteria and white cells and leakage of protein. Indeed, the introduction of more than a critical number of killed bacteria, either Gram positive or Gram negative, into the CSF of an experimental animal is lethal. However, it is increasingly clear that it is not merely the toxic effects of bacterial products, but also the host immune response which causes damage to the central nervous system (see Figure 7.1). Infection results in the release of substances such as tumour necrosis factor (also called cachectin) and interleukin-1 from mononuclear cells, which may damage endothelial cells and lead to raised intracranial pressure and cerebral oedema. Arachidonic acid metabolites from platelets are also probably important in pathogenesis. Levels of prostaglandin E_2, a potent vasocative substance, rise in the CSF in experimental meningitis, and this contributes to cerebral oedema; both the increased levels and cerebral oedema can be blocked by indomethacin (Sande *et al.*, 1987). Complement may be important in opsonizing organisms but can also lyse host cells if bacterial cell-wall products are incorporated into them (Hummell *et al.*, 1985).

Cerebral blood flow is reduced in animal models of bacterial meningitis (Sande *et al.*, 1987); this may be due to focal vasculitis, to raised intracranial pressure or to vasoconstriction. Autoregulation of cerebral blood flow is frequently impaired in meningitis. Thus, cerebral blood flow varies with blood pressure, and hypotension or hypertension will result in cerebral hypoperfusion or intracranial hypertension, respectively. The degree of

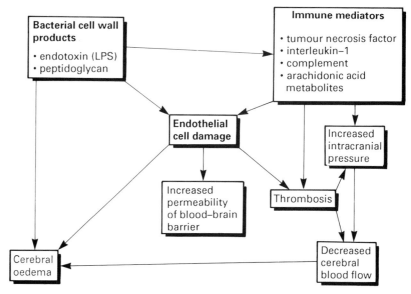

Figure 7.1 Mechanisms in pathophysiology of meningitis

impairment of cerebral blood flow correlates with CSF levels of bacteria and lipopolysaccharide. Reduced cerebral blood flow produces regional hypox-aemia, increased metabolism of arachidonic acid, and anaerobic glycolysis with increased production of lactate and consumption of glucose resulting in low CSF glucose (hypoglycorrhachia).

Intracranial pressure (ICP) is always elevated in bacterial meningitis; the possible mechanisms include cerebral oedema, vasodilatation of cerebral veins and capillaries, loss of autoregulation of cerebral blood flow and impaired circulation of CSF. In a rabbit model of pneumococcal meningitis, methylprednisolone reduces cerebral oedema but not raised intracranial pressure, whereas dexamethasone reduces both (Tauber *et al.*, 1985); this suggests that raised ICP is not due to cerebral oedema alone.

The outcome in neonatal meningitis is generally worse than that in older children. The relatively poor neonatal immune response, permitting rapid bacterial multiplication, is one possible reason. Severe ventriculitis, a hall-mark of neonatal meningitis, is rarely seen outside the newborn period. Fever is relatively uncommon in neonatal meningitis, and this may contrib-ute to the poor outcome as CSF bacterial multiplication in experimental pneumococcal meningitis is far more rapid at normal body temperatures than when animals are febrile (Small *et al.*, 1986).

Pathology

Ventriculitis is common in neonatal bacterial meningitis, particularly Gram-negative meningitis, and there may be collections of pus in the ventricles and subarachnoid space. Subdural effusions are rarely of a sufficient size to cause raised intracranial pressure. Hydrocephalus may develop secondary to pu-rulent exudate obstructing the arachnoid granulations over the surface of the brain, or as a result of exudate in the ventricles obstructing the foramina of Magendie and Luschka or the aqueduct. Intraventricular haemorrhage may occur, and contribute to hydrocephalus. Vasculitis is common and may lead to venous thrombosis; there may be infarcts and focal necrosis. In severe cases there is often widespread neuronal damage which leads to necrotic liquefaction or cerebral atrophy. If abscesses develop they often lack the capsule seen in older children and are multiple.

The most common associated site of infection outside the CNS is the lung (pneumonia or empyema). There may also be otitis or omphalitis (which have occasionally been the original source of sepsis), peritonitis, pyelone-phritis, enterocolitis, osteomyelitis, septic arthritis and abscesses in other organs (skin, liver, etc.).

Clinical features

The classic clinical features of bacterial meningitis are frequently absent and there may be no apparent distinction between the newborn with sepsis with or without meningitis. Klein and Marcy (1990) summarized the clinical signs in 255 neonates with bacterial meningitis in six centres: fever was present in 61%, lethargy in one-half, abdominal signs (anorexia, vomiting, abdominal distension) in one-half, respiratory distress in 47%, convulsions in 40%, irritability in 32%, jaundice in 28%, and apnoea in 7%; 28% had a full or bulging fontanelle and only 15% had neck stiffness. A high-pitched cry may accompany cerebral irritation from any cause, including meningitis.

Diagnosis

Because of the difficulty in making a clinical diagnosis of meningitis it is vital that if sepsis is suspected either an LP is performed or, if the LP is delayed because of the baby's unstable condition, blood cultures are taken and antibiotics started that will adequately cover the organisms likely to cause bacterial meningitis. We have already elucidated in Chapter 5 our reasons for performing an LP in all but the most compromised babies. This is particularly true for late-onset infection, in which a far wider range of organisms may cause infection (including enterococci, *Listeria* and fungi as well as Group B streptococci and Gram-negative enteric bacteria). This wide range makes empirical antimicrobial therapy without a lumbar punc-ture far more difficult. About one-third of all cases of early-onset meningitis are associated with negative blood cultures (Visser and Hall, 1980), so if antibiotics are started for suspected early-onset sepsis without performing a lumbar puncture, this should be done later. However, occasionally menin-gitis may be present with normal CSF microscopy while an intraventricular haemorrhage may complicate the later interpretation of the CSF white cell count.

Interpretation of CSF findings

Information on normal CSF findings in term and preterm infants comes from a number of different studies (Klein and Marcy, 1990). In general, CSF white cell count and protein levels are higher and CSF glucose levels lower in normal neonates than in older children and adults. These differences are even more marked in preterm infants.

In normal preterm infants the mean CSF white cell count is up to 27/µl, about one-half neutrophils, with a range of 0 to 112 (Gyllensward and Malmstrom, 1962). In normal term infants the mean white cell count is lower (~ 5/µl) in most studies but again the range is up to 90 (Naidoo, 1968). Sarff *et al.* (1976) found no difference in CSF findings between term and preterm infants at high risk of infection but without meningitis. The mean CSF white cells counts were 8 and 9/µl and the ranges 0–32 and 0–29 for term and preterm babies, respectively. Sixteen babies with septicaemia without meningitis had a mean CSF white count of 20/µl (range 0–112). Of 21 babies with proven group B streptococcal meningitis and of 98 babies with Gram-negative enteric meningitis, 29% and 4%, respectively, had CSF white counts < 32 (Sarff *et al.*, 1976). This shows that there is considerable overlap between the CSF white cell count in babies with and without meningitis. Bacteria may sometimes be cultured from the CSF of babies with normal CSF microscopy (no white cells and no organisms seen).

The mean CSF protein in preterm babies without meningitis is ~ 100 mg/dl (1.0 g/l) with the normal range ~ 50–290 mg/dl (0.5–2.9 g/l). For term babies the mean is ~ 60 mg/dl (0.6 g/l) and the range 30–240 mg/dl (0.3–2.4 g/l). The CSF protein may be raised in bacterial meningitis, but in one study was within the normal range of 20–170 mg/dl (0.2–1.7 g/l) in 47% of babies with group B streptococcal meningitis and 23% with Gram-negative enteric bacillary meningitis (Sarff *et al.*, 1976). Elevated CSF protein in the absence of pleocytosis may be seen in parameningeal infections, congenital infections and intracranial haemorrhage.

Mean absolute CSF glucose concentrations in normal babies have varied from 50 to 80 mg/dl (2.7–4.4 mmol/l) with a range of 24–100 mg/dl (1.5–5.5 mmol). The CSF glucose is generally low in bacterial meningitis, and may be zero, but in some cases may be higher than the lower limit of the 'normal range'. As CSF and blood glucose concentrations are both lower in healthy newborn infants than in older children, it has been suggested that the ratio of CSF to blood glucose is a useful indicator of neonatal meningitis. In the study by Sarff *et al.* (1976) the mean CSF:blood glucose ratio was 81% (range 44–248) in preterm infants without meningitis and 74% (range 55–105) in term infants. However, 45% of infants with group B streptococcal meningitis and 15% with Gram-negative bacillary meningitis had CSF:blood glucose ratios > 44%, showing that the CSF:blood glucose ratio is relatively poor at discriminating babies with and without meningitis.

Of the 119 babies with neonatal meningitis reviewed by Sarff *et al.* (1976), only one had completely normal CSF microscopy and biochemistry. The Gram's stain reveals organisms in ~ 80% of cases of meningitis. The CSF white cell count is generally higher in Gram-negative enteric bacillary than in group B streptococcal meningitis (median number 2000 and 100 respectively). Although neutrophils usually predominate in bacterial meningitis, the same is also true in early viral meningitis.

In brain abscess there may be a moderate increase in CSF white cell count, with up to a few hundred cells, mostly mononuclear, and raised CSF protein. Organisms are not usually seen on Gram's stain nor grown from the CSF.

Ventriculitis is present in most babies with Gram-negative enteric meningitis and many with group B streptococcal meningitis. The diagnosis can be made by finding > 100 white cells / μl in ventricular CSF obtained by ventricular tap. On the other hand, ventricular taps can result in intracerebral cysts, and ventriculitis is so common that it can almost be assumed to be present, particularly in Gram-negative bacillary meningitis. Ventriculitis can sometimes be diagnosed on cerebral ultrasound imaging by seeing unusual fibrin strands in the ventricles.

In viral meningitis the CSF glucose level is usually normal although low glucose levels may occur, the protein level is often elevated and the mean CSF white cell count is usually < 1000 / μl, although it may be up to 4500 with a neutrophil predominance. Thus, in the absence of organisms on Gram's staining, it can be extremely difficult to distinguish viral from bacterial meningitis.

Management

Clinical assessment

When meningitis is 'proven' (organisms seen on CSF Gram staining) or probable (raised CSF white cell count but no organisms seen), a careful clinical assessment is the first priority. The baby should be examined for a source of infection, notably otitis, omphalitis and osteomyelitis of the skull and also for midline CNS anomalies such as congenital dermal sinuses. These can occur anywhere in the midline from the bridge of the nose, on the scalp under the hairline and down the spine to the sacrum.

Skin rashes – erythematous, maculopapular or purpuric – may accompany bacterial meningitis while a fine, macular rash may occur in enteroviral meningitis. The eyes should be examined for the characteristic retinal or vitreous lesions of fungal meningitis.

The head circumference should be measured, both to see if there has been a marked increase from the last measurement and to act as a baseline for serial measurements during treatment.

A full clinical examination is, of course, essential, both to look for other foci of infection and to assess the overall clinical state. The blood pressure should be measured, but may be artificially maintained due to raised intracranial pressure and peripheral vasoconstriction. Thus an assessment for shock should also include an assessment of peripheral perfusion (capillary return and core–peripheral temperature difference), of pulse character and heart rate and of urinary output.

Antibiotic therapy

The choice of antibiotic therapy will depend on which organisms are seen on Gram staining, either Gram-positive cocci (most probably group B streptococcus, enterococcus or pneumococcus), Gram-positive bacilli (*Listeria*) or Gram-negative bacilli (most likely *E. coli*, *Pseudomonas*, coliforms or *Haemophilus influenzae*), or no bacteria at all. The situation is completely different for infected ventricular shunts and is considered later in this chapter.

It is generally acknowledged that all antibiotics should be given parenterally for the entire duration of therapy of neonatal meningitis. Oral absorption is extremely erratic in the neonatal period and even chloramphenicol, which is well absorbed later in infancy, gives very poor blood levels if given orally to neonates. Aminoglycosides are sometimes given intramuscularly because intravenous boluses can give rise to high serum peak levels, but a slow intravenous infusion of aminoglycoside over 15–20 minutes probably does not exceed the therapeutic range. All other antibiotics used for treating bacterial meningitis should be given intravenously because muscle perfusion may be poor.

For GBS or pneumococcal meningitis, penicillin or ampicillin and an aminoglycoside is the treatment of choice. The recommended dose of penicillin G for treating GBS meningitis is 250 000 units (150 mg) per kg per day (McCracken and Feldman, 1976) because of the high minimum inhibitory concentration (MIC) of some isolates and the poor penetration of penicillin into CSF. Ampicillin should be used at 300–400 mg/kg per day for meningitis. The dose frequency varies with gestational age; the dose and frequency of aminoglycoside is as for systemic sepsis (see Appendix 3).

For meningitis attributable to *Listeria monocytogenes*, ampicillin and an aminoglycoside is the regimen for which there are most data. *Listeria* is susceptible to penicillin *in vitro*, and although there have been a few reports of treatment failures using penicillin G and an aminoglycoside, ampicillin is not always successful either. Penicillin and an aminoglycoside is, therefore, a reasonable alternative regimen. The doses of these two regimens are as for GBS meningitis. The third-generation cephalosporins are inactive against *Listeria*.

There is more controversy over the preferred antibiotic therapy for Gram-negative enteric meningitis. In the United States, ampicillin and an aminoglycoside has been the preferred regimen with which newer treatments have been compared. In 1971–1975 the mortality for 56 infants with Gram-negative enteric meningitis treated with parenteral ampicillin and gentamicin was 30.4% and about one-half the survivors were normal (McCracken and Mize, 1976). The penetration of aminoglycosides into CSF is poor and CSF cultures often remain positive for several days (McCracken, 1972). In order to improve delivery of antibiotics, McCracken and colleagues studied intrathecal and intraventricular administration of aminoglycosides. Intrathecal administration by lumbar puncture did not improve outcome (McCracken and Mize, 1976) while intraventricular aminoglycosides worsened the outlook (McCracken *et al.*, 1980). Nevertheless, the prognosis of Gram-negative meningitis is inversely correlated to the duration of positive cultures (McCracken, 1972); if cultures remained positive after 4–5 days, many authorities would recommend inserting an intraventricular reservoir for aminoglycoside administration.

The third-generation cephalosporins give excellent levels in the CSF, which greatly exceed the MIC of almost all Gram-negative bacilli and it was hoped that these antibiotics would supersede previous therapy. When the combination of ampicillin and one of the third-generation cephalosporins, moxalactam, was compared with ampicillin and amikacin, however, there was no difference in mortality or morbidity between the two treatment regimens (McCracken *et al.*, 1984). It is not clear why this should be. It is possible that rapid killing of bacteria might itself be deleterious, because of release of toxic bacterial products such as endotoxin (Editorial, 1985a).

Moxalactam has now been discredited for the treatment of neonates because it has caused significant bleeding problems. Cefotaxime and ceftazidime are the two third-generation cephalosporins most widely used in the United Kingdom for bacterial meningitis, while ceftriaxone has been used in the USA (Steele, 1984). Ceftriaxone and moxalactam can displace bilirubin from albumin and may cause hyperbilirubinaemia, particularly in babies of very low birth-weight (Robertson et al., 1988), and should be used with caution. There have been anecdotal reports of the efficacy of third-generation cephalosporins, particularly cefotaxime, in treating Gram-negative enteric bacillary meningitis. One report describes the treatment of seven neonates; although the final outcome was said to be good, one baby relapsed, two babies developed cerebral abscesses and two required shunts for hydrocephalus (Naqvi et al., 1985). A recent report suggests that cefotaxime therapy may be associated with a higher than expected rate of relapse of Gram-negative enteric meningitis (Anderson and Gilbert, 1990).

Cefotaxime gives good activity against almost all Gram-negative bacilli although ceftazidime has greater activity against Pseudomonas species. Cefotaxime will also treat Haemophilus influenzae meningitis. The dose is 150 mg/kg per day in three divided doses. As aminoglycosides appear to be surprisingly effective in neonatal meningitis despite poor CSF penetration, perhaps by reducing bacteraemia, it seems sensible to use an aminoglycoside with a third-generation cephalosporin for Gram-negative bacillary meningitis.

Chloramphenicol has been widely used to treat neonatal meningitis in the United Kingdom. In a recent national study by de Louvois and Harvey of nearly 500 cases of neonatal meningitis, 48% received chloramphenicol (J. de Louvois, personal communication). There is little information on the efficacy of chloramphenicol in neonatal meningitis. Heckmatt (1976) reported 36 patients treated for coliform meningitis in Glasgow from 1960 to 1974: most received chloramphenicol; 22 (61%) died, and only nine (25%) were apparently normal. In a more recent study, four of 11 neonates (36%) with Gram-negative bacillary meningitis treated with chloramphenicol died; morbidity could not be assessed from the paper (Mulhall et al., 1983a).

There are strong theoretical reasons for not using chloramphenicol to treat neonatal meningitis. Although chloramphenicol is bactericidal for Haemophilus influenzae, Streptococcus pneumoniae and Neisseria meningitidis and thus is excellent treatment for older infants and children with meningitis, it is bacteriostatic for most Gram-negative enteric bacilli. Thus, chloramphenicol treatment often leads to persistently positive CSF cultures, which would suggest a poor outcome (McCracken, 1972). Most worrying of all, however, is the toxicity of chloramphenicol. In one study, 64 neonates in 10 UK hospitals received chloramphenicol (Mulhall et al., 1983b). Ten babies suffered toxicity: five developed grey baby syndrome (four of these had cardiovascular collapse with cardiac arrest), one other baby became 'very grey' and four had reversible haematological abnormalities. Only one of these babies had been given a dose higher than recommended. Two other babies received a tenfold overdose (due to miscalculation of the dilution of the vial) and 27 babies had elevated serum chloramphenicol levels without signs of toxicity. In a recent study, 20% of babies were started on a chloramphenicol dose higher than recommended (J. de Louvois, personal communication). Although it is easy to say that accidental overdose should never occur, it is more realistic to avoid this possibility by using less toxic drugs. If chloramphenicol is ever used in the newborn period, drug levels should be closely monitored because of the variable metabolism and the danger of under- or overdosing.

When there is CSF pleocytosis but no organisms are seen on Gram staining, empirical antibiotic therapy must be given. Ampicillin and an aminoglyocoside or ampicillin and a third-generation cephalosporin (e.g. cefotaxime or ceftazidime) would appear to be the most sensible combinations, providing effective cover for group B streptococci, *Listeria*, *Pneumococcus*, enterococci and Gram-negative bacilli. Monotherapy with a third-generation cephalosporin will not cover infections with *Listeria* or enterococci and is inferior for GBS infection. Only ∼ 20% of cases of bacterial meningitis have negative CSF Gram stains; CSF pleocytosis may also occur due to viral meningitis, a parameningeal focus such as brain abscess, or following an intraventricular haemorrhage. Thus empirical antibiotics will often be given when there is no bacterial meningitis. This makes it even more important not to use toxic antibiotics such as chloramphenicol.

It is generally accepted that intravenous antibiotic therapy for neonatal meningitis should be continued for at least 21 days, longer if infectious complications supervene or there is delay in sterilizing the CSF.

Supportive therapy

The same basic principles for supportive therapy apply as described for systemic sepsis in Chapter 6. Although inappropriate secretion of antidiuretic hormone (ADH) is common in bacterial meningitis, the first priority is to support the systemic circulation with fresh frozen plasma and, if necessary, inotropic agents. Only when the circulation is adequate should babies be fluid restricted.

Steroids

Although there is some evidence that dexamethasone may be of value in childhood meningitis in preventing hearing loss and possibly other neurological sequelae, this has not been studied in neonates. The rationale for steroids is to diminish a harmful inflammatory response. In newborns it seems likely that a poor immune response and rapid bacterial multiplication are the major problems and there seems little justification at present for using steroids.

Monitoring

Close monitoring of vital parameters is essential in order to minimize morbidity and mortality, and newborns with bacterial meningitis should ideally be looked after in a tertiary referral centre. In shocked babies, continual monitoring of arterial and central venous pressure allows better fluid balance management. Urine output, urine and serum osmolality and serum electrolytes should be monitored to permit anticipation of problems with inappropriate ADH secretion. Haematological parameters, including clotting, should be regularly measured. Sabel and Hanson (1974) found serial serum CRP measurements to be a useful indicator of progress, low levels showing resolution and elevated levels suggesting continuing infection. Drug levels of antibiotics and anticonvulsants may need to be measured. Head circumference should be measured at least daily, as should the baby's weight. Regular neurological examination is, of course, essential. Intracranial pressure (ICP) is rarely monitored invasively in the newborn period but cerebral perfusion pressure (arterial blood pressure minus ICP) may be an important determinant of outcome. The measurement of fontanelle pressure by fontanometer, although non-invasive, is less reliable than invasive ICP monitoring. Invasive monitoring of ICP by subdural catheter or intraventricular catheter is rarely performed in newborns but might be indicated when there is evidence (e.g. rising blood pressure, falling heart rate) of significantly raised ICP. Continuous EEG monitoring, particularly of comatose babies and those receiving muscle relaxants, may reveal clinically unrecognized convulsions which can impair cerebral perfusion. Where this facility is not available, serial EEGs can be helpful.

Repeat lumbar punctures

In neonatal meningitis, unlike meningitis in older children, it is usual to repeat an LP within 48 h of starting antibiotics and often every day until the CSF is sterile to monitor the response to treatment. CSF cultures remain positive in Gram-negative bacillary meningitis (mean 6 days, range 2–11 days) for longer than in GBS meningitis, in which CSF cultures are usually sterile within 2–3 days of starting treatment (McCracken, 1972).

Complications

Small subdural effusions are often seen in bacterial meningitis and do not need any intervention. Larger effusions may cause persistent fever and midline shift of the brain with symptoms of raised intracranial pressure. Such effusions may show up on transillumination of the skull.

Seizures may be evident, may present insidiously with apnoeic attacks or episodes of hypoxia, or may be subclinical and only diagnosed by EEG. In general the presence of seizures is a poor prognostic feature, particularly if they are not controlled by anticonvulsants.

Hydrocephalus is more likely after neonatal meningitis than after meningitis in infancy and later in childhood. Similarly, brain abscess, although still rare, is commoner in the neonatal period, particularly in association with *Citrobacter* and *Proteus* meningitis.

Persisting or recurrent fever may be due to persistence of meningitis, to subdural or intracerebral abscess, to infection in other sites (pleural empyema, septic arthritis, osteomyelitis) or to intercurrent infection.

Recurrences of both Gram-positive and Gram-negative meningitis may rarely occur after stopping apparently successful treatment. A careful search, both clinical and radiographic, should be made for persisting foci of infection, but these are rarely found. We have seen a baby with two recurrences of *E. coli* meningitis despite apparently adequate and successful treatment with cefotaxime; no underlying cause was found and the baby was finally cured using intravenous trimethoprim–sulphamethoxazole.

Mortality and morbidity

The mortality of early-onset meningitis is higher than that for late-onset meningitis and higher in preterm than in term babies. Perhaps surprisingly, the mortality is approximately the same, 25–50%, for all the major bacterial pathogens (Klein and Marcy, 1990). Brain abscess has a mortality of ~ 50%.

Although it is not always clear to what extent meningitis and other predisposing factors such as extreme prematurity have contributed to the outcome, significant neurological sequelae develop in up to one-half of all survivors of neonatal bacterial meningitis caused by any organism. These include major neurodevelopmental handicap, hemiparesis, spastic paraparesis, cranial nerve palsies, hydrocephalus, hearing loss, visual handicap, convulsions, and speech and hearing disorders.

Shunt infections

Infections of ventriculoperitoneal (VP) or ventriculoatrial (VA) shunts should be considered separately from bacterial meningitis. These occur in between 3 and 27% of shunts, with a mean of 11% (Editorial, 1989). Although shunt infections may present like classic bacterial meningitis, they commonly present more insidiously. VP shunt infections cause vomiting, lethargy and irritability with or without fever, whereas VA shunt infections may cause low-grade fever, progressive anaemia, and haematuria and hypertension secondary to shunt nephritis. Infection of a newly placed shunt is highly likely if there is significant infection of the skin overlying the reservoir, a situation that readily occurs in small preterm neonates when the skin of the scalp is stretched over the reservoir.

Coagulase-negative staphylococci, such as *Staphylococcus epidermidis*, are the commonest cause of shunt infections but these may also be caused by *Staphylococcus aureus* and, particularly in babies of low birth-weight, by Gram-negative bacilli (e.g. *Pseudomonas*), by low-grade pathogens such as diphtheroids and by fungi (Editorial, 1989).

The first priority in suspected shunt infection is to obtain a specimen of CSF for microscopic examination by tapping the shunt reservoir. Measurement of serum CRP has been helpful in identifying whether babies with non-specific symptoms have shunt infections. If shunt infection is confirmed the entire shunt must be removed, as the infection will not resolve on antibiotics alone (Schoenbaum *et al.*, 1975). The appropriate antibiotics can be given intravenously. As an intraventricular reservoir or external ventricular drain is usually inserted to drain CSF until the shunt infection is cleared, antibiotics can be given directly into the ventricles (e.g. vancomycin, gentamicin) if there is a problem with severe infection or infection with a multiply-resistant organism. Intraventricular antibiotics can themselves cause a chemical meningitis, so when the CSF is sterile and organisms are no longer seen, intraventricular antibiotics should not be continued merely because of a raised CSF white cell count and protein.

Although one-half of our isolates of coagulase-negative staphylococci are cloxacillin (methicillin) resistant, we start empiric antibiotic therapy of shunt infections in which Gram-positive cocci are seen on the Gram stain of the CSF, using cloxacillin and an aminoglycoside rather than vancomycin because these infections are rarely fulminant and symptoms often resolve simply with removal of the shunt.

There is no evidence that prophylactic antibiotics at the time of shunt insertion reduce the incidence of shunt infections (Editorial, 1989).

Chapter 8

Pneumonia

Introduction

Neonatal pneumonia can be subdivided into four categories, although there is some overlap between them:

1 Congenital pneumonia (transplacentally acquired): as a result of congenital infection with rubella, CMV, *Toxoplasma, Listeria* and *T. pallidum*.
2 Intrauterine pneumonia: autopsy finding of lung inflammation associated with asphyxia and/or infection.
3 Early-onset pneumonia: pneumonia present at birth or soon after, due to infection of amniotic fluid via the maternal genital tract (ascending infection).
4 Late-onset pneumonia: pneumonia presenting at least 48 h after delivery, due to organisms acquired either around delivery or nosocomially.

Definition

Pneumonia is probably the most difficult neonatal infection to define. Even when histological studies are obtained at autopsy, it may be difficult to distinguish between true infection and inhalation of infected amniotic fluid without endogenous infection of the lungs (Davies and Aherne, 1962). This emphasizes the inadequacy of the usual autopsy definition of pneumonia as 'the presence of alveolar and/or interstitial neutrophils'.

In liveborn infants the radiological appearance of early-onset pneumonia may be identical to that of idiopathic respiratory distress syndrome (hyaline membrane disease). In babies on long-term artificial ventilation, particularly those with bronchopulmonary dysplasia, there may be fluctuating consolidation which can be due to pulmonary oedema, haemorrhage, atelectasis or infection.

We have used a working definition of pneumonia in liveborn babies as follows: a clinical picture of respiratory distress associated with chest radiographic changes suggesting pneumonia that persist for at least 48 h. These changes include nodular or coarse patchy infiltrates, diffuse haziness or granularity with air bronchogram, perihilar interstitial streaking and lobar or sublobar consolidation. When there is difficulty distinguishing between pneumonia and hyaline membrane disease we look for additional evidence of sepsis such as neutropenia, abnormal immature-to-total white cell ratio, or chest radiographic appearances not completely typical of hyaline membrane disease. If blood cultures are positive we describe this as 'definite pneumonia'; if negative, as 'probable pneumonia' with the probable causative organism (particularly in early pneumonia) being the organism cultured from the tracheal aspirate or nasopharyngeal aspirate at the onset of symptoms.

Pathogenesis

Congenital pneumonia

In congenital pneumonia the lung infection is part of a generalized fetal infection which has been acquired transplacentally. This infection may have been acquired in the first trimester of pregnancy, as with toxoplasmosis, rubella and congenital CMV infection, or near delivery, as seen in congenital listeriosis and congenital syphilis. Unfortunately, the term congenital pneumonia is often used imprecisely so that there is confusion with intrauterine pneumonia or early-onset pneumonia.

Intrauterine pneumonia

By definition, intrauterine pneumonia occurs in babies who are stillborn or die within 24 h, but there is overlap with early-onset pneumonia. The former is a pathological diagnosis made on the basis of diffuse lung inflammation with infiltration of alveoli by polymorphs, and often round-cell infiltrates of the interstitium of small bronchioles and interalveolar septa (Barter, 1953; Davies and Aherne, 1962). In many ways, however, it is unlike classic bacterial pneumonia in that there is no pleural reaction, little or no infiltration of bronchopulmonary tissue and no fibrinous exudate in the alveoli (Davies and Aherne, 1962).

The possible causes of intrauterine pneumonia include asphyxia and ascending infection of the amniotic fluid. Asphyxia may encourage fetal gasping and aspiration of infected amniotic fluid, with the result that the fetal alveolar neutrophils are from aspirated amniotic fluid (Davies and Aherne, 1962). Naeye and his colleagues have often found histological evidence of chorioamnionitis in cases of intrauterine pneumonia (Naeye et al., 1971, 1977; Naeye and Peters, 1978), but others have found this correlation far less clear-cut and frequently no bacteria are isolated from cases of intrauterine pneumonia (Barter and Hudson, 1974). Benirschke and Driscoll (1967) found histological evidence of chorioamnionitis in 11% of a series of unselected pregnancies, and Siegel and McCracken (1981) have estimated that only 1–6% of infants of mothers with clinical chorioamnionitis become infected. Thus, it is not clear whether intrauterine pneumonia is a true pneumonia or whether it often represents terminal aspiration of infected amniotic fluid in a pregnancy complicated by chorioamnionitis, which itself may have precipitated preterm labour.

Early-onset pneumonia

The pathogenesis of early-onset pneumonia is similar to that for early-onset sepsis. The disease is more likely to occur in association with maternal risk

Table 8.1 Risk factors for sepsis in 35 babies with early-onset pneumonia; Oxford, 1 May 1984–30 September 1987

Risk factor	n	Solitary risk factor
Spontaneous onset of preterm labour	23	17
Prolonged rupture of membranes (> 18 h)	9	2
Maternal fever (> 37.5°C)	3	1
Offensive liquor	2	0
No risk factors	8	—
Total		20 (57%)

factors such as spontaneous preterm onset of labour, prolonged rupture of the membranes and maternal fever (see Table 8.1). The route of infection is by ascending infection from the maternal vaginal tract or perineum which causes a clinical or subclinical chorioamnionitis.

Histologically, the appearance of early-onset pneumonia is unlike that of intrauterine pneumonia, and more closely resembles pneumonia of children or adults. There is a dense cellular exudate with congestion, haemorrhage and necrosis, and bacteria are usually seen. Alveolar hyaline membranes are seen in about one-half of all cases of early-onset pneumonia and, although these have been best described in GBS pneumonia, they occur with equal frequency in pneumonia due to other streptococci and Gram-negative organisms (Jeffery *et al.*, 1977). Although it has been suggested that this represents pneumonia complicating idiopathic respiratory distress syndrome (hyaline membrane disease), it seems more likely that bacterial pneumonia can actually induce hyaline membranes. This picture is seen in term infants with GBS pneumonia and the hyaline membrane may comprise densely packed bacteria (Katzenstein *et al.*, 1976).

Late-onset pneumonia

Most cases of pneumonia occurring after 48 h of age are in babies receiving artificial ventilation. The endotracheal tubes of such babies rapidly become colonized with potential pathogens, and the tubes bypass the mucociliary escalator which is an important defence mechanism against bacteria entering the lower respiratory tract. Aspiration pneumonia is particularly likely to occur in babies with neurological deficit, and those with oesophageal atresia, tracheo-oesophageal fistula or diaphragmatic hernia.

More rarely, organisms acquired at birth can cause pneumonia of later onset. This is more likely with viruses, such as CMV, herpes simplex virus, and enteroviruses, or allied organisms such as *Chlamydia*, than with bacteria.

Epidemiology

Intrauterine and early-onset pneumonia have been diagnosed at autopsy in 15–38% of stillborn and 20–32% of liveborn babies who died (Klein, 1990b). This may be an overestimate of the true incidence of pneumonia because of the problems of definition already outlined. The incidence of early-onset pneumonia over a 41-month period in Oxford, using the definition stated in the earlier section, was 1.78 per 1000 live births (Webber *et al.*, 1990).

In the Collaborative Study of the National Institutes of Health, the incidence of pneumonia in babies who died within 48 h of birth was 27.7% for Black babies but 11.3% for White babies, and this difference was consistent at different birth-weights (Fujikura and Froehlich, 1967). In a study of 1044 autopsies of babies the incidence of pneumonia was higher in Black (38%) than in Puerto Rican (22%) or White babies (20%) (Naeye *et al.*, 1971).

Late-onset pneumonia is commonest in preterm babies who require prolonged artifical ventilation. In the neonatal unit in Oxford there were 41 episodes of late-onset pneumonia affecting 39 babies over a 41-month period: 36 of the babies were preterm and 34 were being artificially ventilated. The mean gestational age at birth was 27.8 weeks (range 23–41) and the mean time to onset of pneumonia was 35 days (range 3–150 days). Of all babies ventilated for more than 24 h, 10% developed late-onset pneumonia (Webber *et al.*, 1990).

In the 1950s and 1960s, outbreaks of *Staphylococcus aureus* infection in neonatal units resulted in many cases of severe staphylococcal pneumonia. Although *S. aureus* pneumonia is now uncommon, outbreaks with other bacteria and viruses, such as respiratory syncytial virus (RSV) and enteroviruses, may still occur and cause pneumonia.

Microbiology

Most microbiological data on pneumonia come from autopsy studies. In a study of neonatal pneumonia, blood cultures were positive in 44% of early-onset cases (Webber *et al.*, 1990). About one-half of the babies with negative blood cultures were heavily colonized with a bacterial pathogen (Table 8.2). Sherman *et al.* (1980) cultured tracheal aspirates taken within 8 h of birth from 320 babies with early respiratory distress and non-specific radiographic changes: 25 had bacteria seen on Gram staining and cultured from the aspirate (Table 8.3), and 14 (56%) were bacteraemic. In a further study the same authors found a similar spectrum of organisms with and

Table 8.2 Bacterial isolates from 35 cases of early-onset pneumonia (presenting before 48 h of age), Oxford, 1 May 1984–30 September 1987

Pneumonia with bacteraemia			Pneumonia with negative blood cultures		
Blood culture	n	Deaths	Endotracheal, nasopharyngeal or surface culture	n	Deaths
Group B streptococcus	11	5	Group B streptococcus	9	2
Streptococcus pneumoniae	3	2	Group F streptococcus	1	0
Haemophilus influenzae	2	1	No organism	9	0
Total	16	8		19	2

Table 8.3 Organisms isolated from tracheal aspirate in 25 babies with probable early-onset pneumonia, Sacramento, 1975–1977

Organism	n	Bacteraemic
Group B streptococcus	14	7
Haemophilus influenzae	3	2
Streptococcus viridans	2	0
Escherichia coli	2	1
Listeria monocytogenes	2	2
Staphylococcus aureus	1	1
Pseudomonas aeruginosa	1	1
Streptococcus pneumoniae	1	—

From Sherman *et al.* (1980), with permission

without bacteraemia, but also *Bacteroides* species (Sherman *et al.*, 1984). *Staphylococcus aureus* is a relatively unusual early-onset pathogen, and the organisms causing early-onset pneumonia are generally covered by the combination of penicillin G or ampicillin with an aminoglycoside.

There has been increasing interest in the role of fastidious organisms that will not grow using conventional bacterial culture techniques. *Ureaplasma urealyticum* colonization of the maternal genital tract is associated with preterm labour. Rudd *et al.* (1986) examined the evidence that *U. urealyticum* might cause pneumonia and found it to be unconvincing. Nevertheless, there are occasional cases of babies dying with pneumonia from whom this is the only organism that can be cultured. The isolation of *U. urealyticum* from endotracheal aspirates was associated with an increased risk of chronic lung disease in a study by Cassell *et al.* (1988), and they suggested that this might be due to pneumonia leading to iatrogenic damage from increased ventilatory requirements. Waites and colleagues (1989) described three babies with persistent pulmonary hypertension associated with *Ureaplasma urealyticum*. There have been no controlled studies using antibiotic treatment effective against *Ureaplasma*, such as erythromycin, so it remains doubtful whether the organism is a true pathogen or a commensal.

Earlier studies suggested that the organisms that caused late-onset sepsis in artificially ventilated babies could be predicted from the organisms colonizing the pharynx or endotracheal tube (Harris *et al.*, 1976; Sprunt *et al.*, 1978). However, recent studies have found such cultures to be poorly predictive (Isaacs *et al.*, 1987a; Evans *et al.*, 1988) and even misleading (Slagle *et al.*, 1989). Concurrent bacteraemia is far less common in late-onset than in early-onset pneumonia: in the Oxford study, seven of 41 episodes (17%) of late-onset pneumonia were bacteraemic compared with 16 (46%) of 35 early-onset episodes (Webber *et al.*, 1990). Furthermore, different organisms from those in the blood were found in the endotracheal or nasopharyngeal aspirate cultures in four of the seven late-onset cases, no organisms in two cases and the same organism in only one case (see Table 8.4). Thus, there must be some doubt that the organisms cultured from the nasopharynx or endotracheal tube are truly those causing late-onset pneumonia.

Table 8.4 Bacterial isolates from 39 babies with late-onset pneumonia (presenting after 48 h of age), Oxford, 1 May 1984–30 September 1987

(a) Definite late-onset pneumonia (7 babies)

Case	Blood culture	Culture from nasopharynx or endotracheal tube
1	Pseudomonas aeruginosa Achromobacter xylosoxidans	No growth
2[a]	Pseudomonas aeruginosa Streptococcus faecalis	No growth
3	Staphylococcus epidermidis	Staphylococcus aureus
4	Staphylococcus epidermidis	Coliform sp. Streptococcus faecalis
5	Pseudomonas aeruginosa	Pseudomonas aeruginosa
6	Staphylococcus epidermidis	Pseudomonas aeruginosa Coliform sp.
7	Staphylococcus epidermidis	Coliform sp.

[a]Baby had cystic fibrosis; died.

(b) Probable late-onset pneumonia (32 babies, 34 episodes)

Cultures of nasopharyngeal or endotracheal secretions		n
Gram-negative bacilli (30)	Coliform sp.	15
	Pseudomonas aeruginosa	12
	Escherichia coli	2
	Proteus mirabilis	1
Staphylococcus aureus		5
Staphylococcus epidermidis		2
Group B streptococcus		1
Haemophilus influenzae		1
No organism		4
Total isolates[a]		39

[a]Multiple isolates common.

In the absence of pneumonia, the mere isolation of a potential pathogen from endotracheal tube aspirate cultures of babies > 48 h old is clearly not an indication for antibiotics. Although babies with late-onset pneumonia have positive endotracheal tube cultures more often than those without pneumonia, such babies are often of very low birth-weight and are receiving prolonged ventilatory support. When they are matched with babies of the same birth-weight who have been ventilated for an equal period, the same proportion of babies are colonized, and colonization of the endotracheal tube occurs at the same rate (Table 8.5). Barter and Hudson (1974) found bacteria almost as frequently in the lungs of babies dying without pneumonia as in those dying with pneumonia.

If there is a pleural effusion, aspiration of this will often give a microbiological cause of the pneumonia. Needle aspiration of the lung has been suggested for the critically ill child with pneumonia or one who has not

Table 8.5 Endotracheal tube colonization patterns in babies with and without late-onset pneumonia artifically ventilated for > 24 h Oxford, 1 May 1984–30 September 1987

(a) Before controlling for gestational age and duration of artificial ventilation

Colonization rate		Significance
Pneumonia present	*Pneumonia absent*	
34/36 (94%)	80/194 (41%)	< 0.001

(b) After controlling for gestational age and duration of artificial ventilation

Colonization rate		Significance
Pneumonia present[a]	*Pneumonia absent[b]*	
28/30 (93%)	25/30 (83%)	NS[c]

[a] Mean time to colonization of endotracheal tube 8 days (range 1–15 days).
[b] Mean time to colonization of endotrachael tube 10 days (range 2–39 days); difference not significant.
[c] NS, not significant.

responded to antibiotics (Klein, 1990b). The mortality from late-onset pneumonia is now very low, however, and needle aspiration is hazardous, while in early-onset pneumonia there is usually less problem in determining the aetiology.

It is not clear how often organisms not cultured by conventional bacterial techniques are responsible for pneumonia or pneumonitis in older babies. In Wilson–Mikity syndrome, babies without initial chest signs or radiographic changes develop these after a few days: an infectious cause or causes has been suspected but not proven. Babies with chronic lung disease often develop exacerbations with increased pulmonary shadowing which might be due to bacteria, viruses (such as CMV which can be acquired perinatally or from blood transfusion) or organisms like *Ureaplasma urealyticum, Mycoplasma hominis, Mycoplasma pneumoniae, Chlamydia trachomatis* or *Pneumocystis carinii.* Stagno *et al.* (1981) found evidence of infection with *Chlamydia trachomatis* (25%), *U. urealyticum* (21%), CMV (20%) and *Pneumocystis carinii* (18%) in 104 Alabama infants aged 1–3 months with pneumonitis but not in controls. However, Rudd and Carrington (1984) could find little evidence of infection with viruses or *Mycoplasma* in a prospective survey of babies in the neonatal unit of the Hammersmith Hospital, London. *Chlamydia trachomatis* is an occasional cause of afebrile neonatal pneumonitis which can be severe enough for the baby to require ventilatory support.

Clinical features

Babies with early-onset pneumonia often present with respiratory distress at or very soon after birth and usually within 24 h. A smaller proportion develop increasing respiratory distress on the second day of life. The signs are identical to hyaline membrane disease with grunting, tachypnoea, tachycardia, flaring of the alar nasi, intercostal recession, sternal retraction and cyanosis. Pulmonary hypertension (persistent transitional or persistent fetal circulation) may mean that cyanosis persists in 100% oxygen; such babies often have a barrel or hyperexpanded chest. If there is associated septicaemia the baby may be shocked and become apnoeic or even have convulsions. Fever only occurs in about half of the babies.

Babies with late-onset pneumonia usually present more insidiously. Most are already receiving ventilatory support and develop increased oxygen requirements, apnoea or tachypnoea if they are on a low rate of ventilation, and may develop abdominal distension and stop tolerating enteral feeds. Those not on ventilatory support may present with grunting dyspnoea, tachypnoea or apnoea, cyanosis, tachycardia and intercostal recession. If pneumonia is unilateral and particularly if there is a large effusion, chest movements may be asymmetrical.

Staphylococcal pneumonia, due to *S. aureus*, is now rare but, when it occurs, babies are extremely ill and usually septicaemic. They may rapidly develop pneumatoceles (Figure 8.1) which can rupture and cause pneumothorax or empyema, ileus is common and there may be staphylococcal enterocolitis with bloody diarrhoea.

About one-half of the babies with chlamydial pneumonitis have a maternal history of vaginal discharge and one-half have, or have had, conjunctivitis. Most babies present between 4 and 11 weeks of age, but sometimes as early as 2 weeks. There is little or no fever; nasal congestion without discharge, tachypnoea, sometimes apnoea, and a paroxysmal, staccato cough are typical. Crepitations may be heard but wheezing is rare. In up to one-half of the babies, the tympanic membrane has a pearly-white appearance. There is hyperexpansion of the chest which is barrel-shaped and associated with bilateral perihilar interstitial infiltrates on the chest radiograph (Beem and Saxon, 1977; Harrison *et al.*, 1978; Tipple *et al.*, 1979).

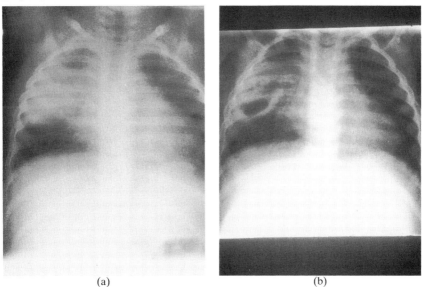

(a)   (b)

Figure 8.1 Staphylococcal pneumonia. (a) Initial radiograph shows right upper lobe consolidation; (b) 12 h later: pneumatocele formation

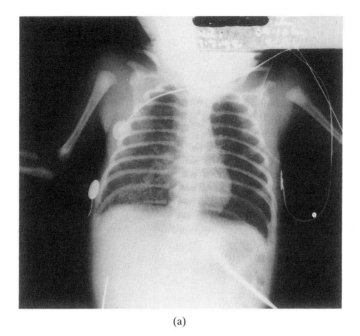

(a)

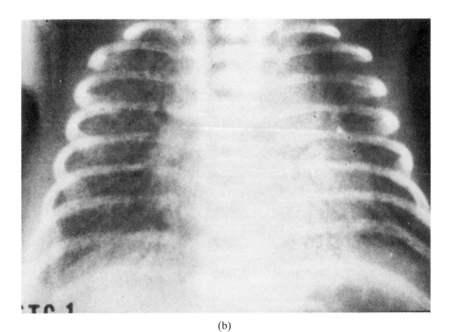

(b)

Figure 8.2 Group B streptococcal pneumonia. (a) Appearance resembling hyaline membrane disease; (b) hypertranslucent lungs, minimal added shadowing

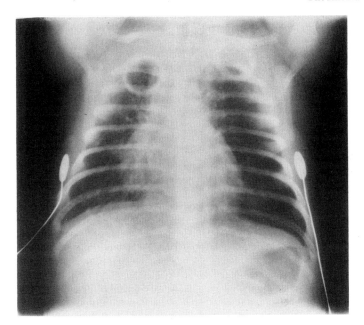

Figure 8.3 Pneumonia due to *Listeria monocytogenes*

Radiology

The chest radiograph in early pneumonia is very variable. In GBS pneumonia more than one-half of the radiographs resemble hyaline membrane disease but pneumonic infiltrates occur in about one-third and most of the rest have radiographs mimicking transient tachypnoea or pulmonary oedema. In babies with pulmonary hypertension the radiograph may show hyperexpanded, hypertranslucent lungs with little or no added shadowing (Figure 8.2), and it may very occasionally be normal early in the illness (Baker and Edwards, 1990). A similar pattern is found with other organisms causing early-onset pneumonia, such as *H. influenzae, Pneumococcus* and *Listeria* (Figure 8.3).

Pleural fluid may be seen (Figure 8.4). If there is doubt about its presence or whether it is too loculated to take a sample by needle aspiration, ultrasound examination of the chest can provide a ready answer. Pneumatoceles may be seen, particularly in staphylococcal pneumonia, but occasionally in pneumonia due to group A streptococci, *Klebsiella* and *E. coli*. Lung abscess may complicate pneumonia; if this diagnosis is suspected on the chest radiograph, CT scan of the lung can be used to distinguish it from an empyema or simple pneumatocele.

A pattern of perihilar interstitial shadowing is seen in *Chlamydia* pneumonitis (Figure 8.5).

Diagnosis

It can be extremely difficult to distinguish early-onset pneumonia from hyaline membrane disease and late-onset pneumonia from pulmonary

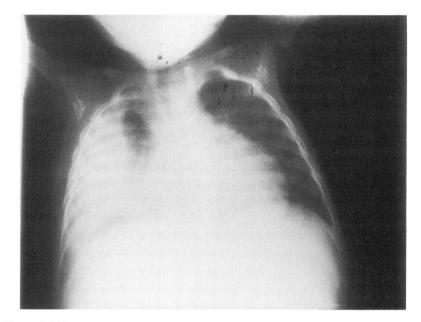

Figure 8.4 Empyema

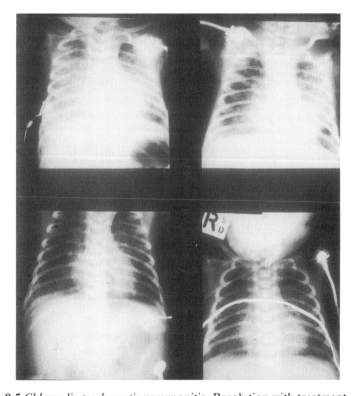

Figure 8.5 *Chlamydia trachomatis* pneumonitis. Resolution with treatment

oedema secondary to a patent ductus arteriosus or other heart lesion, pulmonary haemorrhage (although usually there is tracheal blood) or pulmonary infarct. Not only may the clinical picture be identical but so may the chest radiograph. Often, treatment for pneumonia has to be initiated without any certainty of the diagnosis, and time may resolve best whether the condition was or was not pneumonia. Rapid resolution of pulmonary shadowing within 24–48 h makes a diagnosis of pneumonia less likely since pneumonic shadowing usually persists for several days. We often use the response to a bolus dose of a diuretic in babies with chronic lung disease and new added shadowing to differentiate pulmonary oedema from pneumonia: babies with pulmonary oedema improve rapidly and the chest radiograph improves within hours.

We have found that, when assessing babies with early-onset respiratory distress, junior doctors tend not to recognize spontaneous preterm onset of labour as a risk factor for neonatal pneumonia. Yet this was the commonest risk factor for sepsis in a study of babies with early-onset pneumonia, and in 49% was the solitary risk factor (Table 8.1; Webber *et al.*, 1990).

Some (Yeung and Tam, 1972) but not others (Pole and McAllister, 1975) have found that microscopy of gastric aspirates is useful in the diagnosis of late-onset pneumonia by showing a raised neutrophil count. The limitations of gastric aspirates in early-onset pneumonia and sepsis have been discussed in Chapter 4.

Serology is of very limited value in pneumonia. IgM antibodies can be measured against the TORCH agents (*Toxoplasma*, rubella, CMV and herpes simplex virus) and against *Chlamydia trachomatis*. Antigen-detection tests are widely used for RSV, and increasingly are available for other organisms such as *Chlamydia trachomatis*, group B streptococcus and *Streptococcus pneumoniae*.

Antibiotic treatment

The antibiotic treatment of early-onset bacterial pneumonia is as for early-onset sepsis. Penicillin or ampicillin and an aminoglycoside provide good antibiotic cover against the common early-onset pathogens: in most countries this means not only group B streptococcus, *Pneumoccocus*, untypable *Haemophilus influenzae* and *Listeria monocytogenes*, but also Gram-negative enteric bacilli such as *E. coli*. Staphylococci, both coagulase positive (*S. aureus*) and coagulase negative (*S. epidermidis*), are occasionally reported as early-onset pathogens, although only one case has occurred in 5 years in Oxford (Table 1.3).

For late-onset pneumonia we have already argued that antibiotic treatment based on the organisms known to be colonizing an individual baby can be misleading. We, therefore, treat babies with late-onset pneumonia according to a unit antibiotic policy, which is based on the organisms causing infections (Table 8.4) and the outcome of these infections.

In Oxford we use penicillin and netilmicin for early-onset pneumonia and flucloxacillin and netilmicin for late-onset pneumonia. These are not presented as the correct antibiotic regimens, but merely represent antibiotics that have proved appropriate for our population. Different antibiotic regimens will be appropriate for different populations. We treat pneumonia, whether or not bacteraemia is also present, with 7–10 days of antibiotics, although proven *S. aureus* pneumonia should probably be treated for at least 3–6 weeks.

Supportive treatment

The critical supportive treatment of pneumonia will involve an assessment of whether increased ambient oxygen and ventilatory support are required (or need to be increased) for respiratory failure. Continual monitoring of arterial PaO_2 by skin electrode or arterial saturation by pulse oximeter together with intermittent arterial sampling (preferably via an umbilical or peripheral artery cannula) to monitor pH and PaO_2 allows an assessment of whether ventilatory and metabolic status is satisfactory. Most babies with pneumonia will not tolerate enteral fluids, which anyway can distend the abdomen, impairing respiration, and are in danger of being aspirated if the baby is not intubated. Intravenous fluids are given, therefore, and nothing is given enterally; a nasogastric or orogastric tube is passed to aspirate air and stomach contents. Electrolytes need to be monitored; inappropriate secretion of antidiuretic hormone has been described in older children, although not in newborns, with pneumonia. Supportive therapy for sepsis, as described in Chapter 6, may be needed if the baby is shocked.

Persistent pulmonary hypertension (sometimes called persistent transitional or persistent fetal circulation) may complicate early-onset pneumonia, particularly that due to group B streptococcus, but also *S. pneumoniae* and *H. influenzae*. It is important to maintain a good blood pressure, because if this is lower than the pulmonary pressure, right-to-left shunting will persist. Thus fresh frozen plasma or blood as appropriate and inotropic support such as a dopamine infusion may be needed. The arterial PaO_2 should be kept relatively high and not allowed to dip, as this exacerbates pulmonary vasoconstriction. Pulmonary vasodilators such as tolazoline or prostacycline may need to be infused, but the systemic circulation must first be adequately supported or profound hypotension can occur.

Significant pleural effusions should be aspirated for diagnostic purposes. If these are infected, either they will need to be repeatedly aspirated for therapeutic reasons or a wide-bore intercostal drain should be inserted. Staphylococcal empyema virtually always requires a wide-bore chest drain because the pus is thick with necrotic debris. It is usual to connect the chest drain to a suction pump with underwater drain (closed suction), as pus may be thick. If this fails to drain the empyema adequately, the chest drain may need to be cut short (open drainage) or chest surgery may be needed. For large empyemas it is often necessary to place two wide-bore chest drains, one anterior and one low posterolaterally.

Prognosis

The contribution made by pneumonia to stillbirths and early neonatal deaths is obscure because of the difficulties in defining intrauterine pneumonia and the contribution of other factors. In various autopsy studies from

1922 to 1964, summarized by Klein (1990b), evidence of pneumonia was found in 15–38% of stillbirths and 20–32% of liveborn infants.

The mortality and morbidity in liveborn babies will depend on the population being studied. The mortality is far higher for early-onset than for late-onset pneumonia. In the Oxford study, ten of 35 babies (29%) with early-onset pneumonia died but only one of 39 babies experiencing 41 episodes of late-onset pneumonia (2%) died – a baby with cystic fibrosis (Webber et al., 1990). The mortality of early-onset pneumonia is higher in preterm than in term babies: in Oxford, ten of 23 preterm babies (43%) died, including two with negative blood cultures, but none of the 12 term babies with early-onset pneumonia died.

There is little information about long-term morbidity from pneumonia. It seems likely that the morbidity caused by early-onset pneumonia is higher than that from late-onset pneumonia. The outcome in the very small babies requiring prolonged ventilatory support who develop late-onset pneumonia is mainly influenced by other antenatal and perinatal factors, which confound the results of follow-up studies. Infantile pneumonitis due to Chlamydia trachomatis and other organisms results in recurrent wheezing in almost one-half of the cases, and in lung function evidence of persistent obstructive airways disease (Harrison et al., 1982; Brasfield et al., 1987).

Chapter 9

Osteomyelitis and septic arthritis

Epidemiology

Before antibiotics were widely available, about 10% of cases of septicaemia resulted in osteomyelitis (Dunham, 1933). Neonatal osteomyelitis is a rare condition with a reported incidence of from one in 5000 live births in the UK (Craig, 1962) to one in 15 000 in the United States (Fox and Sprunt, 1978). Certain organisms are more likely to cause osteomyelitis: during the epidemics of neonatal *Staphylococcus aureus* infection in the 1950s and 1960s, there was a higher incidence of neonatal osteomyelitis. Recently, in Sydney, Australia, methicillin-resistant *S. aureus* (MRSA) infections have been associated with an increased risk of osteomyelitis (M. Anthony and P. McIntyre, personal communications). In one unit in Sydney, four of 27 babies with systemic MRSA sepsis developed osteomyelitis during a 2-year period (Table 13.1) and similar rates of osteomyelitis are being seen elsewhere in the city. This high incidence of osteomyelitis is unlikely to be due to increased virulence or inappropriate treatment, as all babies recovered and all received vancomycin. It seems more likely that MRSA has a special tropism for bone (see pages 127–9). Boys are affected more commonly than girls (sex ratio 1.6:1).

Preterm babies may be at increased risk of developing osteomyelitis. Nine of 39 babies with neonatal osteomyelitis weighed < 2000 g at birth (Fox and Sprunt, 1978) although gestational age was not given.

Pathogenesis

Haematogenous spread

This is almost certainly the most common mechanism for osteomyelitis. Neonatal septicaemia, however, is commoner than neonatal osteomyelitis, so other factors must come into play. One of these, as discussed on pages 87–8, is the relative propensity of different organisms to seed to the bone.

In about one-half of all cases of neonatal osteomyelitis there is preceding bacterial infection such as skin sepsis, periumbilical sepsis, otitis media, pneumonia, conjunctivitis, or deep abscess, suggesting that the pathogenesis involves haematogenous spread to the bones. Bacterial osteomyelitis is also a rare complication of neonatal virus infections caused by varicella and herpes simplex viruses.

Umbilical catheters are associated with an increased risk of osteomyelitis (Lim *et al.*, 1977). This may be due to septic emboli from the catheter tip or direct inoculation of organisms from the umbilicus into the bloodstream at the time of catheter insertion. Cases of osteomyelitis have occurred following brief umbilical catheterization for exchange transfusion. *S. aureus* is the commonest organism, but Gram-negative bacilli and fungi can also be responsible. The hips or knees are usually involved, generally on the same side as the catheter tip (Lim *et al.*, 1977).

Haematogenous infection of the long bones usually starts in the most vascular part of the bone, the metaphysis, where there is sluggish blood flow through the arteriolar loops (Ogden and Lister, 1975). From there, infection can spread to the adjacent growth plate (the physis), across the growth plate via transphyseal blood vessels to the epiphysis, or may rupture into the joint space, because in neonates the synovial membrane extends down to the metaphysis (Figure 9.1). The transphyseal vessels which connect the metaphysis with the epiphysis disappear with increasing age and by 1 year of age are absent. In addition, the bone is very thin in neonates and the periosteum loosely attached. Infection of neonatal bone almost always decompresses spontaneously with rupture into the joint, causing concomitant septic arthritis. Lifting of the periosteum occurs, often involving much of the length of the bone, and pus may track through the periosteum to form a subcutaneous abscess.

As bone is very vascular, it heals rapidly. Sequestrum rarely forms; when it does, it is often resorbed. However, the rich blood supply also facilitates infection of the cartilaginous growth plate and epiphysis and the resulting damage to the cartilage is generally irreparable. Neonatal osteomyelitis of the long bones often results in impaired growth of the bone (Trueta, 1959).

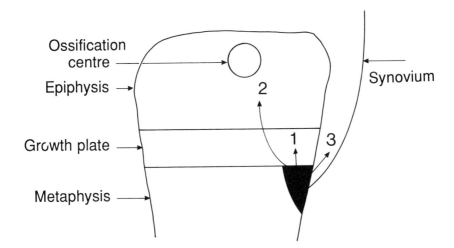

Figure 9.1 Haematogenous osteomyelitis of long bones in neonate. Infection originates in vascular area of metaphysis (shaded area); may spread (1) to involve growth plate, (2) to involve epiphysis, (3) into joint space

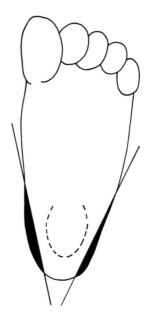

Figure 9.2 Safe area of heel in which to do heel-prick (shaded). Position of os calcis shown to indicate danger of heel-prick on point of heel

Direct inoculation

Heel-pricks should always be done in the fleshy side of the heel; the point of the heel overlies the os calcis (Figure 9.2) and calcaneal osteomyelitis or osteochondritis, commonly due to *S. aureus* or *Proteus mirabilis*, has complicated heel-pricks (Figure 9.3).

Femoral stabs should no longer be necessary in neonatal care. They can cause femoral osteomyelitis, usually due to *S. aureus, S. epidermidis* or *Proteus mirabilis*.

Use of fetal scalp monitors can very occasionally lead to osteomyelitis due to *S. aureus, S. epidermidis*, anaerobes or a variety of other organisms.

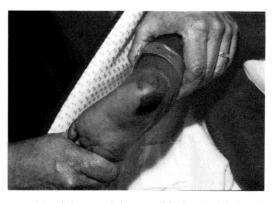

Figure 9.3 Osteomyelitis of the os calcis caused by heelprick into bone

Contiguous spread

Scalp abscesses, usually caused by *S. aureus*, can spread to involve the underlying parietal or occipital bone. Cephalhaematomas may become infected, generally with *S. aureus* or Gram-negative bacilli (*E. coli, pseudomonas*) and extend to involve the parietal bone. Paronychias may occasionally spread to the bone of the underlying finger. Maxillary osteomyelitis may extend from maxillary antral sinusitis, although it can also occur in the absence of sinusitis, presumably due to haematogenous spread.

Transplacental infection

This is the mode of infection in osteitis associated with congenital syphilis. It is an extremely rare cause of bacterial osteomyelitis, occurring in association with early-onset sepsis.

Trauma

Although in many series of babies with neonatal osteomyelitis there has been some association with obstetric trauma, such as forceps delivery, the proportion of babies with osteomyelitis experiencing such trauma has not generally exceeded that of normal babies.

Microbiology

As with older children, *Staphylococcus aureus* is the commonest cause of neonatal osteomyelitis, accounting for > 80% of all cases up to the early 1970s. In one series from the United States, however, eight of 21 infants (up to 52 days old) had osteomyelitis caused by group B streptococcus and only six had staphylococcal osteomyelitis (Edwards *et al.*, 1978). When MRSA is prevalent on the neonatal unit this organism has been found to be an important cause of osteomyelitis (Table 13.1).

Although the organisms causing osteomyelitis might be expected to reflect the organisms causing sepsis, and in particular early-onset septicaemia,

Table 9.1 Organisms causing neonatal osteomyelitis

Staphylococcus aureus
Group B streptococcus
Gram-negative bacilli
  Escherichia coli
  Pseudomonas sp.
  Serratia sp.
  Enterobacter sp.
  Proteus sp.
  Klebsiella sp.
  Salmonella sp.
  Haemophilus influenzae
Group A streptococcus
Miscellaneous
  Coagulase-negative staphylococci
  Neisseria gonorrhoeae
  Treponema pallidum
  Anaerobes
  Fungi

certain organisms seem to have a tropism for bone and occur in the absence of overt septicaemia. Most cases of GBS osteomyelitis occur in previously healthy babies who did not have clinical early-onset sepsis. In contrast, certain organisms that are fairly common causes of sepsis, such as Gram-negative bacilli, are relatively rare causes of osteomyelitis, although they were the commonest cause in a series from India (Kumari *et al.*, 1978). Faecal streptococci, increasingly described as causes of late-onset sepsis, have not been reported to cause neonatal osteomyelitis. *Haemophilus influenzae* is a very rare cause of neonatal and infantile osteomyelitis, although a well-documented cause of infantile septic arthritis. Organisms reported to cause osteomyelitis are given in Table 9.1. In about 5–10% of cases, two or more organisms are isolated from bone (usually *S. aureus* and a beta-haemolytic streptococcus).

In summary, it is clear that in many cases the organisms causing osteomyelitis seed bone at the time of acute septicaemia, which may be of early- or late-onset. Some organisms virtually never cause osteomyelitis despite causing septicaemia; other organisms, such as *S. aureus*, cause osteomyelitis disproportionately often. Thus, the tropism for bone of different organisms varies. In the case of some organisms, such as group B streptococcus, osteomyelitis appears to result from an occult episode of bacteraemia.

Clinical presentation

The onset is either insidious or fulminant. In the insidious form, which is the commoner presentation, the baby is feeding and developing normally and often afebrile. The initial presentation is with swelling of a limb or joint and reluctance to move the limb. Redness is rarely present and 'point tenderness' is absent or difficult to elicit. There may be irritability on handling, for example when having nappies changed. Sometimes the reluctance to move a limb is so severe as to cause a pseudoparalysis, which can be misdiagnosed as nerve palsy (Isaacs *et al.*, 1986a). The classic example is a mistaken diagnosis of Erb's palsy: the main distinction is that Erb's palsy is painless, whereas in osteomyelitis of the clavicle or humerus, movement of the arm is painful (Figure 9.4). Involvement of the femur can cause foot

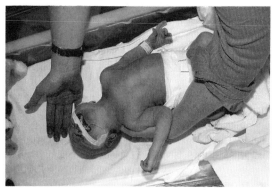

Figure 9.4 Baby with cleft lip and palate and *S. aureus* osteomyelitis of clavicle. Absent left Moro response due to pseudoparalysis mimicking Erb's palsy

drop, and the resulting septic arthritis of the hip may cause the baby to hold the leg flexed, abducted and externally rotated. Pseudoparalysis of a limb may also be caused by the osteitis of congenital syphilis. Oedema may be a prominent feature.

In the newborn period not only is the presentation often insidious, but multiple bones are involved in ~40% of cases. The infection commonly decompresses into the adjacent joint. In contrast, osteomyelitis in older children is acute, with fever; a single bone is most commonly involved, and exquisite local tenderness is the rule.

If the clinical diagnosis of osteomyelitis is not made early, the baby may develop a subcutaneous abscess with more evident inflammation. Thus, retroperitoneal abscesses should suggest vertebral osteomyelitis, whereas an abscess in the thigh, buttock, groin or iliac fossa suggests femoral or pelvic osteomyelitis.

Maxillary osteomyelitis (Figure 9.5) presents with fever, poor feeding, conjunctivitis and erythema and oedema of the eyelid. Proptosis and chemosis are common. The cheek often becomes swollen and inflamed and an abscess may form which can drain below the eye. There is often unilateral purulent nasal discharge and swelling of the hard palate, which may become a draining abscess. The commonest error is to misdiagnose maxillary osteomyelitis as peri-orbital cellulitis.

In the 'fulminant' form of osteomyelitis, signs of bone and joint involvement may occur at the time of, or some time after, signs of sepsis. The babies are malnourished, lethargic with or without fever, do not tolerate feeds, have abdominal distension and jaundice. Multiple bones or joints may be involved (see Case history, below). There is often evidence of abscess formation elsewhere, e.g. liver abscesses or pleural empyema, and babies are gravely ill. The commoner sites of neonatal osteomyelitis are shown in Table 9.2.

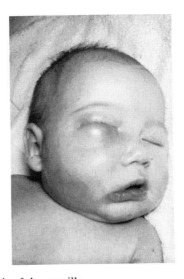

Figure 9.5 Osteomyelitis of the maxilla

**Table 9.2 Commoner sites of neonatal osteomyelitis and
approximate frequency**

Site	Frequency (%)
Femur	35
Humerus	17
Tibia	14
Maxilla	6
Radius	5
Clavicle	3
Phalanges	2
Ulna	2
Skull	2
Ribs	2
Miscellaneous (vertebrae, pelvis, mandible, scapula, sternum, etc.)	12

Case history

A 15-month-old boy was referred for surgery for patent urachus after passing urine through his umbilicus. His umbilicus was not obviously infected, he was afebrile and feeding well. His left thigh was noted to be swollen but not tender or inflamed and he had left foot drop (Figure 9.6). Sciatic nerve palsy secondary to an intramuscular vitamin K injection was diagnosed. The patent urachus was tied off surgically. Two days later, erythematous patches appeared over the right shoulder, wrist and left middle finger (Figure 9.7). Blood cultures, urine and pus aspirated from the thigh, shoulder and wrist grew *S. aureus*. The initial radiograph of his left hip (Figure 9.8a) showed evidence of osteomyelitis with periosteal elevation and bite-like erosions of the metaphysis and epiphysis. At surgery there was septic arthritis of the left hip and extensive destruction of the femoral head.

Infection was eventually controlled with antibiotics and repeated surgical drainage of affected joints. At follow-up the boy has shortening of his left femur (Figure 9.8b), a flexion contracture of the left proximal interphalangeal joint and limited dorsiflexion of the right wrist.

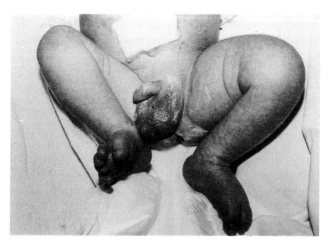

Figure 9.6 Case History: patent urachus. Left thigh swollen, leg externally rotated

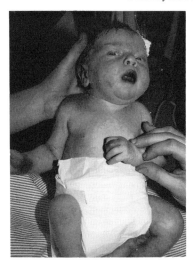

Figure 9.7 Case History: disseminated joint involvement (hip, shoulder, finger, elbow) due to *Staphylococcus aureus*

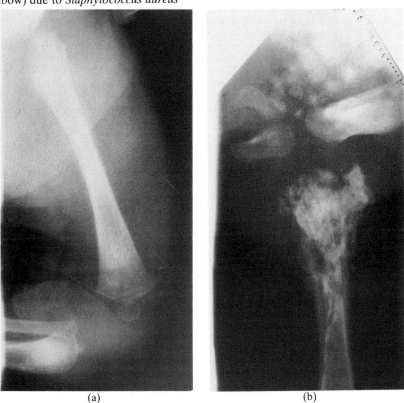

(a)   (b)

Figure 9.8 Case History: staphylococcal osteomyelitis and septic arthritis. (a) Left hip at diagnosis showing 'bite-like' erosions in metaphysis and epiphysis and periosteal elevation. (b) 3 months later there is widespread destruction of left femoral head and neck

Diagnosis

The most important part of making a diagnosis of osteomyelitis is to consider it as a possible diagnosis whenever there is swelling, immobility or redness. The main difference between neonates and older children in confirming a diagnosis of osteomyelitis is the relative importance of radiography and bone scans. In the newborn period, radiographic changes appear early, and are almost always present by the seventh day of illness. In contrast, technetium bone scans are often normal in neonatal osteomyelitis, even in the presence of radiographic changes (Ash and Gilday, 1980), although advances in resolution of cameras have meant that bone scan may be more reliable (Bressler *et al.*, 1984). Gallium scans may be more sensitive than technetium in identifying osteomyelitis but use 5–6 times more radiation (R. Howman-Giles, personal communication). Magnetic resonance imaging of bones is increasingly being used, but is still being evaluated.

Radiographically, there is initial non-specific soft tissue swelling followed by the appearance of metaphyseal, and later epiphyseal, areas of rarefaction which look like bites out of the bone (Figure 9.8a). Metaphyseal lucencies

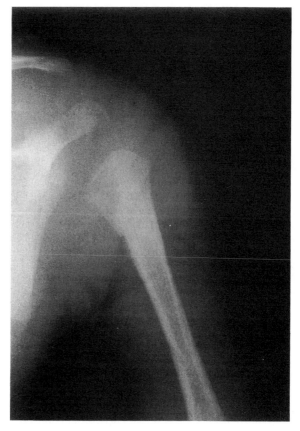

Figure 9.9 Group B streptococcal osteomyelitis of humerus. Punched-out lesion of head

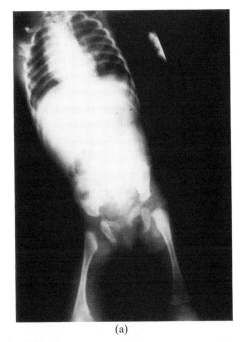

(a)

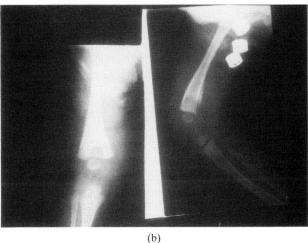

(b)

Figure 9.10a,b Pathological metaphyseal fracture in 4-month-old girl born at 30 weeks' gestation. Originally misdiagnosed as non-accidental injury. *Proteus* osteomyelitis secondary to necrotizing enterocolitis 2 months earlier

surrounded by an area of sclerosis typically occur in *Candida* infection. Concurrent septic arthritis of the shoulder or hip joint may cause lateral displacement and even dislocation of the head of the humerus or femur. Subtle degrees of displacement may be evident only if comparison is made with the opposite side, i.e. a radiograph should be obtained of *both* shoulder or *both* hip joints. There may be periosteal elevation of the shaft of long bones. GBS osteomyelitis typically involves a single bone, causing a punched-out lesion in the head of the humerus or femur (Figure 9.9).

The most difficult differentiation is probably between cellulitis and osteomyelitis. If the initial radiograph is unhelpful, needle aspiration may aid both in identifying the organism and deciding whether there is bony involvement. If this remains in doubt, then serial radiographs may help to resolve the problem. Clinically, cellulitis responds within 24–48 h to antibiotic therapy; a slow response suggests underlying osteomyelitis.

Laboratory tests are of little help. The ESR and serum CRP are usually, but not always, elevated, but these are non-specific and may even be normal in osteomyelitis.

Occasionally, osteomyelitis may present with a pathological fracture; if this is of the metaphysis (Figure 9.10) and there is periosteal elevation, an erroneous diagnosis of non-accidental injury may be made (Isaacs *et al.*, 1986a).

Septic arthritis

As already indicated, septic arthritis is a frequent concomitant of osteomyelitis of the long bones. Occasionally, septic arthritis occurs in the absence of demonstrable osteomyelitis, in which case the pathogenesis is either direct haematogenous seeding of the joint (primary septic arthritis) or secondary to occult osteomyelitis. *Staphylococcus aureus* is the commonest single cause of all cases of primary septic arthritis ($\sim 45\%$) but Gram-negative bacilli (25%) cause proportionately more cases than of osteomyelitis. Other organisms that cause septic arthritis are those described as causing osteomyelitis (Table 9.1). Septic arthritis causes redness and swelling of the joint and paucity of movement of the limb; passive movement of the joint is painful; multiple joint involvement is common. Neonatal gonococcal infection is very rare in the UK, but not in parts of the world where the prevalence of gonorrhoea is high.

Management

In view of the wide range of organisms that can cause neonatal osteomyelitis and septic arthritis, and the long duration of antibiotic treatment, it is particularly important to identify the organism responsible. Pus should, therefore, be aspirated by needle or open drainage from bone, joint or soft tissue abscesses. Blood should always be cultured, because up to 20% of joint aspirates are sterile in septic arthritis, possibly because joint fluid is bacteriostatic or because organisms are limited to the synovium. Urine and CSF should also be cultured, as the likelihood of metastatic spread through bacteraemia is high.

Surgical drainage is necessary for large soft-tissue abscesses, and open surgical drainage of the relevant joint is essential to prevent necrosis of the head of the femur or humerus. Smaller joints can usually be effectively treated by regular aspiration and rarely need open surgical drainage. Because there is spontaneous decompression of infection of the shaft, it is not usually necessary to drill the cortex of the long bones (Fox and Sprunt, 1978) but pus in the bone under pressure should be drained surgically.

Antimicrobial therapy is guided by the Gram's stain on the aspirated pus. If no organisms are seen, or no pus is obtained, empirical therapy might comprise a penicillinase-resistant penicillin (flucloxacillin, oxacillin) to cover staphylococci and streptococci and an aminoglycoside or cephalosporin for Gram-negative bacilli. Anaerobic infection will normally respond to this regimen, but if this seems a likely cause, either the addition of metronidazole (favoured in the UK) or the use of clindamycin (favoured in the USA) is advisable. Initial therapy should be given intravenously. Data concerning older children are accumulating to the effect that treatment can be given orally after a few days. As oral absorption is uncertain in neonates, a change to oral therapy is advised only if the baby can be observed in hospital to monitor clinical progress, weekly serum bactericidal titres (titration of the patient's serum against the patient's organism or a laboratory strain of *S. aureus*; Prober and Yeager, 1979), ESR and serum CRP. Treatment for ≤ 3 weeks results in at least a 15% failure rate, whereas treatment for ≥ 4 weeks or more has a 5% or lower failure rate (Syriopoulou and Smith, 1987); therefore, treatment should be for ≥ 4 weeks.

Early immobilization of the limb and joint is usually necessary, but as soon as there is no further pain, physiotherapy should be started to mobilize affected joints.

Prognosis

The prognosis depends on early diagnosis and effective treatment. The fulminant septicaemic form of osteomyelitis, particularly when there is disseminated infection, has a high mortality. Severe involvement of the joint capsule may lead to permanent damage to the growth plate and resulting disability.

Chapter 10

Urinary tract infection

Definition

A urinary tract infection (UTI) may involve any or all parts of the renal tract, from the kidneys to the bladder. UTI is diagnosed by culturing voided urine or urine obtained by catheterization or by needle aspiration of the bladder. Voided urine is often contaminated with bacteria; as the doubling time of coliform bacteria is only ~ 20 min, delays in transit result in significant increases in the number of organisms cultured.

Conventionally, UTI is defined as the culture of $\geqslant 10^5$ colonies of a single organism from each millilitre of urine. However, this definition is based on Kass' studies of mid-stream urine specimens cultured from adult women who were about to undergo bladder catheterization. The applicability of such diagnostic criteria to neonatal UTI has never been assessed.

Epidemiology

Given the difficulties of making a secure diagnosis, it is not surprising that the reported incidence of neonatal UTI has varied: estimates have ranged from 0.1 to 1% of all infants. The incidence is higher in preterm babies, with figures of 3–10% reported for babies < 2500 g birth-weight (Klein, 1990a). In the newborn period, boys experience between three and eight times as many urinary tract infections as girls (Lincoln and Winberg, 1964a; Littlewood et al., 1969; Bergstrom et al., 1972; Maherzi et al., 1978; Ginsburg and McCracken, 1982), which may partly reflect the increased susceptibility of males to all forms of sepsis (see below).

Pathogenesis

Neonatal UTI is usually thought to occur secondary to bacteraemia. In contrast, UTI in older children usually results from ascending infection. In the neonate, blood cultures are often positive and symptoms of systemic sepsis often precede the appearance of urinary abnormalities, although sometimes the urinary tract is the primary site of infection and bacteraemia occurs secondarily.

Obstructive abnormalities of the urinary tract such as posterior urethral valves, vesico-ureteric or pelvi-ureteric junction stenosis are responsible for only ~ 10% of infections in boys (Bergstrom *et al.*, 1972; Maherzi *et al.*, 1978). Vesico-ureteric reflux (VUR) is found in 30–50% of newborn babies of either sex with UTI (Rolleston *et al.*, 1970; Maherzi *et al.*, 1978). VUR may be a factor in the pathogenesis of UTI, but may also be exacerbated by infection (Schopfner, 1970).

The increased susceptibility to neonatal UTI of boys, who have a three- to eightfold higher incidence than girls, compared with the 1.5- to twofold increase for other forms of sepsis, suggests that other factors may be important. The male prepuce becomes heavily colonized with *E. coli* during the first few days after birth (Bollgren and Winberg, 1976) and uropathogenic P-fimbriated *E. coli* are particularly likely to bind to the foreskin (Fussell *et al.*, 1988). Wiswell and colleagues (Wiswell, *et al.*, 1985, 1987; Wiswell and Roscelli, 1986) have provided compelling evidence, albeit based on retrospective studies, that circumcision reduces the incidence of UTI in boys. Circumcision reduces urethral as well as periurethral colonization with *E. coli* (Wiswell *et al.*, 1988) and *Proteus* (Glennon *et al.*, 1988).

A host factor correlating with susceptibility to UTI is the P-1 blood group antigen, a glycolipid, that is a receptor for the adherence of p-fimbriae. In a study of girls, 97% with recurrent UTI had the P-1 phenotype compared with 75% of controls (Lomberg *et al.*, 1983). Antigens in the P blood group system can also act as epithelial-cell receptors that can bind *E. coli*.

Microbiology

E. coli causes ~ 75% of neonatal UTI and *Klebsiella* ~ 13% (Klein, 1990a). The remainder are caused by miscellaneous Gram-negative organisms (*Proteus, Pseudomonas, Serratia, Enterobacter*) and Gram-positive cocci (enterococci, *Staphylococcus aureus, Staphylococcus epidermidis*). Multiple organisms were found in almost 10% of cases in one series (Maherzi *et al.*, 1978).

Most *E. coli* that cause childhood infections carry one of five capsular (K) antigens (Kaijser *et al.*, 1977), suggesting that this surface polysaccharide may be an important virulence determinant. *E. coli* adhere to uroepithelial cells using fimbriae, and there is much interest in the role of different fimbriae, particularly P-fimbriae, in the pathogenesis of UTI (de Man *et al.*, 1989), and the way their expression is subject to phase variation (being switched on and off). Certain clones seem to be particularly virulent or uropathogenic (Vaisanen-Rhen *et al.*, 1984; Marild *et al.*, 1989).

The urinary tract may be involved by metastatic spread as part of a pattern of disseminated sepsis with *Staphylococcus aureus* or group B streptococcus. *S. aureus* UTI occasionally occurs in isolation, i.e. without evidence of dissemination. Infection with *Proteus* or *Pseudomonas* is more likely to occur in babies with underlying renal tract pathology.

Microscopic examination of the urine sediment can be helpful. However, normal babies without UTI may have up to 50 white blood cells per mm^3 (Lincoln and Winberg, 1964b) while about a quarter of babies with proven UTI do not have pyuria (Klein, 1990a).

Clinical manifestations

UTI may manifest early as part of generalized early-onset sepsis, or may appear late, usually more insidiously. Sometimes UTI may be diagnosed in completely asymptomatic babies who, none the less, have significant bacteriuria.

In early-onset sepsis the signs or symptoms of UTI are non-specific. Over a 12-month period Visser and Hall (1979) cultured urine and blood from 188 babies with suspected early-onset sepsis. Nine babies had bacteraemia but only one of these, with GBS infection, had a positive urine culture. Two babies had bacteriuria with negative blood cultures: one had *Staphylococcus epidermidis* grown from a suprapubic aspirate but recovered without anti-biotics (i.e. the organism was probably a contaminant) and the other grew *E. coli*. Over 5 years in Oxford we have seen positive urines in suspected early-onset sepsis only in association with generalized GBS sepsis (three cases) or as probable contaminants, and we no longer perform suprapubic aspirates as part of the routine cultures for suspected early-onset sepsis.

In infants presenting with late-onset UTI, the main clinical features are failure to thrive (50%), fever (40%), vomiting and/or diarrhoea (40%), jaundice (20%) and irritability or lethargy (20%) (Klein, 1990a). Intolerance of feeds and abdominal distension may be prominent. Although the sudden onset of, or increase in, jaundice is well recognized as suggesting UTI, particularly *E. coli* UTI with septicaemia, jaundice is recorded in less than one-quarter of all cases of UTI. Hepatosplenomegaly may be present. Obstructive uropathy can result in severe hyponatraemia sufficient to cause convulsions. Hypertension is rare.

Renal tract abnormalities may be diagnosed antenatally by ultrasound scan. They are also associated with other congenital anomalies, as for example in the CHARGE (Coloboma, Atresia choanae, Retardation of growth and development, Genital hypoplasia and Ear defects of external ear and hearing) and VATER (Vertebral, Anorectal, Tracheo-Esophageal and Radial anomalies) groups of anomalies. A single umbilical artery is often, although not always, associated with renal tract anomalies, as are abnormalities of the ears. Thus, a full examination is important: the kidneys should be palpated bimanually for abnormalities in size and position; the external genitalia should be examined and the urinary stream observed.

Occasionally, there may be signs of localized sepsis. Suppurative orchitis has been described, caused by various organisms (*Staphylococcus aureus*, *E. coli*, *Pseudomonas*) and prostatitis and epididymitis occur very occasionally. One outbreak of *Serratia* UTI, attributable to contaminated umbilical wash solution, was associated with balanitis. Circumcision can be associated with subsequent UTI.

Diagnosis

The growth of organisms from a suprapubic aspirate (SPA) of urine is the generally accepted 'gold standard' for diagnosing UTI, and it is generally stated that any growth of bacteria is significant. However, even SPA urines can be contaminated with skin bacteria from the baby, or occasionally the bowel can be punctured, although this is less likely if ultrasound is used first to confirm a full bladder. Suprapubic aspiration causes significant haematuria in 0.6% of cases (Saccharow and Pryles, 1969) and is a traumatic procedure for babies, parents and staff. As discussed in Chapter 4, our policy is to reserve SPA for babies in whom UTI seems highly probable and for whom antibiotics need to be started immediately. SPA may also be used to confirm UTI after one or more positive bag urine specimens.

Bag urines are highly likely to be contaminated by the baby's faeces. Clean-catch urines, in which the pot is held poised over the penis or the vagina until the baby urinates, are a decided improvement, although they may require considerable patience. Catheter specimens, particularly from girls, may be less invasive than repeated failed attempts at SPA and could perhaps be used more often.

Management

Antibiotics

The decision whether to initiate immediate antibiotic treatment of UTI while awaiting culture results depends on the level of clinical suspicion of systemic sepsis and whether organisms are seen on Gram's staining of the urine. Although the relative distribution of the different organisms causing UTI differs from that of late-onset septicaemia (more Gram-negative bacilli, fewer staphylococci, rarely enterococci) the range of organisms does not differ substantially. Therefore, if a baby is systemically unwell, and whether or not there is evidence from urine microscopy of a UTI, our policy has been to treat with flucloxacillin and an aminoglycoside, the same antibiotics as for late-onset sepsis. This provides good cover against staphylococci as well as against Gram-negative bacilli. If a baby is known to have renal tract anomalies, is systemically unwell and urine microscopy shows Gram-negative bacilli, we use cefotaxime and an aminoglycoside. On the other hand, if the baby has a positive culture from a bag urine, obtained because of relatively minor symptoms, and is not systemically unwell, we re-assess the baby clinically. If the baby is well, we repeat the bag urine microscopy and culture but do not start antibiotics. If the baby is moderately unwell, we perform an SPA and full septic screen including CSF, and start antibiotics based on the antibiotic susceptibility of the organism from the previous bag urine culture. We repeat urine cultures after 48 hours' treatment to determine whether the urine is sterile, and usually continue treatment for 10 days. Abscesses or complicated infections may require surgical exploration and extended antibiotic treatment.

Supportive treatment

Obstructive uropathy can result in severe hyponatraemia sufficient to mimic salt-losing congenital adrenal hyperplasia. Hypertension is rare but shock may result from systemic sepsis; the blood pressure should always be measured. Haemolytic anaemia can be associated with the jaundice of UTI. The usual supportive measures for sepsis should be employed where

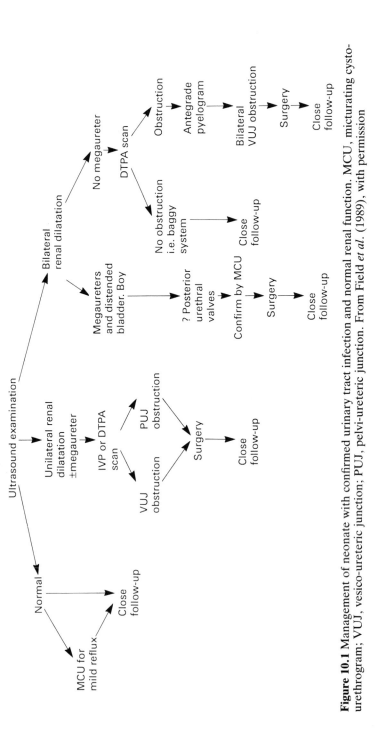

Figure 10.1 Management of neonate with confirmed urinary tract infection and normal renal function. MCU, micturating cysto-urethrogram; VUJ, vesico-ureteric junction; PUJ, pelvi-ureteric junction. From Field *et al.* (1989), with permission

appropriate, as outlined in Chapter 6, and a full blood count and urea and electrolyte levels should be obtained.

Investigation of urinary tract

It is important to detect obstructive lesions early, so it is our policy once UTI is diagnosed to perform immediate investigations of the structure of the urinary tract. The commonest abnormality that can be detected is vesico-ureteric reflux, present in about one-half of all newborns with UTI (Rolleston *et al.*, 1970). Reflux may be exacerbated by UTI so that early investigation may overestimate the severity of reflux. The combination of both intrarenal reflux and urinary infection predisposes to renal damage with scarring, although either alone probably does not cause scarring. Thus, either reflux or further infection must be prevented.

In the past, intravenous pyelography (IVP) and micturating cysto-urethrography (MCU) were used to diagnose structural abnormalities and reflux. IVP has largely been superseded by the use of real-time ultrasound scanning. Ultrasound is very dependent on the skill and experience of the examiner, so ultrasound-based investigation of the urinary tract should be performed only when the appropriate expertise is available. It will detect obstructed systems, showing one or both kidneys dilated with or without dilatation of one or both ureters. Gross vesico-ureteric reflux will also be detected by ultrasound, but not milder degrees of reflux, and most neonatologists would perform an MCU as well as an ultrasound scan in the initial examination. If an ultrasound scan is used as the sole initial radiological investigation and is normal, babies should be closely followed up with regular urine cultures and repeat ultrasound examinations. If UTI recurs, an MCU is indicated because reflux and infection can damage the kidney. On the other hand, if the initial ultrasound scan is abnormal, further investigations will be necessary. A possible scheme of investigation is shown in Figure 10.1. Unilateral renal dilatation is usually due to vesico-ureteric junction (VUJ) or pelvi-ureteric junction (PUJ) obstruction. Marked dilatation of both kidneys suggests mechanical obstruction, severe reflux or a 'baggy' collecting system (congenital mega-ureters or megacalyces). The association of mega-ureters and distended bladder in a boy is usually caused by posterior urethral valves. If there is no mega-ureter, a Tc^{99}-diethylenetriamine penta-acetate (DTPA) isotope scan which measures perfusion and clearance will distinguish an obstructed system from a baggy one.

Babies with moderate reflux not requiring immediate surgery should be followed closely. We start these babies on prophylactic trimethoprim and culture urine samples regularly. Surgery is considered if there are breakthrough infections and persistent moderate to severe reflux.

Chapter 11

Infections of the eye

Definition

It might be thought that the definition of *conjunctivitis* would cause little problem, because inflammation of the conjunctiva should be readily identifiable. In practice, however, it has been difficult to compare different studies of neonatal conjunctivitis because of variation in definitions or even complete failure to define what is meant by conjunctivitis.

Many babies present with 'sticky eyes' caused by purulent discharge, and this can be associated with a varying degree of conjunctival reddening and oedema. Conjunctivitis has been defined as purulent ocular discharge or inflammation of the conjunctivae. The term 'ophthalmia neonatorum' has been used to mean all neonatal eye infections or, alternatively, as synonymous with gonococcal ophthalmitis, the first-described and most serious cause of neonatal conjunctivitis.

Significant inflammation of the nasolacrimal duct is termed 'dacryocystitis', a condition diagnosed by finding a purple swelling lateral to the bridge of the nose from which purulent discharge can be expressed through the lacrimal punctum.

In conjunctivitis there may also be significant involvement of the eyelids and surrounding orbital tissues amounting to cellulitis. Periorbital cellulitis is sometimes subdivided into preseptal cellulitis, with mild inflammation confined to the orbital margins, and orbital cellulitis with severe inflammation beyond the margins of the orbit and often proptosis.

Most eye infections are confined to the conjunctivae but there may be involvement of the cornea, of the inner eye (perforating keratitis and endophthalmitis) or of the whole eye (panophthalmitis).

Epidemiology

Conjunctivitis is the commonest neonatal infection. The incidence in industrialized countries, as judged by prospective studies, has been reported as 2–12% (Johnson and McKenna, 1975; Prentice *et al.*, 1977; Pierce *et al.*, 1982; Sandstrom, 1987). In one study from Belgium, 11% of babies had conjunctivitis by the time of discharge at 7–10 days, and a further 13% developed red or sticky eyes at home before 1 month of age (Fransen *et al.*, 1987). As many babies develop conjunctivitis after leaving hospital, retrospective hospital-based studies will greatly underestimate the incidence.

The incidence of neonatal conjunctivitis depends to a large extent on the incidence of the sexually transmitted organisms *Neisseria gonorrhoeae* and

Chlamydia trachomatis in the adult population. It also depends on ocular hygiene and access to clean water. In developing countries a much higher incidence of neonatal conjunctivitis (15–34%) has been reported, of which gonococcal and chlamydial infection together contribute approximately one-half (Sowa *et al.*, 1968; Otiti, 1975; Maybe and Whittle, 1982; Meheus *et al.*, 1982; Fransen *et al.*, 1986).

A complicating factor is the use of ocular prophylaxis against infection (see below), because the solutions used, particularly silver nitrate, are irritant and cause a chemical conjunctivitis in ∼ 90% of babies. Conjunctivitis is common in babies receiving phototherapy, possibly because of the protective eye-pads or even the lights.

Staphylococcus aureus is an important cause of conjunctivitis, and when there is much spread of staphylococci, as for example when umbilical cord care is not given, epidemics of staphylococcal conjunctivitis may occur.

Eye-wash solutions may become contaminated with water-loving Gram-negative bacilli, such as *Pseudomonas* and *Serratia*, and outbreaks of Gram-negative conjunctivitis in neonatal units have been traced to contaminated eye-wash solutions. Disposable single-use saline sachets have largely prevented this problem.

Microbiology

The three major causes of neonatal eye infections are *Neisseria gonorrhoeae*, *Chlamydia trachomatis* and *Staphylococcus aureus*.

Gonococcal ophthalmitis used to be the commonest cause of blindness, even in developed countries. Three British studies, in which ocular prophylaxis was not given, found no cases of gonococcal ophthalmitis (Prentice *et al.*, 1977; McGill, 1979; Pierce *et al.*, 1982), although 11 of 103 babies with therapy-resistant conjunctivitis in Liverpool had gonococcal infection (Rees *et al.*, 1977). In Britain and the Netherlands, eye prophylaxis has been discontinued and the rare cases of gonococcal ophthalmitis are used as a signal for treating baby and parents. A study from Australia, where a similar approach is used, found that eight (1.4%) of 571 babies with conjunctivitis had gonococcal infection, representing 0.4 per 1000 live births of the population (Johnson and McKenna, 1975). In the United States, where ocular prophylaxis is almost universal, the incidence of gonococcal ophthalmitis is about 0.1 per 1000 live births (Armstrong *et al.*, 1976).

In contrast, *N. gonorrhoeae* has been responsible for between 15 and 44% of all eye infections in studies from Africa. When these figures are combined with the incidence data, they suggest that 2–18% of babies from the African populations studied can be expected to develop gonococcal ophthalmitis.

The incidence of *Chlamydia trachomatis* conjunctivitis in developed countries has generally been reported as approximately 2–4 per 1000 live births (Armstrong *et al.*, 1976; Prentice *et al.*, 1977; Sandstrom, 1987). As the incidence is higher in lower socio-economic groups, the reported incidence will vary according to the socio-economic status of the local population. If much milder cases of conjunctivitis and those occurring after leaving the maternity hospital are included, a much higher incidence of chlamydial conjunctivitis is found. In the United States, such studies have reported an incidence of chlamydial conjunctivitis of 10–63 per 1000 live births (Schachter and Grossman, 1981). This represents up to 43% of all cases of neonatal conjunctivitis (Rapoza *et al.*, 1986). About 60–70% of babies born to mothers with chlamydial infection of the cervix become colonized. Chlamydial conjunctivitis develops in 25–50% of exposed infants and, if untreated, pneumonitis develops in 10–20%.

In Africa a greater proportion of cases of conjunctivitis is probably caused by *C. trachomatis*, with reports suggesting that 13–35% of babies with conjunctivitis, and 2–10% of all babies, have chlamydial conjunctivitis (Maybe and Whittle, 1982; Meheus *et al.*, 1982; Fransen *et al.*, 1986).

Staphylococcus aureus is the commonest organism other than *N. gonorrhoeae* and *C. trachomatis* to cause conjunctivitis. Other bacteria have been isolated from the eyes of babies with conjunctivitis but can also colonize eyes without causing infections. Studies in which appropriate controls have been included have shown that conjunctivitis may be caused by *Pseudomonas aeruginosa*, group A and B streptococci, pneumococci, *Haemophilus influenzae*, meningococci, *Moraxella* (originally *Branhamella*) *catarrhalis*, coliforms, enterococci and *Streptococcus viridans*. Occasional cases due to *Corynebacterium diphtheriae*, *Pasteurella multocida* and clostridia have been reported. Herpes simplex virus, echoviruses, adenoviruses, *candida* and *Mycoplasma hominis* are all rare causes. Dacryocystitis and dacryostenosis are more likely with infections due to *haemophilus* and pneumococci (Sandstrom *et al.*, 1984).

Pseudomonas aeruginosa may cause a mild conjunctivitis or a fulminant panophthalmitis. Other organisms such as group B streptococci, pneumococci, *Staphylococcus aureus* (particularly in the older literature), *H. influenzae* type b, meningococci and *Salmonella enteritidis* may very occasionally cause severe endophthalmitis, probably due to metastatic foci following septicaemia. In a German study, 13 of 16 cases of bacterial endophthalmitis were caused by *Pseudomonas aeruginosa*, two by group B streptococci and one by *Streptococcus pneumoniae* (Lohrer and Belohradsky, 1987).

Clinical features

Gonococcal infection usually presents as an acute severe purulent conjunctivitis, 2–5 days after birth. It may, however, present earlier, be indolent, present later or occasionally be asymptomatic. Typically, the baby develops eyelid oedema, chemosis and a profuse purulent discharge (Figure 11.1). If untreated, corneal involvement with ulceration, perforation and, very occasionally, panophthalmitis occurs and corneal scarring can lead to blindness.

Chlamydia trachomatis usually presents between 5 and 14 days after birth, as infection is predominantly acquired by passage through an infected birth canal. However, early cases occur and there have been occasional reports of babies developing infection despite caesarean delivery with intact membranes. *Chlamydia* causes a more severe conjunctivitis than other organisms except *Gonococcus* (Sandstrom, 1987). A watery discharge rapidly becomes purulent and the eyes are red with oedematous lids (Figure 11.2a). There is marked conjunctival inflammation, sometimes with formation of a

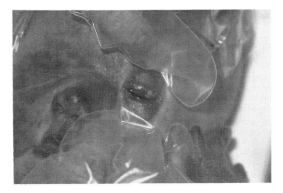

Figure 11.1 Gonococcal ophthalmitis

pseudo-membrane of inflammatory material (Figure 11.2b). Infection may be suppressed, but not cured, by topical antibiotics and will then recur or become chronic. Most untreated cases eventually resolve spontaneously, but chronic infection may lead to conjunctival follicles and even corneal neovascularization (pannus) with 'sheet scarring' or linear scarring as in trachoma.

Pseudomonas conjunctivitis usually appears between 4 and 18 days of age. There may be mild infection limited to the conjunctiva, or lid oedema and erythema. In the fulminant form there is corneal involvement with pannus formation and sometimes perforation, exudate in the anterior chamber and adherence of the iris to the cornea. Although the initial conjunctivitis is usually bilateral, the endophthalmitis is usually (although not always) unilateral (Lohrer and Belohradsky, 1987).

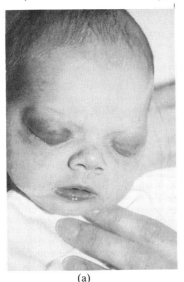
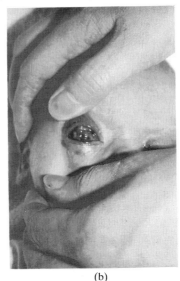

(a)   (b)

Figure 11.2 Chlamydia conjunctivitis: (a) red, swollen lids; (b) exuberant inflammation with pseudomembrane formation

There are no distinctive clinical features to distinguish the other bacterial causes of conjunctivitis (Sandstrom *et al.*, 1984). Herpes simplex causes dendritic or geographic corneal ulcers. *Candida* can cause fluffy infiltrates in the retina or aqueous humour. Maxillary osteomyelitis often presents with purulent conjunctivitis and eyelid oedema before swelling of the cheek develops (Chapter 10).

Diagnosis

A common question in our neonatal unit is how assiduous we should be in trying to diagnose chlamydial conjunctivitis. Routine bacterial conjunctival swabs will not grow *Chlamydia trachomatis*. The diagnosis can be made by culturing the organism on a special cell line, such as McCoy cells, by detecting *Chlamydia* antigen using a rapid technique such as an ELISA, by detecting specific antibodies such as IgA in tears or IgM in serum, or by Giemsa stain of conjunctival scrapings for the classic inclusion bodies. Conjunctival scrapings must include infected cells, so swabs of pus alone are insufficient; this method of identification is used most frequently. Culture is expensive, time-consuming and not widely available. Antigen detection has been well evaluated for cervical specimens but not for eyes. Tear IgA appears late and less than one-half of the cases of chlamydial conjunctivitis have specific serum IgM. We do not look for chlamydial infection in each case of conjunctivitis but only when there is particularly severe infection at 5–14 days, recurrent or chronic infection or a history of maternal vaginal discharge. In Oxford we see one case of chlamydial conjunctivitis on average per year (5000 live births) and one case of chlamydial pneumonitis every 2 years. As $\sim 50\%$ of untreated cases of chlamydial conjunctivitis will develop pneumonitis, we suspect that we are missing about one case a year. Ours, however, is a very low-risk population; in high-risk populations it may be appropriate to screen pregnant women or all cases of conjunctivitis for *Chlamydia*.

Gonococci must be grown in a high concentration of CO_2. If specimens need to be transported for any distance, it is important to inoculate them on to plates and to incubate them in CO_2 in transit to get the maximum yield. Intracellular Gram-negative diplococci seen in the conjunctival pus are usually gonococci but may occasionally be meningococci.

Treatment

Mild conjunctivitis often responds to saline washes alone. Topical antibiotics such as chloramphenicol or trimethoprim–polymyxin will be sufficient to treat most cases of neonatal conjunctivitis.

Gonococcal ophthalmia requires systemic penicillin G: the dose for sensitive organisms is 50 000 units/kg per day 12-hourly, given intravenously (i.v.). Babies infected with resistant penicillinase-producing *Neisseria gonorrhoeae* should be treated with cefotaxime i.v. Frequent eye irrigation is important but topical antibiotics are unnecessary. The baby should be isolated for 24 h as the organism is highly contagious, and both parents should be treated.

Chlamydial conjunctivitis should be treated with topical tetracycline, erythromycin or sulphonamides. Because recurrences are frequent and there is some evidence of a consequent reduction in the incidence of pneumonitis, it is usual to give oral erythromycin 40 mg/kg per day, 6-hourly for 14 days.

Prevention

Credé's prophylaxis with silver nitrate solution, originally 2% now 1%, is extremely effective in preventing gonococcal ophthalmitis. However, it is ineffective against *Chlamydia*, causes a chemical conjunctivitis in up to 90% of all babies, and accidental overdose may occasionally cause blindness. In some countries, such as the Netherlands and the UK, where the incidence of gonococcal infection is very low, the risks of silver nitrate have been found to outweigh the benefits, and isolated cases are diagnosed and treated, as are their parents.

Babies born to mothers with gonococcal infection can be protected with a single i.v. or i.m. dose of 50 000 units penicillin (20 000 units for babies of low birth-weight). Such a regimen has been used as routine prophylaxis for all babies in some North American hospitals. Siegel *et al.* (1980) randomly allocated babies to receive a single dose of penicillin G i.m. at birth, or tetracycline eye ointment. The penicillin group had a lower incidence of GBS infections but a higher incidence of penicillin-resistant enterococcal infections and a mortality rate 2.4 times higher; thus, prophylactic penicillin is not without risks.

Tetracycline eye ointment is effective ocular prophylaxis against both gonococcal and chlamydial infection, and is being used increasingly.

Chapter 12

Intestinal infections

Necrotizing enterocolitis

Definition

Although there is no evidence that necrotizing enterocolitis (NEC) is a primary infection, it is covered in this book because there is circumstantial evidence that microbes are implicated, at least in part, in its pathophysiology. NEC is currently the commonest cause of neonatal peritonitis and a major cause of mortality and morbidity.

Table 12.1 Clinical grading of necrotizing enterocolitis

Grade	Clinical description
I	Bloody stools, no clotting abnormality. No abdominal distension. Tolerate early reintroduction of enteral feeds (within 48 h).
II	Abdominal distension. Suspicious abdominal radiograph without intramural gas. No blood in stools. Tolerate early reintroduction of enteral feeds.
III	Bloody stools, abdominal distension, ileus with dilated small bowel loops on abdominal radiograph, no intramural gas.
IV	Bloody stools, abdominal distension, intramural gas, with or without gas in biliary tree or intestinal perforation.
V	Operative or autopsy diagnosis, histologically confirmed.

NEC is essentially a pathological diagnosis. Classic cases have unique clinical features, such as intramural gas, which are diagnostic. Because of the serious implications, clinicians are often obliged to make a presumptive diagnosis of NEC without firm evidence. Bell and colleagues (1978) suggested a three-step staging system that takes into account the weight of evidence in favour of a diagnosis of NEC. In Oxford we have used a 5-step system, shown in Table 12.1: grades I and II indicate a low probability of NEC but identify occasional cases which progress later to a more advanced grade; grade III is 'probable NEC', whereas grades IV and V represent 'definite NEC'. The Oxford gradings correspond closely to Bell's definitions but allow a more precise clinical description for purposes of comparison.

Epidemiology

The incidence of NEC is greatest in infants of very low birth-weight and lowest in term infants. As the number of cases varies considerably over time within any hospital, it should not be assumed that temporal clustering of cases within a hospital represents an outbreak. Outbreaks of colitis attributable to a number of different micro-organisms may be indistinguishable clinically and histopathologically from NEC. Clustering of cases should therefore be interpreted with caution: in small clusters many of the babies have risk factors for NEC and in larger clusters a search should be made for an infectious cause of colitis.

The reported incidence of NEC ranges from 0.5 to 15 per 1000 live births (Wilson *et al.*, 1981) and develops in ~ 2% (range 1–5%) of babies admitted to neonatal intensive care units (Kliegman and Fanaroff, 1984). The incidence is inversely related to gestational age and birth-weight: Stoll *et al.* (1980) reported NEC in 6.5% of babies with birth-weight < 1500 g, 1% of babies of 1500–2000 g, 0.27% of 2000–2500 g and 0.04% of > 2500 g. Nevertheless, ~ 10% of all cases of NEC occur in full-term infants; 90–95% of cases occur in babies who have received enteral feeds (Kliegman and Fanaroff, 1984).

Pathogenesis

The most likely cause of NEC is an initial episode of intestinal ischaemia, subsequently compounded by bacterial invasion of the disrupted intestinal mucosa. The multiplication of anaerobic (e.g. *Clostridium*) and aerobic (e.g. *E. coli*) gas-forming organisms within the bowel wall is thought to result in the formation of intramural gas (Gall, 1968).

Early reports of associations with NEC were uncontrolled and so did not prove causality. In controlled studies, birth asphyxia, placental abruption, early enteral feeding, patent ductus arteriosus, polycythaemia, exchange transfusion, umbilical vein or artery catheterization and hypothermia have been implicated by some (but not all) workers as significant risk factors (Ryder *et al.*, 1980; Stoll *et al.*, 1980; Kliegman and Fanaroff, 1981, 1984; Yu *et al.*, 1984; Barnard *et al.*, 1985). All these risk factors for NEC could result in intestinal ischaemia and hence local hypoxia. It is interesting that none of them is consistently found to predispose to NEC. It has been suggested that neonates may exhibit the mammalian 'diving reflex' in which cerebral perfusion is protected during hypoxia at the expense of the splanchnic circulation.

NEC almost always develops in association with enteral feeding and it has been suggested that delaying enteral feeding might decrease the risk of NEC. On the contrary, however, La Gamma *et al.* (1985) found in a controlled trial that four of 18 (22%) babies given early enteral feeds developed NEC compared with 12 of 20 (60%) in whom enteral feeds were delayed for 2 weeks, a significant increase in incidence of NEC. Their observations contrast with the sequential but uncontrolled observations of Brown and Sweet (1978) who 'abolished' an outbreak of NEC by delaying enteral feeding.

Lake and Walker (1977) suggested that NEC might result from a breakdown in the intestinal mucosal barrier which would allow absorption of macromolecules. Gray and colleagues (1981) showed an immune complex vasculitis in the damaged intestinal wall of two of four babies with NEC and speculated whether the antigens might be macromolecules. Such an immune complex vasculitis would further contribute to bowel wall ischaemia. The macromolecules might be from milk or alternatively from intestinal micro-organisms. Breast milk appears to be relatively protective compared with feeds based on cow's milk (Kliegman and Fanaroff, 1984). Human breast milk contains immunological factors such as secretory IgA that may be important in protecting against direct bacterial invasion or the action of bacterial exotoxins, whereas cow's milk contains many macromolecules that might contribute to disease.

Is NEC an infectious disease? There have been clusters of cases in associ-ation with a number of different pathogens, including Gram-negative en-teric bacilli (e.g. *Klebsiella*) and anaerobes (e.g. clostridia), and viruses such as rotavirus, coronavirus and enteroviruses (Kliegman and Fanaroff, 1984). No single organism has been consistently isolated in NEC. Clostridia and clostridial toxins are found as commonly in control babies as in those with NEC (Thomas *et al.*, 1984a). Some workers have emphasized that *Klebsiella* species are cultured more frequently and in higher numbers from the faeces of babies with NEC. Lawrence *et al.* (1982) showed that germ-free rats that became colonized with one of a number of single organisms developed NEC: these organisms were *Staphylococcus aureus*, *S. epidermidis*, *Pseudo-monas aeruginosa*, *Clostridia (perfrigens* and *butyricum*) and *Bacillus cer-eus*, all of which produce exotoxins. *E. coli* and *Klebsiella* species alone did not cause NEC. However, if germ-free rats were inoculated with *S. aureus* or *B. cereus*, followed 24 h later and before symptoms by *Klebsiella pneu-moniae*, they developed NEC, and *Klebsiella* outnumbered *S. aureus* by 10 000 to 1. Lawrence *et al.* (1982) suggested, therefore, that bacterial cultures at the time of symptoms may not reveal the causative organism, and they postulated that NEC in the human neonate may be similar to the model infection in the germ-free rat. Exotoxin-producing bacteria could contribute to mucosal damage and this would explain the propensity of NEC to affect the lower ileum where bacterial counts are highest and where macromolecu-lar uptake of bacterial toxins might occur. Such a sequence seems particu-larly likely in the neonatal unit when normal colonization of the intestine is delayed by relatively sterile conditions, by lack of enteral feeding and by

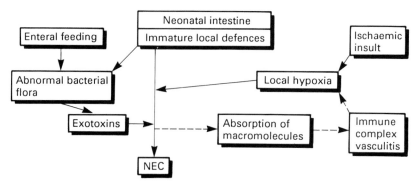

Figure 12.1 Some possible mechanisms in the pathogenesis of necrotizing enterocolitis (NEC)

antibiotics. Scheifele *et al.* (1987) have found an exotoxin produced by coagulase-negative staphylococci in 56% of babies with NEC but in only 6% of controls.

It seems highly likely that NEC is multifactorial. The increased susceptibility of very preterm infants might be due to immaturity of local host defences such as IgA against micro-organisms, to an increased risk of ischaemic injury to the intestine, or to differences in regulation of circulation. Ischaemic injuries have generally been found to be a risk factor for NEC. The enteral flora seems to be an important factor, and it is possible that bacterial exotoxins contribute to NEC (Figure 12.1). Finally, in some cases, particularly those associated with exchange transfusion and the sporadic cases that occur shortly after a blood transfusion has been given to an apparently well infant, NEC is probably caused by emboli.

Pathology

In the early stages there is mucosal oedema, haemorrhage and superficial ulceration but little or no inflammation or necrosis. With advancing disease there is transmural necrosis and an acute inflammatory cellular infiltrate affecting primarily the terminal ileum and ascending colon. In severe cases the entire bowel may be involved; a pseudomembrane of exudate and cell debris may cover necrotic ulcerated mucosa, large vessels may be thrombosed, and perforation of the terminal ileum or colon occurs in up to one-third of cases.

Clinical features

The usual onset of symptoms is at 3–10 days of age, although babies may present on the first day or as late as 2–3 months old. Presentation may be insidious, with apnoea, bradycardia, temperature instability, intolerance of feeds, bilious vomiting and abdominal distension; alternatively, it may be fulminant, with shock, bloody diarrhoea and gross distension of the abdomen, which is red, tense and shiny. Very occasionally, abdominal crepitus may be felt. In the early stages the diagnosis may be difficult to differentiate from sepsis or non-infectious causes of ileus.

The abdominal radiograph may show only distended, centrally placed loops of small bowel or a single, persistently dilated loop. Oedema of the bowel wall leads to separation of small bowel loops. In classic NEC there is pneumatosis intestinalis with a generalized bubbly appearance in the bowel lumen and air visible in the bowel wall (Figure 12.2). Air may be seen in the liver outlining the biliary tree, a sign once thought to be a terminal finding, and one which may appear and disappear over minutes (Figure 12.3). Pneumoperitoneum may be apparent on the plain radiograph but is best seen on a lateral decubitus film with the right side up, when air appears above the liver (Figure 12.4).

Blood cultures are positive at the time of diagnosis in about one-third of patients, mainly with *E. coli*, *Klebsiella* species, *Pseudomonas* species or *S. aureus*. There may be anaemia, neutropenia and thrombocytopenia with disseminated intravascular coagulation. The serum CRP is elevated at the time of diagnosis in >80% of cases (Isaacs *et al.*, 1987d).

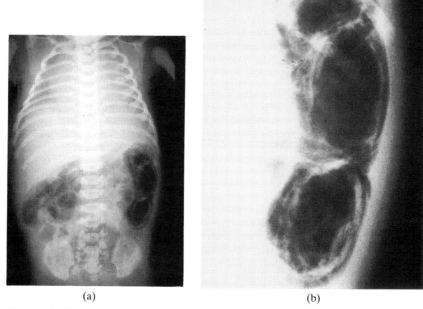

(a)   (b)

Figure 12.2 Plain abdominal radiograph in necrotizing enterocolitis: (a) film showing pneumatosis intestinalis; (b) detail of (a): double shadow of wall of descending colon

Treatment

The most important aspect of treatment is early diagnosis. At the first suspicion of NEC, enteral feeds should be stopped, a nasogastric tube passed to aspirate the stomach contents, and intravenous fluids and antibiotics started after taking blood cultures. The antibiotics used should provide cover against Gram-negative bacilli, *S. aureus* and anaerobes. We use flucloxacillin, an aminoglycoside and metronidazole, but reasonable alternatives would be clindamycin and an aminoglycoside or a third-generation cephalosporin with metronidazole. Faix *et al.* (1988) compared ampicillin and gentamicin therapy with ampicillin, gentamicin and clindamycin and found no difference in mortality but an increase in late strictures in the latter group. We have not found stool cultures very useful, although we always send stools for bacteriology and virology to exclude staphylococcal enterocolitis (see below) and in case other babies develop NEC. Umbilical catheters are removed.

The next priority is vigorous resuscitation, because hypovolaemia is an almost invariable sequel of NEC. Even if the blood pressure is normal there is often a core–peripheral temperature difference of > 3°C, indicating poor perfusion. We almost always resuscitate babies with 10 ml/kg fresh frozen plasma i.v. (or fresh whole blood if there is significant blood loss), as this will support the circulation and replace consumed clotting factors. Close monitoring, as for sepsis, then helps to determine the need for further volume replacement. Ventilatory support is always considered and is often necessary in severe cases.

The necessity for immediate surgical intervention is debatable. Many neonatologists would consider perforation to be an absolute indication for surgery and would often operate when there were signs of peritonism. On the other hand, others, including those at the John Radcliffe Hospital, Oxford, have recently taken a much more conservative approach to surgical intervention. Virtually all babies are initially managed medically. Babies with perforations are resuscitated vigorously and operation delayed until their clinical condition has improved, although almost all later require surgery to remove necrotic bowel and abscess. Babies with gross ascites that is impairing respiration are often managed by inserting an indwelling catheter to drain the ascites. Early diagnosis and a more conservative approach to surgery has kept the mortality from NEC in Oxford to < 10% (Isaacs *et al.*, 1987d).

Continual monitoring of progress is necessary. We have found serum CRP measurements to be a useful adjunct to clinical assessment, as these return to normal in uncomplicated NEC but remain elevated when complications such as stricture of abscess develop (Isaacs *et al.*, 1987d). Babies with probable or definite NEC continue without enteral feeds and with antibiotics for 10 days; earlier reintroduction of feeds has led to relapse. The duration of antibiotics is empirical, and others have stopped these sooner if blood cultures are negative. For more dubious cases of NEC (grades I and II in Table 12.1) we reassess the babies with repeat abdominal radiographs after 48 h. If there has been rapid resolution of any radiographic signs of ileus and NEC seems unlikely, we cautiously reintroduce enteral feeds. Most babies tolerate this, although occasional babies again develop abdominal distension and large aspirates, and are then treated as for probable NEC.

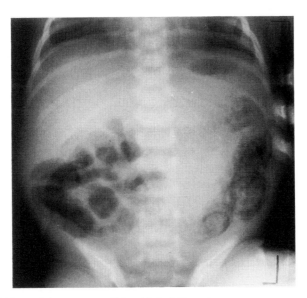

Figure 12.3 Necrotizing enterocolitis. Air in biliary tree

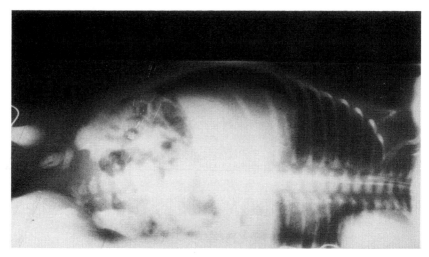

Figure 12.4 Lateral decubitus radiograph showing free air above the liver

Prognosis

The commonly reported mortality rate of NEC is 20–40%, largely attributable to septicaemia, disseminated intravascular coagulation, massive intestinal necrosis and extreme prematurity (Kliegman and Fanaroff, 1984).

Strictures develop in up to 10% of patients, sometimes many days after apparent recovery. Barium studies are necessary, therefore, if intestinal obstruction develops and some centres perform such studies routinely. Many perforations are undiagnosed clinically and abscesses may develop at the site of such perforations. Short-bowel syndrome due to massive resection of necrotic bowel is rare. Recurrences of NEC occur in 3–7% of patients (Kliegman and Fanaroff, 1984).

Prevention

In a randomized controlled trial, Eibl *et al.* (1988) reported a significant reduction in NEC in babies given an enteral immunoglobulin preparation containing IgG and IgA. This was used only for babies for whom breast milk was not available. The use of mother's or pooled banked breast milk is a cheaper and more physiological alternative to oral immunoglobulins.

Oral aminoglycosides have been used as prophylaxis against NEC but their efficacy is, at best, anecdotal and, because of their toxicity and dubious effectiveness, they are rarely used. Standard infection control measures (hand-washing, use of gowns and gloves, cohorting of babies) have been reported to be effective in limiting apparent outbreaks of NEC.

Staphylococcal enterocolitis

Very occasionally, a disease similar to NEC may develop in association with *Staphylococcus aureus* infection. Staphylococcal enterocolitis is characterized by acute onset of bloody or non-bloody diarrhoea with abdominal distension and ileus. In its most severe form there is marked mucosal necrosis and pseudomembrane formation. It is not clear how often this disease is diagnosed as NEC or, indeed, whether it is the same disease. Large numbers of neutrophils and grapelike clusters of Gram-positive cocci are seen on Gram's staining of the faeces and a pure, heavy growth of *S. aureus* can be cultured. The role of staphylococcal toxins in this disease has not been elucidated. An outbreak of four cases in a neonatal unit was described by Gutman *et al.* (1976). We have seen a baby with *S. aureus* septicaemia, diarrhoea and abdominal distension whose abdominal symptoms did not settle with 48 h of appropriate parenteral antibiotics. The baby responded rapidly to oral vancomycin (40 mg/kg per day for 3 days) which is the treatment of choice for staphylococcal enterocolitis.

Hirschsprung's enterocolitis

Babies with Hirschsprung's disease may develop a fulminant enterocolitis with abdominal distension, profuse diarrhoea which is watery but rarely bloody, and shock. Vigorous resuscitation is required before surgery. Babies with Hirschsprung's disease also have an increased incidence of acute appendicitis with perforation (Srouji and Buck, 1978).

Acute appendicitis

This condition is extremely rare in the neonatal period, and only about 50 cases have been reported world wide. The diagnosis is often made late. Most cases occur within 2 weeks of birth and babies present with abdominal distension, bilious vomiting and pain. Fever is variable. The clinical features are generally indistinguishable from NEC or other causes of peritonitis, although the radiograph may show a mass in the right iliac fossa. If peritonitis develops, Gram-negative organisms (*E. coli, Klebsiella* and *Enterobacter* species) predominate but streptococci, *S. aureus* and anaerobes may also be cultured from peritoneal fluid.

Peritonitis

Peritonitis may occur in association with NEC, appendicitis, perforation of the intestine secondary to structural abnormalities, infected omphaloceles or gastroschisis and as a sequel to abdominal surgery. In such cases the infecting organisms are those to be expected from the gut flora. The infected peritoneal fluid often grows multiple isolates of Gram-negative bacilli, *S. aureus* and anaerobes. Boys are more commonly affected.

In contrast, primary peritonitis may occasionally develop in the absence of apparent underlying gastrointestinal pathology. In such cases, as in older children, girls predominate and the organisms responsible are predominantly streptococci (pneumococci and beta-haemolytic streptococci). It is possible that an important route of infection in primary peritonitis is ascending infection from the neonatal vagina.

Gastroenteritis

Outbreaks of gastroenteritis in neonatal units in developed countries are now relatively uncommon.

Escherichia coli is a normal commensal of the neonatal intestine, and although the association of diarrhoea in calves (scours) with certain strains of *E. coli* was recognized in the late nineteenth century it was not until the 1930s that strains of *E. coli* responsible for human neonatal and infantile diarrhoea were distinguished serologically. Enteropathogenic *E. coli* (EPEC), such as strain 0111, were described in association with nursery epidemics and infantile diarrhoea in the 1950s onwards to the mid-1970s in the UK, the USA and Uganda. They do not produce toxins, nor do they invade the mucosa, and the mechanism by which they produce diarrhoea is ill understood. Infection is by the faecal–oral route. EPECs are now a rare cause of neonatal diarrhoea in developed countries, although still important when there is overcrowding and poor sanitation.

Enterotoxigenic *E. coli* (ETEC) produce enterotoxins that are classified as heat-labile (LT) or heat-stable (ST). Although there were reports of outbreaks of ETEC infection in neonatal units in the USA and Scotland in the 1970s, ETEC was a less common cause of neonatal gastroenteritis than EPEC.

Although EPEC and ETEC are more commonly associated with diarrhoea in infants, older children and adults in developing countries, neonatal diarrhoea attributable to these organisms is relatively rarely reported. This may be because of isolation techniques, but also because home delivery is common and breast-feeding, which is protective, is virtually universal. The decline in incidence of neonatal diarrhoea due to these organisms in developed countries may be attributable to improved hygiene, increased use of human breast milk for feeding preterm babies or to a decline in virulence.

In areas of the world where *Salmonella* infection (excluding typhoid, which is extremely rare in neonates) is common or endemic this can be an important cause of neonatal gastroenteritis, albeit accounting for a small proportion of all cases of gastroenteritis. Infection is primarily acquired at the time of birth from ingesting infected faeces or cervical secretions. Outbreaks in neonatal units may occur, with organisms transmitted on the hands of staff, who may themselves develop intestinal colonization. Infection rates in neonatal units have varied from 10 to 85% of exposed babies. Up to one-half may be asymptomatic and the remainder generally have a non-specific gastroenteritis with foul-smelling green 'pea-soup' stools containing mucus and often flecks of blood. About 5% of neonates with non-typhoid *Salmonella* infection have an associated septicaemia, although in some outbreaks the incidence of septicaemia is higher. More neonates than older children develop septicaemia. Septicaemic babies may have rose spots or purpura, but fever may be absent and the symptoms and signs are generally non-specific. Metastatic spread can cause meningitis, osteomyelitis, septic arthritis, pericarditis, pneumonia, empyema, pyelonephritis, cholecystitis, endophthalmitis and skin sepsis. Very occasionally, the metastatic manifestations may be the presenting symptom. Many infected neonates will develop a carrier state for many months, which is generally asymptomatic, although chronic *Salmonella* enteritis with intractable diarrhoea has been described. Oral antibiotics prolong the carrier state and increase the risk of relapse, yet neonatal salmonellosis may be associated with septicaemia and the risk of metastatic spread. Blood, urine and CSF cultures should be taken from newborns with *Salmonella* gastroenteritis, and intravenous ampicillin (100 mg/kg per day) started if there is fever, toxicity or severe diarrhoea.

Shigella is now a relatively uncommon cause of neonatal diarrhoea in developed countries, although in the 1930s it was an important neonatal pathogen. It still causes neonatal diarrhoea in the Indian subcontinent. Septicaemia may very occasionally occur due to *Shigella*, and meningitis even more rarely, but septicaemia may also be caused in *Shigella* dysentery by other enteric organisms that penetrate the inflamed mucosa. Ampicillin resistance is now common and co-trimoxazole is the preferred antibiotic for uncomplicated shigellosis.

Campylobacter jejuni and *Campylobacter fetus* have both been associated with nursery outbreaks of diarrhoea in which the index case acquired the infection from the mother at delivery. Outbreaks have also been associated with the use of unpasteurized milk. The index case in an outbreak is generally born preterm and presents within 12–24 h of birth with fever, respiratory distress, vomiting, diarrhoea, cyanosis and convulsions. Septicaemia progresses rapidly to meningitis. Secondary cases have diarrhoea, often with mucus, pus and blood, but rarely fever unless they develop septicaemia with or without meningitis. Oral erythromycin is the treatment of choice for enteritis but intravenous chloramphenicol (25–50 mg/kg per day 6-hourly) and an aminoglycoside is probably the regimen of choice for meningitis. However, in a report of a nosocomial outbreak when 11 babies developed *Campylobacter jejuni* meningitis, Goossens *et al.* (1986) successfully treated them with ampicillin and gentamicin although a beta-lactamase-producing strain was isolated. One baby had mild hydrocephalus but the rest recovered uneventfully.

A number of different viruses has been associated with neonatal gastroenteritis. Most of these are detected by electron microscopy of stools or by antigen detection but cannot be cultured; enteroviruses (echo-, coxsackie- and polioviruses), on the other hand, can be detected only in tissue culture: thus, both electron microscopy and culture for viruses should be performed.

Rotaviruses, the commonest cause of gastroenteritis world wide, are a rare cause of neonatal gastroenteritis, although outbreaks in neonatal units have been described. Often rotavirus is found to be endemic in neonatal units, with up to 50% of the babies excreting the virus without developing symptoms.

Other viruses that have caused outbreaks of neonatal gastroenteritis include Norwalk agent, coxsackieviruses, echoviruses, astroviruses and coronaviruses. The most important of these are the enteroviruses, because they can cause other systemic manifestations such as meningitis and myocarditis (see Chapter 15).

Infection control measures, above all hand-washing, preferably with alcohol-based rubs, are of prime importance in the prevention of spread of gastroenteritis. Treatment, with the exceptions outlined previously in terms of antibiotics, is primarily symptomatic. Oral rehydration is rarely successful in preterm neonates, and dehydration and electrolyte imbalance can develop rapidly, so intravenous rehydration is usually needed. Antispasmodic agents can cause severe ileus and should not be given to newborns.

Chapter 13

Infections with specific bacteria

Group B streptococcus

Group B streptococci are the most important cause of early-onset sepsis in developed countries, are an important cause of late-onset sepsis with meningitis, and are beginning to be described as an important cause of sepsis in some developing countries (Macfarlane, 1987). The first reported case of neonatal group B streptococcal (GBS) sepsis was in 1939 but it was not until after 1970 that the increasing incidence became apparent in the United States and Europe.

The main route of neonatal infection is undoubtedly from a mother who is colonized rectally or vaginally. About 15–20% of women are colonized at the time of delivery, although reported colonization rates have varied from 5 to 30%. Colonization rates are higher in sexually experienced women, during the first half of the menstrual cycle, women with an intrauterine device, women < 21 years of age and women with lower parity (Baker and Edwards, 1990). GBS colonization is *not* a sexually transmitted disease, an important point in talking to parents of infected babies: colonization does not increase with the number of sexual partners, with oral contraceptive use, with vaginal discharge or with gonococcal infection (Baker and Edwards, 1990). If colonized women are treated with antibiotics during pregnancy the organism may be temporarily suppressed but organisms can usually be cultured again once therapy is discontinued. Maternal colonization is associated with an increased risk of preterm delivery and of premature rupture of membranes. Colonized preterm babies have a greater risk of systemic GBS sepsis with a poorer outcome than full-term babies. Thus, although it has been shown that treatment of colonized mothers with oral penicillin for the last 2 weeks of pregnancy can reduce colonization, failures do occur and such a strategy presupposes that most colonized mothers will deliver at term.

Without intervention, 40–70% of babies of colonized mothers become colonized, and of these about 1% become infected (Figure 13.1). Early-onset disease, associated with ascending infection and in most cases with the maternal risk factors outlined in Chapter 1, is responsible for about two-thirds of the cases of sepsis. The incidence of early-onset GBS sepsis is about 0.3 per 1000 live births in the UK but 3–4 per 1000 in the USA, despite similar rates of maternal colonization. Using a definition of early-onset disease as sepsis occurring in the first 5 days after birth, Anthony and Okada (1977) found that 60% of early-onset cases presented before 24 h of age, while Stewardson-Krieger and Gotoff (1978) found more than one-half of their cases were symptomatic at birth. About one-third of early-onset cases present with pneumonia and septicaemia, one-third with septicaemia alone and one-third with meningitis. Although 74% of cases of early-onset disease are associated with maternal risk factors, this still means that one-quarter of cases occur in term infants in the absence of maternal fever or prolonged rupture of the membranes (Boyer *et al.*, 1983). The mortality is highest in preterm babies but morbidity from meningitis remains high at all gestational ages.

Pregnant women are colonized approximately equally commonly with serotypes I, II or III. In early-onset sepsis without meningitis the same frequency distribution of serotypes is seen. In contrast, > 90% of cases of late-onset sepsis and 85% of cases of early-onset meningitis are caused by serotype III group B streptococci. This supports the concept that different pathogenetic mechanisms are involved in early and late sepsis and in meningitis. In early sepsis, group B streptococci infect the amniotic fluid and have direct access to lung tissue, so that the relative virulence of the different serotypes are less important. In late sepsis the organism has not only to survive in the baby's nasopharynx, but to invade the mucosa, to survive and multiply in the bloodstream and to invade the meninges. Thus, serotype III appears to have increased virulence compared with the other serotypes, and is more likely to cause meningitis.

Late-onset GBS sepsis primarily occurs in the second, third and fourth week with approximately equal frequency, and thereafter with decreasing frequency to 12 weeks of age. Infection after this time is rare, although it may occur up to 3–5 months of age (Anthony and Okada, 1977).

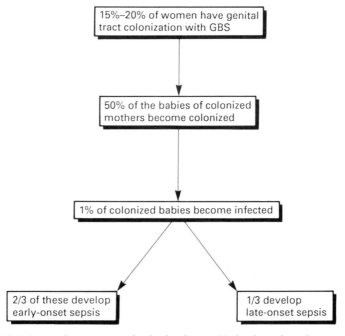

Figure 13.1 Approximate rates of colonization and infection of mothers and babies with group B streptococci

Most cases of late-onset infection probably result from GBS colonization of the nasopharynx at birth, secondary to maternal colonization, with later invasion of the bloodstream. Nosocomial colonization has been well described and, although subsequent infection is rare, sporadic cases and even neonatal unit outbreaks (Noya *et al.*, 1987) of nosocomial GBS sepsis have been described. The great majority of cases of late-onset meningitis occur in full-term babies.

Meningitis is the commonest manifestation of late-onset GBS sepsis, occurring in ~ 85% of cases (Anthony and Okada, 1977; Baker and Edwards, 1990); recent data suggest that the proportion of GBS cases with meningitis has fallen to ~ 50%. Other manifestations are bacteraemia without an established source of infection, osteomyelitis and septic arthritis. Rarer presentations include facial cellulitis, which causes unilateral swelling and erythema of the cheek, submandibular or preauricular region; pleural empyema; endophthalmitis; breast abscess; endocarditis and suppurative pericarditis.

The mortality from early-onset sepsis is ~ 20% and has remained high despite early recognition of symptoms and prompt treatment, often from birth. The mortality from late-onset sepsis is 10%, but about one-half of the survivors of GBS meningitis have neurological sequelae, mostly severe (Edwards *et al.*, 1985).

Prevention

Many babies with early-onset GBS sepsis are septicaemic at birth, and it seems unlikely that further advances in antibiotic or supportive treatment will greatly affect the mortality or morbidity. What then of prevention? The possible strategies are to attempt to reduce maternal colonization during pregnancy, to treat all babies from birth, to attempt passive protection of the baby by giving antibodies to the mother or by actively immunizing her, or to attempt to reduce maternal–fetal transmission during labour. Screening all women for GBS carriage during pregnancy and treating carriers with oral antibiotics during the third trimester has proved impractical because women usually become recolonized once antibiotics are stopped and because the highest mortality is in preterm babies. Siegel and colleagues (1980) apparently reduced the incidence of early-onset GBS sepsis in preterm and full-term babies by giving a single dose of penicillin G i.m. at birth. However, no cultures were obtained before treatment, so the results are difficult to interpret. There was an increase in infections with penicillin-resistant enteric bacilli and the mortality rate was 2–4 times higher in the treated than in the control group. Pyati and colleagues (1983) found that i.m. penicillin at birth did not reduce the incidence or mortality of early-onset GBS sepsis in babies < 2000 g. Whether they develop early- or late-onset sepsis, it has been found that babies who become infected with serotypes II and III group B streptococci have absent or very low levels of maternally acquired opsonic IgG antibody against the type II or III capsular polysaccharide, compared with babies who do not become infected. Baker *et al.* (1988) immunized 40 pregnant women with the type III capsular polysaccharide to try to produce protective antibody levels. Only 20 (57%)

of the 35 with low levels responded to the vaccine although, if they did respond, IgG crossed the placenta. Those women who fail to produce antibodies in response to natural colonization with group B streptococci *do* respond to the vaccine (Baker *et al.*, 1990), but polysaccharide vaccines are unsatisfactory because of the low proportion of women who respond. It is likely that protein–polysaccharide conjugate vaccines will improve the immune response. An alternative not yet tried is to give specific immuno-globulin to the mother during labour, but this would require high-titre preparations, as standard i.v. preparations contain low levels of IgG antibodies.

The approach to prevention of early-onset GBS sepsis that has proved most successful is the use of intrapartum antibiotics. Boyer and Gotoff (1986) screened women for GBS carriage at 26–28 weeks' gestation. They randomized 160 women who had fever ($>37.5°C$), premature onset of labour (<37 weeks) and/or prolonged rupture of membranes ($>12\,h$) to intrapartum ampicillin $2\,g$ i.v. at once, then $1\,g$ i.v. 4-hourly until delivery, or no treatment. Maternal fever was reduced by ampicillin from 21 to 8%, colonization of babies was reduced from 51 to 9% and there were five cases of early-onset sepsis in the control group but none in the treatment group. Cephalosporins are an alternative in penicillin-allergic women. This ap-proach will not protect the 26% of cases of early-onset GBS sepsis with no risk factors, although in Chicago these accounted for only 6% of all fatal cases (Boyer *et al.*, 1983). It also relies on a single screening culture for carriage, which will fail to identify $\sim 8\%$ of women colonized at delivery (Boyer *et al.*, 1983).

It is arguable whether such an approach is practical in the UK, where GBS infection rates are currently so much lower than in the USA. An alternative would be to treat all women who have perinatal risk factors with intrapartum i.v. ampicillin without knowledge of their carriage status, but >500 women in Oxford would need to be treated to prevent a single case of GBS sepsis. Another possibility would be to use a rapid GBS antigen detection test, such as a latex agglutination test, on vaginal secretions from parturient women with risk factors and to treat only those who were positive. There have been practical problems in persuading laboratory staff to provide such a service on a 24-hour basis, although the tests are so simple that even doctors can do them.

In the UK screening of pregnant women for GBS carriage has been done for research purposes only. Screening may also be important, however, in preventing some cases of preterm labour. Maternal GBS colonization is associated with an increased risk of preterm labour (Regan *et al.*, 1981; Moller *et al.*, 1984). In Denmark, screening has been performed by culturing urine as opposed to cervical secretions. Thomsen *et al.* (1987) cultured urine from 4122 women at 27–31 weeks' gestation, and randomly allocated the 69 colonized women to oral penicillin (10^6 units 8-hourly for 3 days) or placebo, repeated if colonization recurred. Penicillin reduced the incidence of pre-term delivery from 12 of 32 (38%) to 2 of 37 (5%) and increased the mean gestational age from 36.2 to 39.6 weeks. If oral penicillin can really avoid 10 preterm deliveries a year in 4000 deliveries, this strengthens the argument for routine screening of pregnant women.

Is it possible to prevent late-onset GBS sepsis by treating asymptomatic babies who are colonized with GBS? Paredes *et al.* (1976) showed that even i.v. penicillin treatment did not eliminate nasopharyngeal carriage in babies with GBS sepsis. Although it is possible that this selected group of babies was unrepresentative, it is generally acknowledged that penicillin does not eradicate colonization nor prevent late sepsis. Indeed, Pyati *et al.* (1983) found that i.m. penicillin prophylaxis was associated with an increase in the incidence of late-onset GBS sepsis from 0.5 to 1.5 per 1000 live births. Penicillin treatment will alter normal flora and may cause moniliasis. There is no evidence that penicillin treatment can prevent late-onset GBS infection in asymptomatic, colonized babies, and it may be disadvantageous.

Nosocomial transmission of group B streptococci is most likely when there is overcrowding, and can be prevented by hand-washing (Baker and Edwards, 1990). We do not isolate babies with GBS sepsis or colonization, but do re-emphasize the importance of hand-washing.

Treatment

Penicillin G or ampicillin are the antibiotics of choice for GBS sepsis. An aminoglycoside is often given initially because of synergy *in vitro* rather than any proven clinical efficacy. The recommended dose of penicillin G has been increased because of the high MIC of the organism and poor CSF penetration (McCracken and Feldman, 1976). The dose for bacteraemia without meningitis is 200 000 units/kg per day for 10 days (150–200 mg/kg per day of ampicillin) and for meningitis is 400 000 units/kg per day (300–400 mg/kg per day of ampicillin) for at least 14 days. Endocarditis is treated with 300 000 units/kg per day for at least 4 weeks. Relapses or recurrences of meningitis occasionally occur; these may be caused by ventriculitis or arguably occasionally by tolerant organisms with a much higher minimum bactericidal concentration (MBC) than minimum inhibitory concentration (MIC), suggesting that they might be suppressed but not killed by antibiotics. However, tolerance can also be demonstrated in populations of group B streptococci that respond rapidly to antibiotic treatment. The outcome from early-onset GBS sepsis is worse in babies of low birth-weight with neutropenia, acidosis, apnoea or pleural effusion (Payne *et al.*, 1988).

Listeria monocytogenes

Listeria monocytogenes is a Gram-positive rod that causes serious infections especially in fetuses and newborns, pregnant women, elderly and immuno-compromised individuals. It is an intracellular organism; cellular immunity is probably critical in recovery, therefore, although the incidence and severity of infection is not greatly increased in HIV infection. It causes monocytosis in rabbits (hence the name), although not usually in humans. Listeriosis was originally thought to be primarily a zoonosis because 50 species of animals can be infected and there is little person-to-person spread, but there is increasing evidence of food-borne spread. *Listeria* can exist in soil and can contaminate crops. Most cases are sporadic, but outbreaks of listeriosis have occurred. One outbreak in Canada was caused by eating coleslaw, made with cabbage that had been fertilized with sheep manure

(Schlech *et al.*, 1983). Listeria readily contaminates both fresh and frozen poultry carcasses, and will survive the 'cook–chill' process (Kerr *et al.*, 1988). In an investigation of 154 sporadic cases of listeriosis, Schwartz *et al.* (1988) found that ~ 20% of the cases could be attributed to eating uncooked hot dogs or undercooked chicken. Both cow's and goat's milk may contain *Listeria*; not only is unpasteurized milk a vehicle of infection, but one outbreak implicated pasteurized milk (Flemming *et al.*, 1985). Milk products such as cheese, and particularly soft cheeses from endemic areas such as France and Switzerland, may contain high concentrations of *Listeria* and have caused outbreaks. Belgian paté has been implicated in an outbreak in Britain and possibly shellfish in New Zealand. The organism can be isolated from salami and continental sausage (Hall *et al.*, 1988). It might seem that there is little that is safe for the pregnant woman to eat, but prudent dietary advice might include the avoidance of unpasteurized milk, soft cheeses, pre-packed salads, patés and undercooked meat, particularly 'cook–chill' poultry. The organism grows well at refrigerator temperatures (4°C) but is killed by thorough cooking.

The incidence of congenital listeriosis is highest in Germany, Holland, Switzerland and France, but is rising in America (Broome *et al.*, 1986) and Britain (Hall *et al.*, 1988). Although the reported UK incidence of perinatal listeriosis is 1 in 20 000 live births (McLaughlin, 1987), in Oxford from 1987 to 1989 the incidence (on small numbers) is 1 in 2000 live births. In our neonatal unit *L. monocytogenes* is now the second commonest cause of early-onset infection after the group B streptococcus.

Early-onset neonatal infection probably results primarily from bacteraemic infection of the mother, with infection of the placenta and transplacental spread. The placenta is often covered with miliary granulomata such as are seen in the baby (granulomatosis infantiseptica). On the other hand, some babies present with pneumonia without granulomata, a picture more suggestive of ascending infection. Most cases of early-onset neonatal listeriosis are associated with symptomatic maternal illness (Becroft *et al.*, 1971; McLaughlin, 1987) suggesting that maternal bacteraemia is probably an important predisposing factor. However, extensive maceration of the fetus may be found soon after maternal symptoms and in some instances the infected fetus may serve as a reservoir of infection, and infect the mother.

Pregnant women present with a febrile illness in which sore throat, headache and chills are prominent. Diarrhoea, pyelitis and backache have all been reported. Blood and urine cultures are usually positive, as well as vaginal swabs. Symptoms generally resolve even without treatment, although *Listeria* meningitis develops in a small number. Infections before 24 weeks' gestation generally result in spontaneous abortion, whereas later infections may cause stillbirth even at term or spontaneous preterm onset of labour. Meconium staining of the liquor (which is thin and may in fact be a pigment rather than true meconium) during preterm labour is highly suggestive of *Listeria* infection and rarely occurs otherwise: Becroft *et al.* (1971) reported it in 9 of 13 cases of congenital listeriosis.

Neonatal infection, as for group B streptococcus, may be of early or late onset. Most early-onset cases present at, or soon after, birth (Becroft *et al.*, 1971; Teberg *et al.*, 1987). Respiratory distress is the most consistent finding,

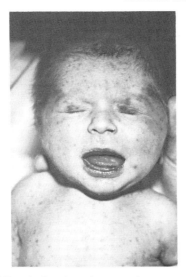

Figure 13.2 Congenital listeriosis: pin-point granulomata

with a radiographic appearance that may mimic hyaline membrane disease or be more suggestive of pneumonia (Figure 8.3). Other presenting features include hepatosplenomegaly, apnoea, convulsions, hypo- or hypertonia, vomiting, and mucous stools sometimes with blood. The classic rash is rarely present but consists of tiny white or pink pin-point granulomata on the face, trunk and notably the posterior pharyngeal wall (Figure 13.2). This rash is frequently misinterpreted as petechial. Meningitis occurs in ∼ 30% of early-onset cases: there may be a significant preponderance of mononuclear cells (mainly monocytes and macrophages) in the CSF. Very occasionally, all the cells are mononuclear, but the associated clinical features and a raised CSF protein and low CSF glucose level should distinguish it from viral meningitis. When organisms are seen on Gram's staining they are not infrequently misinterpreted as Gram-negative rods (*Haemophilus influenzae*) or Gram-positive cocci (group B streptococci).

Late-onset infection presents at 1–4 weeks of age, almost exclusively with non-specific features of meningitis. In > 90% of cases there is no history of maternal illness (McLaughlin, 1987) and it is thought that late-onset infection results from nasopharyngeal colonization at birth, from a mother with asymptomatic perineal carriage, with later invasion of the bloodstream. McLaughlin (1987) reported that 12 of 50 cases of late-onset infection were probably due to cross-infection. An outbreak in a newborn unit has been reported in which the mode of transmission may have been a communal rectal thermometer, while cross-contamination has occurred in a delivery suite, and an infected mother, whose baby with known congenital listeriosis was on the neonatal unit, infected a term baby on the maternity ward. Thus, it is wise to isolate both mother and baby in cases of proven or suspected congenital listeriosis.

The accepted treatment of choice is ampicillin and an aminoglycoside, because this regimen has been most widely employed and gives the best survival rates in animal models. There is, however, little evidence in human neonates that ampicillin and an aminoglycoside is superior to penicillin G and an aminoglycoside, although high-dose penicillin must be used because of the higher MIC. The addition of an aminoglycoside has a synergistic effect both *in vitro* and in animal models of *Listeria* meningitis, where ampicillin therapy alone is associated with a high relapse rate. *Listeria* is resistant to cephalosporins. Because of the intracellular nature of *Listeria* we treat septicaemia for 14 and meningitis for 21 days, although we stop the aminoglycoside after 7 days, and in treating meningitis often change to oral ampicillin after 14 days if the baby is well. Most US practitioners use 10 days of i.v. therapy for *Listeria* sepsis and 14 days for meningitis (C. Baker, personal communication). These regimens are purely empirical. In our experience about one-third of the babies with clinical congenital listeriosis are colonized with *Listeria* but have negative blood and CSF cultures and normal CSF microscopy; we treat them as for *Listeria* septicaemia.

The mortality from early-onset *Listeria* sepsis is up to 50%, although considerably lower for late-onset meningitis. Survivors of meningitis may develop hydrocephalus, ptosis, strabismus and other neurological sequelae. There are no large studies of the outcome of neonatal *Listeria* infection.

Streptococcus pneumoniae

Early-onset infection with pneumococcus, acquired by ascending infection from the maternal genital tract, is relatively uncommon. The clinical features are identical to those of early-onset GBS infection. Babies often have the same risk factors as for GBS infection, and present early with respiratory distress, a chest radiograph showing pneumonia or mimicking hyaline membrane disease, and with hypotension and leucopenia (Bortolussi *et al.*, 1977). The infection is often fulminant with a poor outcome. Meningitis can be present in early-onset sepsis, but babies may also present at 2–4 weeks of age with meningitis. Although pneumococcal meningitis is generally considered to be rare in the neonatal period, the neonatal incidence in the USA is 3 per 100 000 population, which is greater than that at any age after one year (Klein and Marcy, 1990).

Haemophilus influenzae

Early-onset *Haemophilus influenzae* infection is rare but apparently increasing in incidence in both the USA (Wallace *et al.*, 1983) and the UK (Milne *et al.*, 1988). In both countries the incidence of septicaemia is ~ 0.1–0.23 per 1000 live births. The clinical picture may resemble that of hyaline membrane disease, or early conjunctivitis may be the presenting feature with or without septicaemia (Milne *et al.*, 1988). Most cases are associated with maternal chorioamnionitis and preterm labour. The great majority of cases are due to non-typable *Haemophilus influenzae* and ampicillin resistance is rare. Only ~ 1% of women have vaginal carriage of *H. influenzae* (Klein and Marcy, 1990).

H. influenzae is a rare cause of late-onset meningitis, which then occurs mainly in term babies and is attributable to *H. influenzae* type b.

Staphylococcus aureus

S. aureus is a rare cause of early-onset sepsis but an extremely important cause of late sepsis. Outbreaks of staphylococcal infection in neonatal units have been described since 1889, with epidemics in the 1920s, 1950s and early 1970s. Although outbreaks are now rare in developed countries, they are still a major problem in developing countries. When routine umbilical cord care (topical chlorhexidine) was inadvertently stopped in Oxfordshire, a small outbreak of omphalitis and bullous impetigo was a potent reminder that *S. aureus* is still ubiquitous and no less virulent.

S. *aureus* may be carried on the hands of staff, and overcrowding of neonatal units has been shown to be a major factor in spread to babies (Haley and Bregman, 1982). *S. aureus* can also be carried in the nose or rectum of members of staff, which may sometimes be an important mode of transmission. Nevertheless, hand-washing as opposed to elimination of nasal and rectal carriage has consistently been shown to be a better way of limiting outbreaks. There is little doubt that the application of topical antiseptics (hexachloraphane, chlorhexidine, gentian violet, triple dye) or alcohol to the umbilical stump is important in preventing infection, although bathing of babies in hexachloraphane has been abandoned because of worries about neurological toxicity from absorption through the skin. Eichenwald *et al.* (1960) identified four babies with asymptomatic echovirus 20 infection who showered *S. aureus* into the surrounding air. Such 'cloud babies' may occasionally contribute to spread of staphylococcal infection.

Colonization of the umbilicus, nose and skin occurs early, with up to 40–90% of babies colonized by 5 days of age. The commonest manifestation of *S. aureus* infection is probably conjunctivitis. Skin infections of various sorts are, however, common. Bullous impetigo presents with yellow blistering lesions (Figure 13.3) round the umbilicus, nappy area, neck or axilla. The bullae contain clear yellow fluid that can easily be aspirated and shown by Gram's stain to contain numerous neutrophils and Gram-positive cocci. Strains of phage type II are particularly associated with bullous impetigo. Other skin manifestations include skin abscesses, often at the site of cannulas, paronychia (Figure 13.4), cellulitis (often periumbilical), and staphylococcal scalded-skin syndrome (Figure 13.5). The last of these, sometimes called Ritter's disease or (erroneously) toxic epidermal necrolysis, is the result of an exotoxin produced by *S. aureus*. A scarlatiniform rash progresses to wrinkling of skin and then widespread desquamation which can be produced by rubbing the skin gently (Nikolsky's sign). Toxic shock syndrome is exceedingly rare in newborns. Babies with microabscesses (septic spots) can sometimes be managed by rubbing the heads off the spots with an alcohol-based swab. All the other skin manifestations described above require a systemic antistaphylococcal antibiotic such as flucloxacillin. Although bullous impetigo is a superficial infection, it may be associated with septicaemia, as may any of the above infections.

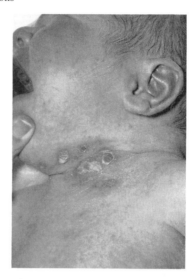

Figure 13.3 Bullous impetigo

S. aureus may cause a wide range of systemic manifestations. Septicaemia may be primary without an obvious focus, or secondary to a focus of infection. Infection may be localized to the skin, lungs (pneumonia often with pneumatoceles and/or empyema), bone, joint, kidneys, heart (endocarditis), or gut (enterocolitis). Meningitis is rare in the absence of an intraventricular shunt, although it may occasionally arise following an intraventricular haemorrhage or by metastatic spread in disseminated disease. Staphylococcal endocarditis is extremely rare, except in association with intravascular catheter-associated thrombus. The other diseases are described in the relevant chapters. Disseminated staphylococcal infection with metastatic spread to bone, joint, skin, kidneys, liver, spleen, lung and (very occasionally) CNS, has a grave prognosis, the mortality being ~ 50%.

Methicillin-resistant *S. aureus* (MRSA) has become an increasing problem in adult and neonatal intensive care units world wide. The resistance genes code for a penicillin-binding protein that prevents the action of

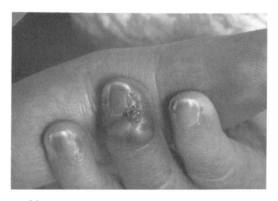

Figure 13.4 Paronychia

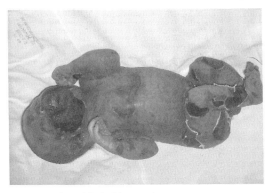

Figure 13.5 Staphylococcal scalded-skin syndrome

beta-lactam antibiotics on cell wall synthesis. They are usually chromoso-mally mediated rather than plasmid-mediated. The gene alters the bacterial cell wall and appears to render the organisms more stable (Editorial, 1985b). The spread of MRSA within units occurs mainly via the hands of staff and can be controlled by improved hand-washing and cohorting of colonized babies (Davies *et al.*, 1987; Millar *et al.*, 1987). Nasal mupirocin (pseudo-monic acid) may eradicate nasal and skin carriage but recurrence is common (Davies *et al.*, 1987). Colonization is more common than symptomatic infection, but in a prolonged outbreak in Sydney (Table 13.1), 19% of colonized babies developed systemic infection, 23 with septicaemia and four with osteomyelitis (M. Anthony, personal communication). There were no deaths. MRSA can cause conjunctivitis, pneumonia, endocarditis, menin-gitis and skin sepsis as well as bone infections and septicaemia. The treat-ment of MRSA infection is with systemic vancomycin which, provided that it is infused over 1 h, is generally extremely well tolerated.

Table 13.1 Occurrence of methicillin-resistant *Staphylococcus aureus* (MRSA) in the neonatal unit, Children's Hospital, Sydney, January 1986–December 1987

Babies	n
Admitted	898
Colonized	140 (16%)
With nosocomial MRSA colonization	108 (12%)
With systemic MRSA sepsis	27 (19% of colonized babies)
Septicaemia	23
Osteomyelitis	4
Died from MRSA sepsis	0

Staphylococcus epidermidis

S. epidermidis, or more precisely coagulase-negative staphylococci, are increasingly being recognized as a cause of late-onset neonatal sepsis, par-ticularly in preterm babies. In the John Radcliffe Hospital, Oxford and many other neonatal units in the UK and world wide, they are now the leading cause of late-onset sepsis. The organism has a particular predilection for synthetic plastics in cannulas and shunts, eroding into the plastic and possibly thereby obtaining nourishment. Some of the colonies thus formed secrete a glycocalyx or 'slime' layer around them, which may protect them against host defences and antibiotics. Septicaemia may be associated with indwelling umbilical catheters or silastic central lines although half the babies with *S. epidermidis* septicaemia in Oxford had never had such a line. In a study of seven babies with long-standing umbilical catheterization who developed *S. epidermidis* sepsis, the isolates from the blood were the same as those from the catheter site in only four of the babies (Valvano *et al.*, 1988). *S. epidermidis* is the leading cause of infections of intraventricular shunts.

S. epidermidis is a frequent contaminant of blood and CSF cultures, contamination occurring from the skin of the baby or the person taking the cultures, or alternatively in the laboratory. There is always a problem, therefore, in distinguishing contamination from true septicaemia. Clinical features of infection and the presence of an umbilical catheter or a central line may be highly suggestive. Serum CRP may be elevated in *S. epidermidis* septicaemia, although usually not to such a high level as that in septicaemia caused by other bacteria, and the immature-to-total white cell ratio may be elevated. Quantitative or semi-quantitative blood cultures show low colony counts in presumed contaminated cultures and high colony counts in presumed sepsis. Such cultures are time-consuming, however, and rarely available as a routine service. In septicaemia, organisms tend to grow more quickly (within 24–48 h) and often in both aerobic and anaerobic blood culture bottles, although neither of these can be taken as an absolute indicator of true sepsis.

The features of sepsis with *S. epidermidis* are non-specific, and often more insidious and less fulminant than with other organisms. In one study, 14 of 29 babies with *S. epidermidis* sepsis had pneumonia (Hall *et al.*, 1987). Thrombocytopenia is found in about one-half of the babies, and we have found the trend in platelet counts to be a useful way of monitoring the response to antibiotic treatment in those babies with sepsis and a central line in whom we have attempted to leave the central line in place (Chapter 6). In general, it can be expected that *S. epidermidis* septicaemia in the presence of a central line will often resolve with antibiotics and without removing the line (Sadiq *et al.*, 1987), but shunt infections never resolve without removing the entire shunt tubing.

Endocarditis is a rare complication of *S. epidermidis* septicaemia, almost always in a structurally abnormal heart. Meningitis in the absence of an intraventricular shunt, or rarely an intraventricular haemorrhage, virtually never occurs. Shunt infections can present insidiously or as fulminant meningitis. Infections of ventriculoperitoneal shunts may cause peritonitis, whereas infections of ventriculoatrial shunts can cause a chronic nephritis ('shunt nephritis') with microscopic haematuria, anaemia, failure to thrive and hypertension. *S. epidermidis* is one of the organisms described as causing persistent bacteraemia, which may be symptomatic (Patrick *et al.*, 1989) or asymptomatic (Albers *et al.*, 1966).

Multiple antibiotic resistance of *S. epidermidis*, including resistance to methicillin/flucloxacillin, is increasing. In many units vancomycin is used, with an aminoglycoside or cephalosporin, as empirical treatment for suspected late-onset sepsis. Our policy has been to treat suspected catheter-associated sepsis with flucloxacillin and an aminoglycoside and to consider removing any umbilical catheter or central line, although increasingly we are attempting to preserve these. Blood cultures are taken from the catheter or central line and from a peripheral vessel. In our experience, babies infected with *S. epidermidis* that is reported as flucloxacillin-resistant have often responded to flucloxacillin and an aminoglycoside and/or removal of the catheter by the time that sensitivity results are available. If the baby is not improving, and especially if the platelet count is falling, we would start vancomycin and again consider removing the catheter. We have had no deaths and no long-term complications from *S. epidermidis* sepsis. On the other hand, *S. epidermidis* can be fatal, particularly in very preterm babies, and many authorities would advise a more aggressive approach to *S. epidermidis* sepsis.

Gram-negative bacilli

Escherichia coli, and to a lesser extent other enteric bacilli, has always been an important early-onset neonatal pathogen. However, in the 1970s, widespread colonization of babies in neonatal units with Gram-negative enteric organisms was described. Organisms such as *E. coli*, *Klebsiella*, *Enterobacter* and *Serratia* became responsible for an increasing proportion of episodes of late-onset sepsis such as bacteraemia, meningitis, pneumonia and skin sepsis (Freedman *et al.*, 1981). In the UK, but not the USA, *Pseudomonas* became an important late-onset pathogen (Isaacs *et al.*, 1987a). A similar increased incidence in cases of Gram-negative sepsis occurred simultaneously in adult intensive care units. Initially, most organisms were sensitive to ampicillin, but plasmid-mediated beta-lactamase resistance rapidly emerged. In addition, several outbreaks of infection due to organisms resistant to aminoglycosides and other antibiotics, such as the third-generation cephalosporins, have now been described (Nelson, 1983). Outbreaks of infection with less well-known Gram-negative bacilli such as *Acinetobacter* have also occurred (Stone and Das, 1985).

Most of these organisms are water-loving and, therefore, readily colonize humidified endotracheal tubes and incubators, indicating the need for frequent changes of sterile water in ventilators, incubators and resuscitation equipment. Although *Pseudomonas* may be found on taps and in sinks, careful typing of isolates suggests that these are an infrequent source of colonizing organisms and that most babies become colonized from their mothers or from other babies through poor hand-washing by staff (Adams and Marrie, 1982; Morrison and Wenzel, 1984; Isaacs *et al.*, 1987a). Gastrointestinal colonization of neonates may be an important reservoir of organisms that can be carried to other babies on the hands of staff. Nasojejunal tube feeding rapidly leads to abnormal colonization of the jejunum with coliform bacilli (Challacombe, 1974). The use of antibiotics for > 3 days is also associated with increased nasopharyngeal colonization with Gram-negative bacteria and bowel colonization with *Klebsiella*, *Enterobacter* and *Citrobacter* (Goldmann *et al.*, 1978).

Gram-negative bacillary septicaemia may accompany necrotizing entero-colitis and urinary tract infections. Like *S. epidermidis*, Gram-negative bacillary septicaemia may occasionally persist. Affected babies may be asymptomatic: Albers *et al.* (1966) described two babies, one with *Klebsiella* and one with *Proteus* bacteraemia which persisted for 3–5 days in the absence of symptoms. Babies may have persistent symptomatic Gram-negative bacteraemia despite apparently appropriate antibiotic therapy, and in the absence of a demonstrable focus of infection. We have seen two extremely preterm babies with NEC and *Klebsiella* bacteraemia whose bacteraemia persisted after successful resection of necrotic gut. Both babies remained bacteraemic and unwell for over 7 days, despite appropriate antibiotic therapy, had a laparotomy which showed no gut ischaemia, and multiple investigations which failed to locate a focus; the infections eventu-ally resolved.

There are no specific features of infections with Gram-negative bacilli. Although the skin lesions of ecthyma gangrenosum have been associated with *Pseudomonas* infection, they may also be seen with other organisms including fungi. All the Gram-negative bacilli have the potential to cause meningitis. They may also cause ascending cholangitis and, very occasion-ally, pneumonia. Osteomyelitis attributable to Gram-negative enteric ba-cilli is rare, but if it does occur it is often insidious in onset and presentation.

Enterococci (faecal streptococci)

The enterococci or faecal streptococci, such as *Streptococcus faecalis*, *Strep-tococcus faecium* and *Streptococcus bovis*, are usually but not always Lance-field Group D streptococci. Their importance as neonatal pathogens, particularly as a cause of late-onset sepsis, is being recognized increasingly. Coudron *et al.* (1984) reported an outbreak of *S. faecium* in which the mode of transmission was thought to be via the hands of staff. Luginbuhl *et al.* (1987), describing an enterococcal outbreak, found that bowel resection and the presence of and duration of central venous catheters were risk factors for enterococcal sepsis. Enterococcal colonization may be selected by the use of cephalosporins, but Dobson and Baker (1990) reported increasing numbers of sporadic cases of enterococcal sepsis despite rarely using cephalosporins.

Dobson and Baker (1990) reported 56 cases of enterococcal sepsis over 10 years in Houston (1977–1986), and noted an increased incidence from 1983 to 1986. Before 1983 the incidence was 0.1–0.4 per 1000 births, but from 1983 it was 0.6–0.8 per 1000. Thirty-six of the babies developed their infection after 7 days of age (defined as late-onset) and 20 before this. Twelve of the episodes were associated with necrotizing enterocolitis (10 late, 2 early). The babies with early-onset sepsis tended to be older (mean gestational age 36.9 weeks); two-thirds of them had recognized perinatal risk factors for sepsis, such as prolonged rupture of membranes, maternal fever or spontaneous preterm labour. There were no cases of maternal chorioamnionitis. Eight of the babies developed enterococcal sepsis on the first day of life.

Late-onset enterococcal sepsis occurred mainly in babies of very low birth-weight (mean gestational age 29.5 weeks) who had undergone multiple invasive procedures. Focal infections were common: 15% had meningitis, 15% pneumonia and 23% scalp abscess, while 23% of infections were catheter-related.

Early-onset sepsis caused mild respiratory distress with apnoea and oxygen requirement, but not usually requiring intubation, and not usually with chest radiographic changes. Four of 18 (22%) had diarrhoea. Late-onset sepsis caused severe apnoea and bradycardia, circulatory collapse and increased ventilatory requirements.

Enterococci are relatively resistant to penicillin and the cephalosporins, but are sensitive to ampicillin and vancomycin although neither are bactericidal. The addition of an aminoglycoside to ampicillin or vancomycin gives synergy *in vitro*. Infected catheters must be removed to clear catheter-related enterococcal bacteraemia (Dobson and Baker, 1990). The prognosis of enterococcal sepsis is generally good, with most babies responding rapidly to therapy. In the series of Dobson and Baker (1990) the mortality was 6% for early sepsis, 8% for late sepsis and 17% for sepsis associated with NEC.

Tuberculosis

Virtually all cases of neonatal tuberculosis (TB) result from TB of the mother, although occasionally the baby may be infected by a household contact or even by a member of staff with open TB. The mother most commonly has active pulmonary TB, often asymptomatic, and infects the baby postnatally by the respiratory route. Alternatively, she may have uterine TB which can be due to adjacent spread, such as from tuberculous peritonitis, or due to blood-borne spread to the fallopian tubes; the baby may then aspirate tubercle bacilli *in utero* or at the time of delivery. If the mother is infected during pregnancy, the placenta may be infected, with resultant infection of the amniotic fluid, and the fetus may be infected by transplacental blood-borne spread or by aspiration of contaminated amniotic fluid.

Congenital TB due to early intrauterine infection is very rare and usually results in abortion or stillbirth. Transplacental fetal infection through the portal vein can cause a primary complex in the liver and infection of the portal nodes, leading to hepatomegaly usually accompanied by jaundice, lymphadenopathy, splenomegaly and meningitis. Most affected babies, however, are normal at birth, though may be of low birth-weight. The mother may have fever before, at or soon after delivery. The baby may fail to thrive and by 3 weeks of age be listless, irritable and anorexic. Very occasionally, however, the baby is well but has changes visible radiographically (see Figure 13.6). There may be patchy pneumonic changes on the chest radiograph, which progress to mediastinal and hilar lymph node enlargement, with segmental or lobar collapse due to the extrinsic pressure of the nodes. The baby develops respiratory symptoms with tachypnoea and cyanosis, often intermittent. Acid-fast bacilli are best seen in the gastric aspirate but may also be found in trachael aspirates or urine; however, the sensitivity of these tests is < 10%. Liver ultrasound and biopsy are helpful if the primary lesion is in the liver. The tuberculin response is unreliable. The mother should be examined and a chest radiograph, tuberculin skin test and other relevant investigations performed if neonatal TB is suspected.

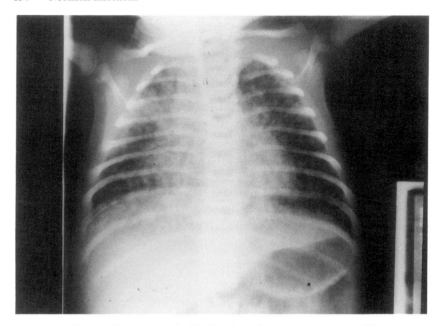

Figure 13.6 Neonatal tuberculosis. Mother found to have sputum-positive pulmonary TB 3 weeks *post partum*. Baby had cough but was otherwise well. Chest radiograph showing large nodular lesions and right upper lobe consolidation. Gastric aspirate: acid-fast bacilli seen

As it is difficult to prove that the baby has TB, treatment often has to be started empirically, especially when maternal TB has been diagnosed. All the antituberculous drugs are potentially toxic but neonatal tuberculosis can be devastating and meningeal involvement has a high morbidity. In symptomatic infants, treatment should be started with isoniazid (10 mg/kg per day) and rifampicin (15 mg/kg per day). Pyrazinamide (20 mg/kg per day), should be added for miliary TB or tuberculous meningitis. If the mother has active TB but the baby is asymptomatic at birth, the options are to give the baby BCG vaccine (Kendig, 1969), or to give isoniazid-resistant BCG and treat the baby with isoniazid (10 mg/kg per day) prophylactically (Dormer *et al.*, 1959); both approaches have been shown to be successful. If the mother has only just been diagnosed, the Red Book of the American Academy of Pediatrics recommends separating her from the baby until she is sputum negative, which occurs rapidly on treatment. Whether separated or not, she should be treated for TB and encouraged to breast feed, expressing her milk if necessary. Neonatal unit staff should be screened for TB when starting work, because a single member of staff with open TB can expose or infect a very large number of babies.

Case history

A 3-week-old White baby boy was referred by the chest physicians because they had just diagnosed his mother as having sputum-positive pulmonary tuberculosis. The baby had been feeding slightly less well for 2 days, but had good weight gain. He had a staccato cough but was not tachypnoeic or dyspnoeic and was afebrile. The remainder of the physical examination was normal. A chest radiograph (Figure 13.6) showed large nodular lesions and right upper lobe consolidation. A Mantoux test was negative, and CSF was normal. A gastric aspirate smear contained acid-fast bacilli. He was treated with rifampicin and isoniazid for 9 months. Mother and baby made complete recoveries.

Syphilis

Untreated latent maternal infection with *Treponema pallidum* in the first 2 years after infection causes fetal or perinatal death in 20% of pregnancies, preterm delivery in 20% and, if pregnancy goes to term, congenital syphilis in ~ 40%, with resulting handicap (Stray-Pedersen, 1983). In most developed countries, syphilis serology is included in routine antenatal care; congenital syphilis is seen only, therefore, in the babies of women who do not attend for antenatal care, women who are inadequately treated or those who become reinfected during pregnancy. In many developing countries, congenital syphilis is still one of the commonest and most serious congenital infections.

The mother may often be in the asymptomatic latent stage of syphilis. Infection of the placenta and transplacental spread to the fetus can cause miscarriage, abortion, fetal death, hydrops fetalis, preterm labour and intrauterine growth retardation. The placenta is often enlarged. Babies may be asymptomatic at birth and develop symptoms only later, or may have a wide range of manifestations including fulminant sepsis. The characteristic skin lesion is a maculopapular eruption over the buttocks, back, thighs, soles, palms and perioral area. It is pink, becoming brown and there may be indurative erythema or desquamation of the soles and palms. Sometimes the lesions are bullous (pemphigus syphiliticus) and mimic impetigo, and the desquamation is thought wrongly to be staphylococcal scalded-skin syndrome. There should not be confusion with the vesicular lesions of herpes simplex virus infection. The skin on the trunk is often dry and flakes off when rubbed. Rhinitis ('snuffles') develops between 1 week and 3 months of age and is initially clear, becoming more purulent or even blood-stained. Ulceration of the nasal mucosa can lead to a 'saddle nose' deformity. Laryngitis may cause a hoarse or aphonic cry. Mucous patches may be seen on the lips, tongue and soft palate. Hepatosplenomegaly is present in up to 90%, and about one-half also have generalized lymphadenopathy. Haemolytic anaemia and thrombocytopenia are common and there may be jaundice with unconjugated and/or conjugated hyperbilirubinaemia. Osteitis of the long bones is usually asymptomatic at birth, although later pain or a pathological fracture may cause pseudoparalysis of a limb (pseudoparalysis of Parrot). Neurological and renal manifestations are rare at birth, although severely affected babies may have signs of meningitis and eye involvement (chorioretinitis, glaucoma, uveitis, chancres of the eyelid). Untreated babies are at risk of late manifestations of syphilis: keratitis, deafness, teeth abnormalities and scarring as a result of earlier lesions.

The most common problem in developed countries is the interpretation of tests in pregnancy before and after treatment, and the management of an asymptomatic baby. The various tests employed to diagnose syphilis are shown in Table 13.2. IgM tests are, unfortunately, still experimental, and

Table 13.2 Tests for syphilis

Type of test	Name of test	
	Abbreviation	Description
Non-specific screening tests (detect antibodies to cardiolipin)	VDRL	Venereal Disease Research Laboratory
	WR	Wassermann reaction
	RPR	Rapid plasma reagin
	RST	Reagin screen test
Specific antibody tests (detect antibody to *T. pallidum*)	FTA-ABS	Fluorescent treponemal antibody absorption (absorbed with non-pallidum treponemes)
	FTA-ABS DS	Fluorescent treponemal antibody absorption double staining
	MHA-TP	Microhaemagglutination assay for *T. pallidum* antibody
	TPHA (or HATTS)	Haemagglutinating antibody
	RIA	Radioimmunoassay
	ELISA	Enzyme-linked immunosorbent assay
Direct examination of lesion or tissue	DFA-TP	Dark-field microscopy Direct fluorescent antibody test for *T. pallidum* Silver stains
	H & E stains	Haematoxylin and eosin

the antibody tests described detect mainly IgG; this, of course, means that antibody detected in the baby is almost exclusively transplacentally acquired maternal antibody.

Pregnant women who are seropositive for syphilis, i.e. have positive specific antibody tests, should be treated with penicillin. Even if they give a history of supposed penicillin allergy, skin tests should be performed to confirm this and desensitization performed; penicillin is the only acceptable therapy for syphilis during pregnancy (Centers for Disease Control, 1988a). Maternal erythromycin treatment results in many failures and many cases of congenital syphilis due to poor transplacental passage.

Diagnostic evaluation of the newborn baby of an affected woman should always include a full physical examination and serology on a serum specimen (not cord blood, which may give false-positive reactions). Radiological examination of the long bones for osteitis and CSF examination should be performed for all babies of women not treated before 20 weeks' gestation, for all symptomatic babies and probably for all babies with a positive Venereal Disease Research Laboratory (VDRL) test. The CSF of babies with neurosyphilis may have a raised white cell count and protein. A positive CSF VDRL test is diagnostic of neurosyphilis, even if the white cell count and protein level are normal. There is no information on whether false-negative CSF VDRL tests occur, but babies with negative CSF VDRL tests but CSF abnormalities of cells or protein should be treated for neurosyphilis. Fluorescent treponemal antibody (FTA) tests on CSF have given conflicting results in adults and have not been adequately studied in congenital syphilis. Other tests in the evaluation would include full blood count, liver function tests and urinalysis.

Congenital syphilis is confirmed if *T. pallidum* is identified by direct examination of specimens from lesions, placenta or umbilical cord. Congenital infection is likely if the baby has a positive specific antibody test and is symptomatic or was stillborn, if the baby has a positive CSF VDRL test, if the mother was inadequately treated or if the baby has a fourfold increase in antibody levels over 3 months' follow-up; it is unlikely if the baby has negative specific serology, if positive tests become negative by 6 months or if the mother was effectively treated (titre fell fourfold or more) and the baby's titre is at least four times lower than the mother's (Centers for Disease Control, 1988a).

Treatment of definite or probable congenital syphilis should be with i.v. or i.m. aqueous crystalline penicillin G (50 000 units/kg per day 12-hourly) or with i.m. aqueous procaine penicillin G (50 000 units/kg once daily), given for at least 10 days. Babies in the 'unlikely' category, as defined in the previous paragraph, need not be treated if close follow-up is certain; if it is not, they should be treated as if 'definite'. This treatment is effective against neurosyphilis. There is no proven alternative antibiotic to penicillin.

Close follow-up of treated and untreated babies, at 3, 6 and 12 months at least, is essential, and serological tests should be repeated until they become negative. Persistently elevated titres over several months are an indication for re-treatment. Patients with neurosyphilis should also have serum and CSF serology repeated every 6 months for at least 3 years. Re-treatment should be considered if clinical signs persist or recur, if there is a persistent fourfold rise in a non-specific antibody test, or if a high titre fails to decrease fourfold within a year (Centers for Disease Control, 1988a).

Case history

A one-day-old baby boy was referred with suspected congenital herpes simplex virus infection. Mother was 21, single and had received no antenatal care. She reported no problems in pregnancy. The baby weighed 2080 g at birth at full term. He had desquamation over the trunk and limbs and the skin peeled with pressure. Bullae containing mucopurulent fluid were present over both ankles, wrists and the abdomen (Figure 13.7a,b). The palms and soles were bright red and indurated. The baby had hepatosplenomegaly. The VDRL test was positive on mother and baby's serum. The baby's CSF contained 30 lymphocytes and was VDRL, *Treponema pallidum* Haemagglutinating Antibody (TPHA) and FTA positive, with specific IgM to *T. pallidum* detected. Radiographs of the long bones showed periostitis (Figure 13.7c). The baby was successfully treated for neurosyphilis and the mother for syphilis. No contacts could be traced.

Tetanus

Neonatal tetanus is probably the single most important cause of neonatal mortality in developing countries, causing 30–60% of all neonatal deaths, an estimated 800 000 deaths a year (Galazka *et al.*, 1987; Hinman *et al.*, 1987). It is called 'eight day disease' both in the Punjab and on the Hebridean island of St Kilda, because babies die at this age, and 'no suck' disease in Nepal because trismus prevents sucking. The disease is caused by contamination of the umbilical stump with *Clostridium tetani* spores, which are found in animal faeces and survive in the soil. Most cases have been ascribed to the

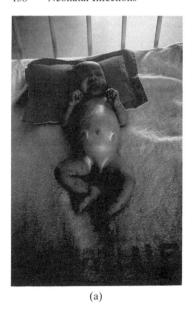

(a)

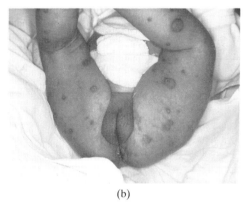

(b)

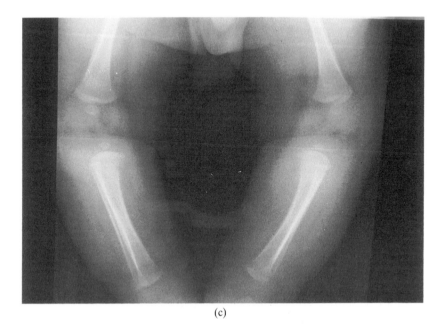

(c)

Figure 13.7 Congenital syphilis: (a, b) peeling of skin over abdomen and bullous lesions on legs (courtesy of Dr Heather Jeffery); (c) radiograph showing periosteal elevation of femora and bilateral erosions of the medial tibial epiphyses (Wimberger's sign)

use of mud on the umbilicus. A study from Pakistan showed a significant association between neonatal tetanus and repeated applications of ghee, clarified butter made from the milk of cows or water buffalo (Traverso *et al.*, 1989). On St Kilda the disease was caused by anointing the cut umbilical cord with ruby-red oil from a seabird, the fulmar, which was stored in the dried stomach of a solan goose (Woody and Ross, 1989); when this practice was stopped, neonatal tetanus promptly disappeared.

Neonatal tetanus presents at 3–14 days, with muscle rigidity mainly involving the masseter (causing trismus or lockjaw), the facial muscles (risus sardonicus), the abdominal and spinal muscles (causing opisthotonus). There are characteristic intermittent muscle spasms which increase in frequency and severity and may be precipitated by loud noises or painful stimuli. Respiratory muscle involvement leads to respiratory failure. The mortality can be as high as 60–90% (Athavale and Pai, 1965; Salimpour, 1977) although if artificial ventilation and muscle relaxants are available it can be reduced to 10% (Smythe *et al.*, 1974). Conventional treatment is with penicillin G, tetanus antitoxin which can only neutralize unbound toxin, and supportive treatment.

The main hope lies in prevention. Education about birth practices and umbilical cord hygiene is obviously important. Women who have been fully immunized against tetanus virtually never have an affected baby. Thus, the main strategy of the World Health Organization has been to eradicate neonatal tetanus by ensuring that all women of child-bearing age are fully immunized with three doses of tetanus toxoid (Galazka *et al.*, 1987).

Whooping cough

There is some controversy whether maternal antibodies against *Bordetella pertussis* are able to cross the placenta. Cohen and Scadron (1943) found that babies of women immunized during pregnancy were protected against infection when exposed to *B. pertussis*. It seems likely that babies whose mothers have had natural pertussis infection are more likely to be protected than babies whose mothers were immunized in childhood (Bass and Zacher, 1989).

A particular problem arises if the mother or a sibling has whooping cough around the time of delivery. About one-half of the babies might be expected to develop pertussis (Cohen and Scadron, 1943), which can be life-threatening in infancy. Granstrom *et al.* (1987) treated 32 of 35 mothers who had peripartum pertussis infection with oral erythromycin (250–500 mg, 8-hourly for 10 days) and 28 of their babies with oral erythromycin ethyl succinate (40 mg/kg per day, 8-hourly for 10 days). Other family members with pertussis were also given erythromycin for 10 days. None of the babies developed clinical or laboratory evidence of pertussis infection. These observations, although uncontrolled, suggest that it may be possible to decrease the serious risk of neonatal pertussis infection using erythromycin.

Chapter 14

Fungal infections

Introduction

As the survival of babies of very low birth-weight has improved, fungal infections have become an increasing problem. Fungi are ubiquitous organisms found in soil and decaying organic matter and commonly found colonizing animals, birds and man. They are organisms of low pathogenicity; they may cause local disease in the face of normal or marginally reduced immunity, but systemic disease usually indicates a profound immune defect.

Candidiasis

Candidus is Latin for 'dazzling white', the colour of colonies of Candida. Candida exists mainly as oval yeast cells (blastospores), which bud asexually and can form true filamentous hyphae and chains of elongated budding cells called pseudohyphae, which are seen in tissues during infection. *Candida* species possess a cell wall. There is limited evidence that they can elaborate toxins which could contribute to pathogenicity. *C. albicans* is the most pathogenic, but other species (*C. parapsilosis, C. krusei, C. tropicalis, C. pseudotropicalis, C. lusitaniae* and *C. guilliermondii*) are occasional human pathogens. The most important characteristics associated with virulence seem to be the ability to form pseudohyphae, attachment to epithelial cells of the buccal and vaginal mucosa, and secretion of acid proteinases (Odds, 1981).

Candida albicans and other *Candida* species are the most important causes of neonatal fungal infections. Oral candidiasis affects ~4% of all babies (Kozinn *et al.*, 1958), many of whom will develop dermatitis of the napkin area, and is particularly likely in babies who have received antibiotics (Seelig, 1966).

Immunity

Immunity against deep candidiasis and other deep fungal infections is predominantly mediated by neutrophil leucocytes, and persistently leucopenic patients are at increased risk of systemic fungal infection. T cells are important in mucosal immunity: patients with the most profound T-cell defects, as for example those with AIDS, get severe mucosal candidiasis but systemic infection is rare. Opsonization of *Candida* can be mediated with great efficiency by the alternative pathway of complement in the absence of antibody. *Candida* will elicit secretory and humoral antibodies in adults.

The greatly increased susceptibility of infants of very low birth-weight to systemic fungal infection is not completely understood. It probably results from defective function of a number of host defence mechanisms, notably relatively impaired opsonization and less efficient neutrophil phagocytosis.

Epidemiology

Candida species have been demonstrated as commensals and pathogens in many animals and birds, although spread from these to humans has not been described. The organisms readily colonize mucous membranes and skin, but are not found in the air (Nilsby and Norden, 1949). Transmission of *Candida* usually requires direct proximity of a mucous membrane or skin to a colonized site. Adults are frequently colonized without developing overt disease: about one-third carry *Candida* in the mouth, gastrointestinal tract, vagina or on intertriginous areas of skin. Pregnancy is associated with an increased incidence of colonization with *Candida* (Pedersen, 1964). Infection ascending from the vaginal tract, which is frequently colonized in the last trimester, can cause disseminated or mucocutaneous infection in the fetus. Placental infection may occur but transplacental haematogenous transmission is not thought to occur commonly, if at all. *Candida* may be acquired during parturition or from sucking on an infected nipple. *Candida* can contaminate feeding bottles and dummies and can be carried on the hands of staff, although nosocomial infection is probably far less common than infection following colonization from birth. Bottles of intravenous fluids have occasionally been contaminated in hospital pharmacies by the use of air pumps, and this has resulted in outbreaks of nosocomial candidaemia.

Neonatal systemic candidiasis is increasing in frequency. Weese-Mayer *et al.* (1987) described 21 patients in their neonatal unit over a 7-year period with systemic candidiasis, representing 0.9% of all admissions. Significant risk factors are shown in Table 14.1. The most important of these, apart from birth-weight which was not specifically evaluated, was duration of previous antibiotic therapy. The presence of intravascular catheters for intravenous feeding is a risk factor for systemic candidiasis, but the duration of central venous or umbilical artery catheterization was not a risk factor in the study of Weese-Meyer and colleagues (1987). Other studies have shown that babies < 1500 g are at increased risk of systemic candidiasis, with an incidence of ~ 3–4% (Baley *et al.*, 1984a; Johnson *et al.*, 1984; Loke *et al.*, 1988). Fat emulsions such as Intralipid may encourage growth of *Candida*, although they have been particularly associated with infection with another fungus, *Malassezia furfur*. *Candida* will grow well in parenteral nutrition

Table 14.1 Risk factors for the development of neonatal systemic candidiasis

Very low birth-weight (< 1500 g)
Prolonged antibiotic therapy
Prolonged total parenteral nutrition
Prolonged use of fat emulsion in parenteral nutrition
Prolonged artificial ventilation

After Weese-Mayer *et al.* (1987)

fluid containing 20–40% glucose. Prolonged parenteral nutrition, particularly when fat emulsions are used, is an independent risk factor for systemic candidiasis (Weese-Meyer *et al.*, 1987).

The mechanism by which antibiotics increase susceptibility to fungal infections is not clear. Although the suppression of normal flora permitting proliferation of fungi is often quoted, even relatively narrow-spectrum antibiotics may lead to fungal infection. Other possibilities are that antibiotics might remove competition for nutrients or might remove antifungal substances elaborated by bacteria. The suggestion that antibiotics might stimulate fungal growth by some unknown direct effect has never been substantiated experimentally.

Pathology and pathogenesis

Candida blastospores attach to the mucosa or skin and pseudohyphae – chains of elongated yeast forms – develop. Invasion of the mucosal surface or epidermis results in formation of a pseudomembrane of epithelial cells, leucocytes and *Candida* yeast cells, both blastospores and pseudohyphae. Ulcers may form on mucosal surfaces, and have a sharp edge and a base of granulation tissue with fibrin, neutrophils and *Candida*.

When disseminated infection occurs there may be haematogenous spread to multiple sites with the formation of microabscesses in brain, lung, liver, spleen and kidney. Endocarditis may occur. Organisms may embolize to bone or joint, causing osteomyelitis or septic arthritis. Deep subcutaneous abscesses, indistinguishable clinically from staphylococcal abscesses, may develop in neonates; these contain abundant hyphae. Granulomata are rare in *Candida* infections.

The mechanism by which *Candida* causes damage is poorly understood. Some workers have proposed that surface proteins may stimulate histamine release, and others have emphasized the role of putative toxins from the organisms, but no cause of tissue damage has been shown consistently. What is clear is that *Candida* is of low pathogenicity in normal hosts. Neonates seem to be at particular risk because of their impaired host defences and possibly also because they may be exposed to a large number of organisms.

Clinical features

Congenital candidiasis occurs as a result of ascending infection from the maternal vaginal tract. There may be prolonged rupture of the membranes, but the organism can cross intact membranes. Babies may be covered in vesicular or pustular skin lesions with an erythematous base. There may be involvement of the oral mucous membranes. Aspiration of infected amniotic fluid can cause pneumonia, which may be severe and even fatal (Dvorak and Gavaller, 1964). Spread to distant sites including liver microabscesses may occur; this could be due to transplacental haematogenous spread or, more probably, to secondary haematogenous spread following primary ascending infection. In babies born at or near term, congenital skin and even lung lesions due to *Candida* may resolve rapidly without specific antifungal treatment. In babies born more prematurely, antifungal therapy is advisable.

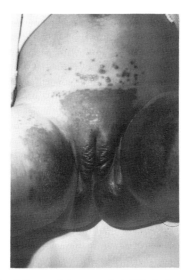

Figure 14.1 Candidiasis of the napkin area. Satellite lesions can be seen

Oral candidiasis, which often appears at about a week of age, causes distinctive white plaques with underlying erythema on the tongue, buccal, palatal, gingival and pharyngeal mucosa. Candidiasis of the skin is common, causing vesicles or pustules which frequently coalesce to form patches of thickened skin. These are commonest in the napkin area (Figure 14.1), but may occur also around the umbilicus, in skin folds such as the axillae and over the trunk and face. The angry red napkin rash often has a white edge, involves the skin creases and discrete satellite lesions may be seen.

Systemic involvement usually presents acutely and the signs and symptoms may mimic bacterial sepsis. One or several organs may be involved. *Candida* meningitis may be present in babies without obvious neurological impairment and LP should always be considered. Isolated renal candidiasis may lead to huge fungal balls in the pelvis of one or both kidneys, causing obstruction: if bilateral, the baby may present with oliguria or anuria and renal enlargement. Fundoscopy should always be performed in suspected candidiasis, because endophthalmitis may be present, causing fluffy white exudates in the retina or floating in the vitreous humour (Baley *et al.*, 1984a). Skin abscesses may develop as the first presenting sign and resemble staphylococcal abscesses, so that fungal infection can be diagnosed only by microscopic examination and culture of the pus. Arthritis, osteomyelitis and endocarditis are very occasionally described. Brain abscess has been described in the absence of meningitis, usually as an autopsy finding. Pulmonary candidiasis can occur as part of congenital candidiasis. However, babies may also develop later pulmonary infection which presents as pulmonary consolidation with increasing ventilatory requirements. These features are very non-specific and *Candida* is a common commensal isolate in endotracheal cultures, perhaps from oral contamination. Nevertheless, *Candida* pneumonia has been shown at autopsy to be present in some cases (Loke *et al.*, 1988).

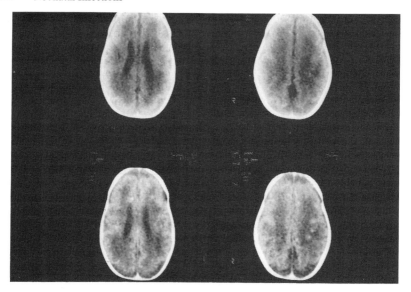

Figure 14.2 CT brain scan from baby with *Candida* meningitis showing lesions due to *Candida* in brain substance, ventricular dilatation and early cerebral atrophy (courtesy of Dr Albert Lam)

Case history

A 27-week gestation, 660 g boy developed respiratory distress from birth, requiring artificial ventilation. He was extubated and in air by 7 days. On day 14 he developed a fluctuant swelling above the left ankle, not involving the joint. The aspirated pus contained neutrophils and Gram-positive cocci and grew MRSA and a few colonies of *Candida albicans*. He was treated with i.v. vancomycin. Four days later he became systemically unwell with increasing apnoea and bradycardias. His CSF contained $90 \times 10^9/l$ WBC (72% neutrophils) and $10 \times 10^9/l$ RBC. No organisms were seen on Gram's staining but the CSF grew a scanty growth of *Candida albicans*. Blood cultures were sterile but urine contained yeasts and grew a heavy pure growth of *Candida*. Cerebral ultrasound scan and computerized tomographic (CT) scan of the brain (Figure 14.2) showed rounded lesions in the brain parenchyma, ventricular dilatation and early cerebral atrophy. Renal ultrasound showed similar lesions in both kidneys. He was treated with i.v. amphotericin B and flucytosine for 30 days with no toxicity, and with clinical and radiological resolution of his meningeal, cerebral and renal lesions.

Diagnosis

As the clinical features of candidiasis are non-specific, a laboratory diagnosis should be made whenever possible by obtaining clinical specimens. *Candida* species grow readily on Sabouraud dextrose media; they will also grow in blood culture bottles.

Scrapings or swabs from skin or mucosal lesions should be examined for fungal elements using a potassium hydroxide preparation. Some laboratories use calciflor white instead of KOH to stain for yeasts. Cotton-wool swabs are not the best to use as *Candida* sticks to the cotton wool. Pus from skin abscesses and 'septic' arthritis should always be examined by wet-mount microscopy and cultured for fungi. *Candida* meningitis causes a CSF pleocytosis and fungal elements are usually seen on Gram's staining or wet-mount microscopy.

There are particular problems with the clinical diagnosis of *Candida* pneumonia and UTI. The isolation of *Candida* from an endotracheal aspirate is probably clinically significant only when there is associated radiological and clinical deterioration. Even when the baby has clinical pneumonia and *Candida* is found in endotracheal secretions, it may not be the cause of the pneumonia. Confirmation should be sought by obtaining cultures of any pleural fluid present and of blood and urine before starting treatment. Similarly, bag urine specimens may frequently become contaminated with *Candida*, and urine cultures positive for *Candida* should be repeated, with a very low threshold for suprapubic aspiration of urine. Indeed, if renal candidiasis is suspected, this is the investigation of choice.

Candida is a rare contaminant of blood cultures in neonates. In neonates, it is extremely unwise to ignore the growth of *Candida* from a blood culture, even if taken through an umbilical or central catheter. Repeat blood cultures may be negative, yet the baby progresses to fulminant systemic *Candida* infection (Weese-Mayer *et al.*, 1987). We, too, have mistakenly dismissed growth of *Candida* from one of two blood culture bottles as a contaminant, and have been reassured by a sterile repeat blood culture, only for the baby to develop *Candida* meningitis one week later. In suspected fungaemia, blood cultures should always be performed, and a single positive culture is a strong indication for starting antifungal treatment. Ascuitto *et al.* (1985) detected fungal elements in Gram's stains of buffy coat smears from three babies with fungaemia.

Antibody tests and skin tests are of no value in deciding whether or not a baby is infected with *Candida*. Antigen detection has occasionally been of value (Schreiber *et al.*, 1984) but remains to be more completely evaluated.

Prevention

It is our policy to give prophylactic oral nystatin to at-risk babies (those on prolonged antibiotics or receiving prolonged parenteral nutrition). This reduces mucocutaneous colonization with *Candida* (Sims *et al.*, 1988), although prevention of systemic candidiasis has not been confirmed. The most important aspect of prevention is to minimize risk factors by judicious use of antibiotics and invasive procedures.

Treatment

The treatment of local skin conditions and mucocutaneous candidiasis in the neonatal period is with topical and oral preparations of nystatin, miconazole or clotrimazole. Oral ketoconazole is effective against chronic mucocutaneous candidiasis, as seems to be a relatively new antifungal drug, fluconazole, but neither have been evaluated in newborns. Whenever possible, antibacterial antibiotics should be stopped when candidiasis, either local or systemic, is diagnosed.

Systemic candidiasis is usually treated with amphotericin B, with or without flucytosine (5-fluorocytosine). Amphotericin B has to be given by intravenous infusion, although it can be effective topically for some local infections. Amphotericin causes significant renal toxicity in a proportion of patients. In the study by Baley *et al.* (1984b), seven of 10 babies of very low birth-weight treated with amphotericin developed 'severe renal toxicity' defined as oliguria (< 1 ml/kg per hour) or anuria for 18 h, while five had a rise in serum creatinine and five (all of whom died) had hypo- or hyperkalaemia. On the other hand, some of the babies had renal candidiasis, the criteria for severe renal toxicity were somewhat dubious and only two babies had raised urea levels. Faix (1984) reported similar renal toxicity but other workers have reported far less toxicity with amphotericin (Johnson *et al.*, 1984; Loke *et al.*, 1988), although anaemia and hypokalaemia may occur as well as renal toxicity. In older children and adults it is recommended that a test dose of 0.1 ml/kg be given. If no reaction occurs, treatment is begun at 0.25 mg/kg per day then increased by daily increments of 0.25 to 1.0 mg/kg per day, at which dose it is continued. This is because adverse reactions such as fever, chills, headache, nausea and vomiting often develop. These have not been reported in neonates, however, and we begin treatment at the full dose of 0.5–1 mg/kg per day without a test dose. Baley *et al.* (1990) have examined the pharmacokinetics and toxicity of amphotericin and have come, via a more scientific approach, to the same conclusion. If renal toxicity does develop, we reduce the dose or stop the drug, but in our experience significant toxicity is extremely rare. Loke *et al.* (1988) used a lower daily dose of 0.3 mg/kg amphotericin. Amphotericin B must be diluted in 5% dextrose, because saline causes precipitation; it should be infused over 4–6 h and the solution should be protected against the light. It is recommended that a total dose of 25–30 mg/kg amphotericin be given, equating with about 4 weeks' treatment.

Flucytosine, also called 5-fluorocytosine (5-FC), is an antifungal agent that is well absorbed orally and which has excellent CSF penetration, with CSF levels up to 88% of serum levels (Steer *et al.*, 1972). It cannot be used alone, as resistance rapidly develops. It can accumulate and cause bone marrow toxicity with neutropenia and also hepatotoxicity. For this reason blood levels should be monitored during treatment, usually weekly.

We would always use flucytosine as well as amphotericin B for treating *Candida* meningitis because of the superior CSF penetration of flucytosine. If flucytosine is also used there is no need to use intrathecal amphotericin, as sometimes advocated, which can cause marked toxicity. For fungaemia without meningitis, amphotericin alone may suffice. Butler *et al.* (1990) have used amphotericin alone for all neonatal fungal infections and report results similar to those reported by others who use flucytosine.

Miconazole has occasionally been used to treat systemic candidiasis, but experience is extremely limited compared with that of amphotericin B and flucytosine. Clarke *et al.* (1980) reported intermittent ventricular tachycardia which resolved when miconazole was stopped and did not recur when the drug was re-started. McDougall *et al.* (1982) reported its use in two babies, one of whom relapsed after stopping miconazole, although only 10 days' treatment was given, and the other who deteriorated on miconazole. Both babies responded to amphotericin B and flucytosine.

It is generally felt that it is not possible to treat systemic fungal infections successfully without removing intravascular catheters, because these are always colonized during fungaemia (Sadiq *et al.*, 1987). It has sometimes been thought sufficient to remove central venous or umbilical artery catheters in babies with isolated fungaemia and not to start antifungal treatment. The number of days that catheters were in place was not a risk factor in the study of Weese-Mayer *et al.* (1987) although their presence or absence could not be assessed as a risk factor. The same authors removed catheters without initial fungal treatment in 12 babies out of 21 with confirmed fungaemia: nine of these were cured, and the authors felt it was particularly successful in babies with birth-weight > 2000 g and those not critically ill. However, two of the three babies unsuccessfully managed this way died from systemic fungal infection and one relapsed 36 days later. Most reports of neonatal fungal infection have emphasized that the high mortality was in part attributable to delayed diagnosis and failure to recognize the seriousness of positive fungal cultures.

Prognosis

The mortality from systemic candidiasis is high, in part at least because of the high-risk population with compounding problems. The mortality from untreated disease is nearly 80%, whereas that from disease treated with antifungal agents is ∼ 25–30%, although it is > 60% for babies of very low birth-weight (Baley *et al.*, 1984a; Johnson *et al.*, 1984). In up to 30% of cases the diagnosis of fungal infection is not made until autopsy. Long-term renal damage from renal candidiasis is not usually a major problem. Survivors of *Candida* meningitis may have hydrocephalus or neurological impairment but other factors may contribute to the adverse outcome.

Other fungi

There have been few reports of other fungi causing problems in the neonatal period. *Malassezia furfur* appears to thrive on fat emulsions and has been associated with total parenteral nutrition. Murphy *et al.* (1986) reported an outbreak of colonization and infection with *Hansenula anomala*, a yeast usually encountered as a contaminant in the brewing industry. The origin of the outbreak was never established. Seven of eight babies with systemic infection weighed < 1500 g and all had multiple problems of prematurity. *Coccidioides imitis*, which is endemic in parts of North, Central and South America, is a very rare neonatal cause of patchy pneumonic infiltration and disseminated coccidiomycosis. *Cryptococcus neoformans*, which is found world wide, is an equally rare cause of disseminated disease: it can cause hepatosplenomegaly, jaundice, hydrocephalus, intracranial calcification and chorioretinitis, a spectrum of disease suggesting congenital infection, although the mother is usually asymptomatic. Fewer than ten neonatal cases of infections with each of these organisms have been documented. Infections due to the bread moulds often found in refrigerators – the zygomycetes (which include *Mucor*, *Absidia* and *Rhizopus*) – are equally rare. Dennis *et al.* (1980) reported isolating *Rhizopus* from the plaster dressing on an abdominal wound. The zygomycetes are ubiquitous and can cause enterocolitis with diarrhoea, often bloody, and abdominal distension. *Aspergillus* infection, resulting in pneumonia and disseminated aspergillosis involving the brain and most other organs, has been described in only seven babies, aged 2–7 weeks.

Chapter 15

Viral infections

Introduction

Viruses cause relatively few neonatal infections, yet these can be severe and often fatal. Their recognition is important because of the increasing potential to prevent or treat such infections and because the diagnosis may have important implications for the management of other babies in the nursery.

Herpes simplex virus infection

Herpes simplex virus (HSV), like the other herpesviruses, has the ability to remain latent for months or years and to reactivate periodically. HSV is a DNA virus. Two major sub-types, HSV-1 and HSV-2, are recognized: HSV-1 primarily causes oral and pharyngeal lesions, whereas HSV-2 usually affects genital areas and is thus a commoner cause of neonatal infections, but both subtypes can affect the genital area and cause neonatal infections.

Transmission

The great majority of severe neonatal HSV infections occur secondary to maternal genital infection. The virus is acquired by passage through an infected birth canal or, more rarely, by ascending infection after rupture of the membranes. There have been occasional cases of babies developing rashes in the first 24 h after caesarean section with apparently intact membranes. Some cases of local and disseminated neonatal infection have been associated with fetal scalp monitors. Transplacental infection is exceedingly uncommon (see Clinical Features, page 150).

Acquisition of the virus postnatally from an oral or skin infection in the mother, another relative or member of staff or from another infected baby is rare. Light (1979) reviewed the literature from 1951 to 1977 and found only 24 reported cases of nosocomial neonatal HSV infection, despite countless exposures. Thirteen babies, seven of whom died, had apparently acquired infection from a mother with oral herpes or serological evidence of infection, but some mothers may have had genital infection, as this was not excluded. Nine babies, of whom seven died, had acquired infection from other relatives or staff and two babies were cross-infected from other infected babies. Since then, a small number of limited neonatal unit outbreaks have been described in which DNA fingerprinting was used to prove that the isolates were identical (Linneman et al., 1978; Halperin et al., 1980; Hammerberg et al., 1983).

Epidemiology

The incidence of neonatal HSV infection is considerably higher in the USA than in the UK, even allowing for varying levels of awareness and recognition. In the USA, rates as high as 0.5 per 1000 live births have been reported (Nahmias et al., 1983), whereas in the UK the estimated rate is about 2 per 100 000 (Hall and Glickman, 1988).

Risk of infection

Infants born to mothers with *active primary* genital herpes are at greatest risk of infection, with transmission rates of ~50% if delivered vaginally (Nahmias et al., 1971; Brown et al., 1987). Caesarian section, if performed within 24 h of membrane rupture, greatly reduces the risk of HSV transmission to the neonate, to < 10% (Nahmias et al., 1983). Maternal reactivations of genital herpes are less likely to result in neonatal herpes infection, although such cases are well documented (Whitley, 1990). Prober et al. (1987) studied 34 babies of women with recurrent genital HSV. The babies were delivered vaginally; viral cultures on maternal vaginal secretions and the babies' oropharyngeal secretions showed that the babies had been exposed to HSV at the time of delivery. None was treated and none became infected. The difference between these babies and other babies studied previously, who became infected, was that the babies of mothers with recurrent genital HSV had high titres of neutralizing antibody to HSV, whereas infected babies generally had low or absent titres. Similar observations were made by Brown et al. (1987). An additional risk factor is that mothers with primary genital infection shed more virus, and for longer.

Babies with high antibody titres to HSV, indicating recurrent maternal HSV infection, do occasionally become infected but tend to be older and have more localized infection (Prober et al., 1987).

Clinical features

Very few babies have been reported with features such as microcephaly and keratoconjunctivitis that are suggestive of true congenital HSV infection attributable to transplacental transmission (Nahmias et al., 1983). There is an increased risk of spontaneous abortions in mothers with genital herpes, and HSV has occasionally been isolated from abortuses.

Neonatal HSV can present as infection: (1) localized to the skin, eye or mouth: (2) generalized, involving the liver, adrenals, lungs and many other organs including the brain as well as skin, eye and mouth; (3) localized to the lung (pneumonitis), or (4) localized to the central nervous system (meningoencephalitis).

Involvement of the skin, eye or mouth may be an isolated finding or part of disseminated disease. It can present at, or soon after, birth and usually in the first week of life. If untreated, up to 80% of cases of localized disease will progress to involve the CNS or other organs (Nahmias et al., 1983). With improved awareness, an increasing proportion of babies are being diagnosed with localized infection, and early recognition and treatment of localized disease has been paralleled by a fall in the proportion of infected babies with disseminated disease (Whitley et al., 1988).

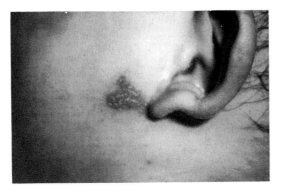

Figure 15.1 Herpes simplex virus infection. Vesicular skin lesions

Skin involvement is the commonest manifestation of HSV infection. There may be only one or two vesicles, or crops of vesicles that sometimes are quite large and bullous (Figure 15.1). Rarer skin lesions are zosteriform eruptions, which are easily misdiagnosed as due to varicella–zoster virus, a generalized petechial rash, areas of denuded skin or erythema multiforme.

The most common eye lesion is keratoconjunctivitis with characteristic dendritic conjunctival or corneal ulcers. Chorioretinitis may be seen at birth or complicating keratoconjunctivitis. Uveitis and cataracts may also develop. Microphthalmia and optic atrophy have been described as sequelae of eye infection.

The mouth, tongue, palate and occasionally the larynx may be involved with classic herpetic ulceration, which is also often seen as part of disseminated disease.

Disseminated disease usually presents in the first week of life, although occasionally at birth or even after 2 weeks of age. The presentation is usually non-specific with fever, vomiting, lethargy and poor feeding. Other variable features are jaundice, hepatomegaly, purpura or generalized erythema, apnoeic episodes, acidosis, cyanosis and respiratory distress. Convulsions or irritability may be the presenting feature if there is concomitant CNS involvement, which is present in about one-half. Pneumonitis may be the presenting feature, usually at 3–7 days. About one-quarter develop a bleeding diathesis with disseminated intravascular coagulopathy (DIC) and shock, which usually is rapidly fatal. The disease is often fulminant with death within hours, and before specific antiviral therapy the mortality was > 80% (Nahmias *et al.*, 1983); even with the newer antiviral drugs (acyclovir and vidarabine) the mortality is 15–20%.

Localized meningoencephalitis presents later, with a mean age of 11 days but a range of 7–30 days (Nahmias *et al.*, 1982, 1983). The clinical features are those of meningitis, although *focal seizures and absent gag reflex are particularly suggestive of HSV encephalitis.* The seizures rapidly become generalized and intractable. The CSF usually contains only 50–200 white cells per ml, mostly lymphocytes, though occasionally up to 2500. Red cells in the CSF are only occasionally found, suggesting haemorrhagic necrosis, but no more commonly than in other forms of neonatal meningoencephalitis. The CSF protein is usually high and glucose normal or slightly low. HSV can be grown from the CSF in ~50% of cases of meningoencephalitis (Whitley *et al.*, 1980).

Diagnosis

Considering the high rate of dissemination if localized HSV infection is untreated (~80%) and the high mortality of disseminated disease, early diagnosis is essential, especially as effective antiviral therapy is now available.

HSV infection often resembles bacterial sepsis clinically. However, the timing of symptoms may suggest a diagnosis of HSV infection. *A history of primary or recurrent HSV infection or clinical evidence of maternal genital infection is obtained in <30% of cases of neonatal HSV infection* (Yeager and Arvin, 1984).

The timing of symptoms may help to distinguish HSV infection from bacterial sepsis. Pneumonitis presents at 3–7 days with respiratory deterioration and perihilar streaky shadowing progressing to a 'white-out'. Disseminated disease tends to present somewhat later than early-onset bacterial sepsis. Focal fits and absent gag reflex may suggest HSV encephalitis. The baby should be examined carefully with special reference to skin, eyes and mouth.

If vesicular lesions are seen in isolation or as part of generalized disease, every effort should be made to obtain some vesicle fluid for electron microscopy or immunofluorescence and viral culture. Electron microscopy will not distinguish HSV from other herpesviruses, such as varicella–zoster virus, but in the absence of a history of maternal chickenpox, neonatal zosteriform eruptions should be presumed to be due to HSV. The presence of intranuclear inclusions and giant cells on Papanicolau staining of cell scrapings from the base of skin vesicles, oral ulcers or the cervix is only 60–75% sensitive in diagnosing HSV infection (Nahmias *et al.*, 1983). If the roof of a vesicle is removed with a needle, the base can be vigorously swabbed and the swab smeared on a slide for immunofluorescent staining. Immunofluorescence is more sensitive than electron microscopy and has replaced it in many laboratories. The same swab can be used for viral culture but must be placed in viral transport medium, not Stuart's medium.

Viral cultures take 1–4 days to show the classic cytopathic effect and can be extremely useful. Cultures should be taken from the nasopharynx in all suspected cases and from any skin lesions, the conjunctiva and CSF where clinically indicated.

Serology is generally unhelpful. Serum IgM responses are often delayed: Sullender *et al.* (1987) found an IgM response in neither of two babies tested < 10 days after onset of symptoms, in three of six tested at 10–12 days, and in 13 of 17 tested after 14 days. Serum IgG can be used only to attempt to make a retrospective diagnosis of HSV infection and neonates often produce no IgG antibodies or the titre does not rise four-fold (Kahlon and Whitley, 1988). The use of CSF antibodies to HSV is controversial because IgG may diffuse passively into the CSF rather than being synthesized intrinsically (Nahmias *et al.*, 1982). However, occasionally HSV-specific IgM may appear early in the CSF, allowing rapid early diagnosis (Dwyer *et al.*, 1986). Antigen detection using ELISA, DNA probes or amplification of DNA by polymerase chain reaction is still being evaluated but may allow rapid diagnosis to become more widely available.

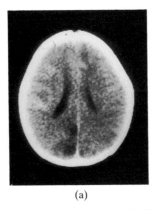 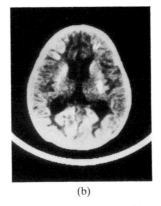

(a)   (b)

Figure 15.2 Herpes simplex encephalitis. Computerized tomographic brain scans: (a) at presentation: loss of grey-white matter differentiation; focal area of attenuation in right parietal lobe: (b) 2 weeks later; unenhanced scan showing dystrophic gyral calcification and cerebral atrophy

Brain biopsy has been advocated by some experts as the surest way of confirming HSV encephalitis and excluding other diagnoses. On the other hand, the clinical picture and CSF findings may be supported by an EEG showing a temporal or parieto-temporal focus, albeit a non-specific finding, and many neonatologists would treat on suspicion of HSV encephalitis without performing a brain biopsy. The CT scan is often normal early in the disease but within days may show unilateral or bilateral temporal lobe changes, cerebral atrophy and loss of grey–white matter differentiation. The CT scan may rarely progress to calcification of the gyrae (Figure 15.2). CSF antibodies may take 6–8 weeks to rise, so repeat LP for a retrospective diagnosis should be postponed until then.

Treatment

Acyclovir and adenosine arabinoside (vidarabine, ara-A) are equally effective in neonatal HSV infection (Whitley *et al.*, 1991). The daily dose of both drugs is 30 mg/kg per day, acyclovir being given intravenously 8 hourly and vidarabine 12 hourly, for 10 to 14 days. Whitley *et al.* (1991) found no difference in mortality, morbidity or drug toxicity for acyclovir and ara-A in treating babies with localized, disseminated disease or encephalitis. Eye lesions should also be treated with topical antivirals such as 1% idoxuridine (IDU) under the supervision of an ophthalmologist.

Even with early treatment, which has been shown to reduce significantly the mortality from HSV infection, one-half of the survivors of meningoencephalitis and 86% of the survivors of disseminated disease have major sequelae. Relapses can occur after stopping treatment. Acyclovir-resistant HSV have been reported, either naturally occurring and apparently of low virulence, or after prolonged acyclovir therapy. So far there have not been any failures of therapy of neonatal HSV infection attributed to acyclovir-resistant strains.

The prognosis of babies with disseminated disease and those with intractable convulsions from meningoencephalitis is so poor that failure to respond rapidly to treatment should be seen as grounds for considering withdrawing intensive care.

Prevention

Babies of women with active genital herpes lesions are at greatest risk. If the mother has a history of recurrent genital lesions no immediate intervention seems indicated (Prober *et al.*, 1987), and women can be delivered vaginally and the baby observed for skin or oral lesions. It should be emphasized that this recommendation is controversial and some would recommend caesarean section. If the mother has active, primary genital herpes, a caesarean section should be performed as soon as possible after membrane rupture and certainly within 6 h, if possible. Nasopharyngeal viral cultures should be taken after 24 h to identify infected babies. Should a mother with active primary genital herpes deliver vaginally, especially after prolonged rupture of the membranes, strong consideration should be given to starting the baby on anticipatory (prophylactic) acyclovir. Treatment of the symptomatic mother around the time of delivery with acyclovir has not been evaluated but Greffe *et al.* (1986) have documented modest transplacental passage of acyclovir.

The Committee on the Fetus and Newborn of the American Academy of Pediatrics (1980) recommended performing cervical cultures for HSV during the last few weeks of pregnancy of women with a history of genital infection, and advised caesarean section for those with positive cultures within a week of delivery. However, this would identify only $\sim 20\%$ of at-risk pregnancies (Prober *et al.*, 1988) and would cost $\sim US\$1.8 \times 10^6$ for every case of neonatal herpes averted, as well as resulting in more than one maternal death due to complications of caesarean section for every 10 neonatal cases prevented (Binkin *et al.*, 1984).

Neonates with confirmed or suspected HSV infection should be isolated whenever possible and vigorous attention paid to hand-washing. Staff or mothers with cold sores present particular problems. We recommend that the lesions be treated with topical 35% IDU in DMSO cream 5–6 times a day for up to 3 days. Staff are not allowed to handle babies for 24 h. Mothers are not separated from their babies but wear a mask for 24 h. These recommendations are empirical and based on the potential severity of infection.

Case history

Twins, a boy and a girl, were born at 35 weeks' gestation by vaginal delivery. The mother had no history of genital lesions and cervical examination was normal. The girl had a small bruise on her back. The babies were initially well. At 5 days of age the girl developed some small blisters over the site of the bruise. These spread over the next few days to involve a slightly wider area of skin. On day 13 she had two severe apnoeic episodes. She had meningitis (CSF: 250 WBC), but viral and bacterial cultures were sterile. A swab of the base of a skin vesicle was positive for HSV by immunofluorescence and later grew HSV-2. EEG and brain scan were normal. She improved rapidly with intravenous acyclovir, but at follow-up at 6 months was worryingly hypertonic.

Her brother was well until day 11 when he developed unilateral conjunctivitis and photophobia. He became lethargic and anorexic over the next 48 hours. The CSF was equivocal (225 WBC). Ophthalmological examination showed iridocyclitis and keratoconjunctivitis. Serum IgM specific to HSV-2 was detected. Ultrasound and CT scan showed a thalamic infarct. He responded well to intravenous acyclovir and at follow-up at 6 months of age had defects in the iris but no detectable neurological abnormality. Recognition of the girl's shin lesions as being herpetic could have prevented both twins developing encephalitis.

Varicella–zoster virus

Only ~ 5% of women of child-bearing age have not had chickenpox. Varicella-zoster virus (VZV) infection affects ~ 0.7 per 1000 pregnancies (Sever and White, 1968). Its effects on mother, fetus and baby can sometimes be disastrous.

Effect on mother of gestational chickenpox

A high incidence of life-threatening pneumonitis in women with gestational chickenpox (but not zoster) has been reported (Paryani and Arvin, 1986), but such reports tend to be highly selective. It is not clear whether the risk is greater than that for normal adults.

Long-term effects of exposure *in utero* to varicella–zoster virus

There is very limited evidence that intrauterine chickenpox could lead to an increased risk of leukaemia (two fatal cases in 270 exposures; Adelstein and Donovan, 1972) and of other cancers. Fine *et al.* (1985) reported the incidence of cancer to be 2.3-fold greater than expected in a follow-up study of babies exposed *in utero* to VZV or CMV. The basis for this slight increase in risk of malignancy could be the chromosome abnormalities, usually transient, that VZV can induce *in vitro* in tissue culture and *in vivo* in peripheral blood leucocytes from children with chickenpox (Aula, 1964).

Congenital varicella syndrome

First-trimester maternal chickenpox may result in characteristic congenital malformations sufficient to be termed a syndrome (Alkalay *et al.*, 1987). There are cicatricial skin lesions of a limb, usually the leg (Figure 15.3), often with hypoplasia of that limb. Brain (microcephaly, cortical atrophy, cerebellar hypoplasia) and eye lesions (microphthalmia, optic atrophy, lenticular cataracts, chorioretinitis, nystagmus) are usual. The risk of congenital varicella syndrome in the baby of a mother with first-trimester chickenpox has been estimated from prospective studies at 2.2% with a range of 0–9% and 95% confidence intervals of 0.5–6.5% (Siegel, 1973; Enders, 1984; Paryani and Arvin, 1986: Preblud *et al.*, 1986). As studies with negative or less dramatic findings might not have been published, the true risk may be somewhat lower than this, although it seems wise to counsel parents using this figure. The risks with first-trimester maternal zoster and second- or third-trimester chickenpox are almost certainly far lower (Enders, 1984; Paryani and Arvin, 1986; Preblud *et al.*, 1986), although isolated cases of congenital varicella following these infections have been reported (Brice, 1976; Webster and Smith, 1977; Bai and John, 1979).

Pregnant women, particularly those in the first trimester, who are in

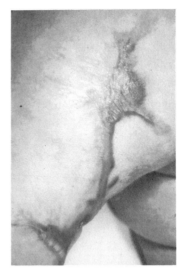

Figure 15.3 Congenital varicella syndrome. Cicatricial scarring of the leg

contact with chickenpox and have no past history of having had chickenpox, should be given varicella–zoster immune globulin (ZIG). The rationale is to modify the severity of disease in the mother and to decrease the risk of congenital varicella syndrome.

Perinatal maternal chickenpox

The spectrum of illness in the neonatal period varies from a well baby with a few spots to a fulminant illness with rash, visceral lesions and pneumonitis with extensive exudation of fluid from the lungs followed by pulmonary necrosis (Figure 15.4).

When maternal chickenpox occurs around the time of delivery, the baby may develop life-threatening illness. Only about one-quarter of the babies whose mothers develop chickenpox at any time during the last 21 days of pregnancy will be infected (Myers, 1974); however, the timing of illness in mother and baby is critical to the severity. Erlich *et al.* (1958) noted that if the baby's rash was present at birth or appeared within 4 days, the baby survived; if, however, the baby's rash developed 5 or more days after birth, fatalities occurred (Table 15.1).

The incubation period for congenital varicella (time between mother's and baby's rash) is ~ 9–15 days, although if maternal viraemia is massive this

Table 15.1 Timing of chickenpox in mother and baby in relation to severity

Onset of mother's rash in relation to delivery	Onset of baby's rash in relation to delivery (days after)	Died (n)	Survived (n)	Neonatal mortality (%)
5–21 days before	0–4	0	27	0
4 days before to 2 days after	5–10	7	16	30

From De Nicola and Hanshaw (1979)

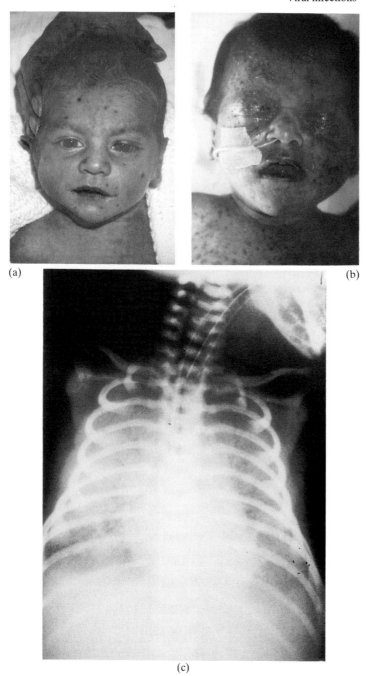

(a)   (b)

(c)

Figure 15.4 Perinatal chickenpox: (a) baby born with maternal antibody and rash but well; maternal chickenpox 10 days before delivery; (b) baby born well, developed rash on day 5 with fatal pneumonitis, despite ZIG and acyclovir; maternal chickenpox 3 days before delivery; (c) chest radiograph of (b) showing varicella pneumonitis

Table 15.2 Timing of mother's chickenpox rash in relation to presence of antibody in babies

Time, before delivery, of mother's rash (days)	Proportion of babies with detectable vzv antibody (IgG titre ≥ 32)
0–2	0 of 26
3–5	11 of 23
> 6	18 of 18

From Miller *et al.* (1989)

may be shortened to 3 days or the baby's rash may very occasionally occur simultaneously with the mother's. The corollary of the timing of the baby's rash is that, if the mother's rash appeared 5 or more days before delivery, the baby survives, whereas if the mother's rash appeared 4 days before to 2 days after delivery, then without intervention the mortality is ~ 30% (Table 15.1, and de Nicola and Hanshaw, 1979).

The reason for the importance of timing appears to be that severely affected babies acquire a large transplacental inoculum of virus before maternal antibody has crossed the placenta. Babies whose mother's rash develops 6 or more days before delivery all have detectable antibody, whereas if the mother's rash develops earlier, antibody is often not present (Table 15.2).

Zoster immune globulin (ZIG), an immunoglobulin preparation from donors with a high antibody titre to VZV, is generally effective in ameliorating the severity of infection, although it does not actually prevent infection. Hanngren *et al.* (1985) gave ZIG to 95 babies with perinatal exposure and 45 (50%) developed chickenpox. Of the 41 babies in the maximum risk group (mother's chickenpox 4 days before to 2 days after delivery), 21 became infected, of which two cases were severe. ZIG has not been standardized and the effective dose is not known. When 100–125 mg was being given in the UK, three fatalities occurred in 5 years, despite early prophylactic ZIG (Holland *et al.*, 1986) and the recommended dose has been increased to 250 mg.

Which babies should be given ZIG? The serological data of Miller *et al.* (1989) suggest that babies whose mothers developed their rash 6 or more days before delivery do not need ZIG, whereas those whose mother's rash was 0–5 days before delivery should be given ZIG. There are less data for babies whose mother's rash develops after delivery: their babies have no antibody but the viral inoculum may not be as great, although the mother may well have been viraemic before delivery. Rubin *et al.* (1986) reported a case of severe neonatal varicella in a baby aged 15 days whose mother developed varicella 8 days after delivery. It is, perhaps, reasonable to give ZIG to babies whose mother's rash develops up to 15 days after delivery although there are no data to support such a recommendation.

The antiviral treatment of babies with severe varicella infection is with acyclovir (60 mg/kg per day, 8-hourly, i.v.), but this is not always successful (Holland *et al.*, 1986).

Given the importance of the timing of the maternal rash, it may be worth attempting to delay labour for a few days when a mother has had recent chickenpox. This is obviously easier in spontaneous or elective preterm labour but consideration could be given to trying to prevent spontaneous term labour from progressing.

There have been no controlled studies of acyclovir treatment for mothers with peripartum chickenpox. In view of the report of Greffe *et al.* (1986) that acyclovir may sometimes cross the placenta, this approach, aimed at decreasing maternal and fetal viraemia, may be worth further study.

Babies exposed perinatally to chickenpox, even if they do not have clinical infection, have an increased risk of developing zoster infection early in childhood.

Postnatal exposure to chickenpox

Neonates exposed to chickenpox postnatally as opposed to perinatally, usually when a sibling develops the infection, may be at slightly increased risk of severe infection if the mother has not had chickenpox (Preblud *et al.*, 1984, 1985; Rubin *et al.*, 1986), although the risk is difficult to quantify because of selective reporting.

A common situation is that a sibling at home has chickenpox at the time that a well mother and term baby are due to be discharged from hospital. If the mother has had chickenpox, preferably documented by finding VZV IgG in her serum, there is virtually no risk, and mother and baby should be sent home. If the mother has no antibodies to VZV it seems reasonable to give the baby ZIG and to send mother and baby home. The alternatives are to split up the family or not to intervene at all, in which case the baby will almost certainly develop chickenpox with a risk of severe infection (Rubin *et al.*, 1986).

Nursery outbreaks

Most nursery outbreaks are characterized by very little spread of chickenpox, probably because of the high proportion of babies with maternal antibody and very mild disease. However, one baby with Turner's syndrome exposed at 7 days developed fatal chickenpox pneumonitis at 21 days despite maternal antibody (Gustafson *et al.*, 1984). Very preterm babies (less than 30 weeks' gestation) are likely to have low or undetectable levels of antibody even if the mother has had chickenpox; if such babies are exposed to chickenpox they should probably be given ZIG, as should other preterm babies with no maternal history of VZV infection. Infected babies and mothers should be isolated and nursed by immune staff.

Enteroviruses

The enteroviruses (echoviruses, Coxsackieviruses and polioviruses) are small RNA viruses for which man is the only natural host. Spread in older children and adults is primarily by the faecal–oral route, although respiratory spread may also occur. However, in the neonatal period, aspiration or ingestion of infected maternal blood or cervical secretions at the time of delivery seems to be the most important route of infection.

Transmission

There is some evidence that polioviruses can cross the placenta, particularly late in pregnancy, and cause abortion, stillbirth or neonatal infection. First-trimester intrauterine infection probably does not occur. Live oral polio vaccines given in the first trimester have not caused congenital abnormalities. It has been suggested that Coxsackieviruses can cause placental and transplacental infection in the third trimester, although probably not in the first or second trimesters. Echoviruses probably do not cause transplacental infection to the same extent as the other enteroviruses, although occasional cases have been described.

The most common mode of neonatal echo- and Coxsackievirus infection, based on the time of presentation, is almost certainly contact with infected maternal blood or cervical secretions during delivery. Following oral or respiratory acquisition there is local spread to regional lymph nodes within 24 h. After about 3 days there is minor viraemia with spread to multiple sites. Symptoms start when viral multiplication occurs in these sites at 4–5 days and leads to major viraemia. Some infections have followed caesarean delivery, even with intact membranes, suggesting that infection has occurred from maternal blood or that the viruses can cross intact membranes.

Outbreaks of echovirus and Coxsackievirus infections frequently occur on neonatal units. Usually a baby presents with the features of perinatally acquired ('vertical') infection and spread occurs to other babies ('horizontal' infection) via secretions carried on the hands of staff or when staff members become infected. Sometimes there is no clear index case and infection presumably started with an ill member of the family or the staff. Horizontal infections are nearly always far milder, presumably because the babies receive less virus and perhaps also because many have passively acquired maternal antibody.

Epidemiology

In temperate climates, enterovirus infections peak in the summer and autumn months although they may occur at any time of the year. Neonatal poliomyelitis is rare in both developed and developing countries. Echovirus and Coxsackievirus infections have been reported world wide, although Coxsackievirus infections have been described in South Africa in particular (Editorial, 1986). The incidence of neonatal enterovirus infection is unknown because many cases are asymptomatic and because often the appropriate viral cultures are not performed. Prospective studies carried out in neonatal units over 1–2 years may detect no cases of enterovirus infection, whereas in other years there may be an outbreak with several cases. We have detected 18 enterovirus infections in Oxford in 5 years in babies with symptoms or well contacts of symptomatic babies, which is an incidence of 0.7 per 1000 live births, and almost certainly an underestimate.

Clinical manifestations

It is now clear that babies infected at delivery (vertical infection) generally have a different and more fulminant clinical course than those infected horizontally.

Echoviruses

Babies with vertically acquired echovirus infection tend to present at 3–5 days, although very occasionally at birth or as late as 7 days. In about one-half of the cases there is a history of peripartum maternal illness that may be fever, coryza, gastroenteritis or severe abdominal pain, which is often misdiagnosed as placental abruption and precipitates urgent delivery. The most common neonatal clinical manifestation is a sepsis-like picture, sometimes with rash, progressing rapidly to fulminant hepatic necrosis with a severe bleeding disorder due to disseminated intravascular coagulopathy (DIC) and decreased clotting factors (Modlin, 1986). The liver may be enlarged and ascites, often heavily bloodstained, develops. Bleeding becomes generalized and may cause haemopericardium. The haemoglobin concentration often falls by several grams in a few hours. The mortality from this condition is ~ 80%. Liver histology post mortem shows centrilobular necrosis suggestive of ischaemia rather than hepatitis, a picture also seen in yellow fever. As most babies who die have had catastrophic bleeding and hypotension, ischaemia is not surprising, and virus can be readily grown from the liver. It is not clear whether the primary insult to the liver is infection (hepatitis) or ischaemia or perhaps both.

In fulminant echovirus infection there may also be meningitis, myocarditis, pneumonitis and gastroenteritis, and virus can easily be cultured from stool, throat swab or nasopharyngeal aspirate as well as urine, CSF, ascitic fluid, pleural fluid and multiple organs including the adrenal glands.

In contrast, horizontal infection is usually relatively mild, even in very preterm infants (Isaacs *et al.*, 1989). More than one-half of the babies are symptom free. Most babies present after 7 days of age and often after 14 days. Babies may develop meningitis (with a presentation similar to that of bacterial meningitis), myocarditis, pneumonia, gastroenteritis, or a non-specific illness with fever, irritability and apnoeic episodes.

Any echovirus serotype can probably cause severe infection, although the most commonly reported serotypes are echoviruses 11, 6 and 7, presumably reflecting their frequency of circulation in the population.

Coxsackieviruses

A less clear distinction has been drawn between vertical and horizontal Coxsackievirus infections than for echovirus infections, although as for echoviruses, horizontal infections are usually milder than vertical infections (Kaplan *et al.*, 1983). In South Africa there have been neonatal unit outbreaks in which babies who were thought to be horizontally infected developed fatal myocarditis (Editorial, 1986). Neonatal Coxsackie A virus infections have rarely been reported. Coxsackie B virus infections most commonly result in either meningitis or myocarditis or sometimes both. A macular rash, occasionally petechial, is a common accompaniment. Rarer manifestations include hepatitis, pancreatitis, enterocolitis, fever, paralysis and bronchitis.

Babies with myocarditis present suddenly with listlessness, poor feeding, tachycardia and fever. Murmur is often absent or unremarkable and the diagnosis is made by finding cardiomegaly and ECG changes and by echocardiography. Babies may recover gradually, may die rapidly from circulatory failure, may make an apparent recovery but then collapse in terminal heart failure or may deteriorate relentlessly despite inotropic support (Kaplan *et al.*, 1983). Occasionally, pericardial calcification develops. The presentation of Coxsackievirus B meningitis is clinically similar to that of bacterial meningitis.

Polioviruses

Probably > 90% of neonatal poliovirus infections are asymptomatic. Bates (1955) described 58 cases of symptomatic infections: about one-half were secondary to maternal infection, 15% were due to nosocomial infection and the rest were of unknown origin. The initial presentation was non-specific with fever, anorexia and irritability, although rarely diarrhoea. All but one of the 44 with adequate clinical data developed paralytic poliomyelitis, of whom one-half died, one-quarter recovered and one-quarter had residual paralysis.

Diagnosis

The diagnosis of neonatal enteroviral infections is largely based on appropriate viral cultures. If there is a suspicious peripartum maternal illness, stool and throat swabs from the mother should be cultured, and at least stool and nasopharyngeal aspirate or throat swab from the baby. A viral cytopathic effect is usually seen in tissue cultures within 2–4 days. Rapid viral diagnosis is not readily available. Probes have been developed which can detect enterovirus genome but this is very much a research tool at present. Serology is not generally helpful because of the large numbers of serotypes that can cause similar disease. However, specific IgM against Coxsackie B viruses may be detected in myocarditis, as only B2–B5 have been associated frequently with myocarditis.

Treatment

The treatment of severe enterovirus infections is supportive. Immunoglobulins are highly unlikely to modify the illness once established. We have unsuccessfully given intravenous human immunoglobulin in a vain attempt to treat babies with massive bleeding from hepatic necrosis. Blood transfusions and replacement of clotting factors with fresh frozen plasma and vitamin K are the mainstay of attempted management for hepatic necrosis. Myocarditis may require digitalization and possibly additional inotropic support if heart failure develops or progresses, and anti-arrhythmics for arrhythmias. Digitalis should be used with caution and initially at low doses because of possible increased sensitivity during enterovirus infection.

Prevention

It has been advocated that, when there is evidence or even suspicion of an outbreak of enterovirus infection on a neonatal unit, the unit should be closed to outside admissions and all babies in contact with infected babies, including all new admissions, should be given prophylactic immunoglobulin (Nagington *et al.*, 1983). We have questioned the wisdom of such a policy, because (a) most horizontal infections are relatively mild, (b) closing units may lead to babies receiving suboptimal care, and (c) human immunoglobulins, being blood products, are not completely without risk. In an outbreak in Oxford there were two simultaneous 'index' cases, both with meningitis and both thought to have been horizontally infected (Isaacs *et al.*, 1989). At this time spread had already occurred to eight other babies, all but one being of 27–30 weeks' gestation. Five were symptom-free and one each had pneumonia, gastroenteritis and apnoeic episodes. With no intervention other than to reinforce the importance of hand-washing there was further spread to only two babies, both symptom-free.

Because of the evidence that horizontal infections with Coxsackieviruses are more severe than horizontal echovirus infections, Coxsackievirus outbreaks should probably be managed more aggressively. In a Coxsackievirus outbreak, especially if there is more than one case of myocarditis, it would seem appropriate to give i.m. or i.v. immunoglobulins to all babies to attempt to lessen the severity of subsequent infection.

When perinatal enterovirus infection is strongly suspected on clinical grounds (we were recently consulted on twins delivered to a mother with hand, foot and mouth disease) or if virus has been isolated from the mother, the baby should be given 300–400 mg/kg of immunoglobulin by i.v. infusion. Poliovirus infections are preventable by immunization. Whenever possible, we isolate babies with known or suspected enterovirus infection and cohort the staff.

Prognosis

Vertically transmitted echovirus infection has a high mortality ($> 60\%$) and if hepatic necrosis develops the mortality is $> 80\%$ (Modlin, 1986). Horizontal echovirus infections have occasionally been fatal in neonates, as they have in infants, older children and adults. In general, however, death from horizontal infection is extremely rare. There have been contrasting reports on the long-term outcome of enteroviral meningitis with estimates of the incidence of residual neurological sequelae ranging from none (Bergman *et al.*, 1987) to up to 15% (Farmer *et al.*, 1975; Sells *et al.*, 1975; Wilfert *et al.*, 1981). Myocarditis usually responds to conservative management or digitalization. Coxsackievirus myocarditis has a high mortality, particularly if the disease is vertically acquired (Kaplan *et al.*, 1983).

Hepatitis B virus

Hepatitis B virus is a highly infectious DNA virus which can cause severe to fulminant hepatitis, but also has the important ability to cause a chronic carrier state lasting many years. There are > 200 million carriers in the world. Carriers are at greatly increased risk (approximately tenfold) of cirrhosis and hepatocellular carcinoma.

Structure

The hepatitis B virus comprises an inner core which contains the DNA, a DNA polymerase and an antigen called the core antigen (HBcAg) and an outer coat of lipid, glycoprotein and the surface antigen (HBsAg). An additional antigen, the e antigen (HBeAg) is seen during acute infections but also in some asymptomatic carriers and is an important marker of infectivity (Figure 15.5).

Epidemiology

In Taiwan, China, South-East Asia, Japan and parts of Africa, hepatitis B infection is endemic, with up to 15% of the population being chronic carriers (surface antigen positive). In the United Kingdom, Europe and America it is people whose families originate from those areas who are most likely to be chronically infected with hepatitis B. Other high-risk groups are intravenous drug abusers, male homosexuals, people regularly receiving blood or blood products such as those on haemodialysis (particularly if the donors are not screened), and medical and nursing staff. There is increasing evidence of spread occurring within families, mainly to siblings (Szmuness *et al.*, 1973).

Transmission

The most important method of transmission of hepatitis B virus in the neonatal period is vertical transmission from an infected mother. This is also

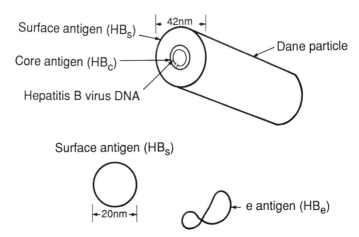

Figure 15.5 Diagrammatic representation of electron microscopic appearance of the hepatitis B virus. (From Forfar and Arneil (1991) with permission)

the most common method of transmission world wide, being the major factor in maintaining endemicity in Asian populations. Transmission could be transplacental or at the time of delivery. The success of immunoglobulin and vaccine in preventing transmission suggests that most neonatal infections occur around delivery, presumably by contact with infected maternal secretions.

The e antigen is an important determinant in transmission to neonates and particularly in the development of the chronic carrier state. Babies of asymptomatic carrier mothers who are e antigen positive and have no detectable antibody to the e antigen (HBeAG+) nearly all become infected and 85% will become chronic carriers (Stevens et al., 1975, 1979). In contrast, babies of mothers with antibody to e antigen (HbeAb+) virtually never become carriers. Polakoff (1985) found that none of 71 babies of HBeAb+ mothers became carriers, while Stevens et al. (1979) found 3 of 14 such babies were infected but none became carriers.

In South-East Asia a high proportion (up to 50%) of surface-antigen-positive carrier women of child-bearing age are e antigen positive with no antibody, whereas in the UK, Europe and America most carriers are either e antibody positive or have no detectable e antigen or e antibody (i.e. they are just surface antigen positive). This explains the fact that the vertical transmission rate in Japan, Taiwan and South-East Asia from all surface-antigen-positive mothers is 40–80% whereas in Britain, Europe and the USA the transmission rate is usually < 5%.

Some babies become infected and may develop acute hepatitis (although they do not become carriers) despite their mothers being e antigen negative or e antibody positive. It may be that the demonstration of hepatitis B virus DNA in the mother's blood will prove a good indicator of whether such neonatal infection is likely to occur (de Virgilis et al., 1985).

If women develop acute hepatitis B infection in pregnancy or up to 2 months after delivery, about one-half of their babies become infected (Schweitzer et al., 1972). Neonatal infection is most likely (> 70%) if the mother's hepatitis is in the third trimester or early puerperium but only 10% in the first or second trimesters (Schweitzer et al., 1973).

Hepatitis B surface antigen can be detected in breast milk by radioimmunoassay, but not by less sensitive techniques. Studies have not shown any difference in transmission rates between breast-fed and bottle-fed babies, so breast milk is probably an uncommon mode of transmission. It is not known, however, whether breast milk infects a small number of babies who would not otherwise have been infected. Transmission of hepatitis B from breast milk could be important where wet nursing is practised.

Diagnosis

Traditional diagnostic tests for hepatitis B antigens were superseded initially by radioimmunossay and subsequently by enzyme-linked immunosorbent assays (ELISAs), which can also be used to detect antibody. Hepatitis B virus DNA can be detected by hybridization (Scotto et al., 1983) and, although this is primarily a research tool, the presence of hepatitis B virus DNA may correlate with those babies who develop infection (de Virgilis et al., 1985).

Clinical features

Most babies who become chronic carriers are asymptomatic, although they may have persistently elevated serum transaminases and liver biopsy may show chronic persistent or chronic active hepatitis (Schweitzer *et al.*, 1973).

Acute icteric hepatitis develops in a small number of infected babies, but does not usually present until 2–5 months of age (Dupuy *et al.*, 1975). This may be fulminant with massive hepatic necrosis, or may progress to cirrhosis.

Prevention

Ideally, all pregnant women should be screened for HBsAg, but if this is impossible, women with risk factors for hepatitis B, as outlined above, should be tested.

Passive immunization with hepatitis B immunoglobulin is 70–80% effective in preventing perinatal transmission of hepatitis B from both e-antigen-positive and surface-antigen-positive mothers (Beasley *et al.*, 1981, 1983a). The first dose needs to be given within hours of birth.

Active immunization with plasma-derived vaccines has a similar success rate (70–80%) in preventing perinatal transmission (Maupas *et al.*, 1981; Beasley *et al.*, 1983b). The newer hepatitis B vaccines derived by recombinant DNA technology, such as the recombinant yeast vaccines where yeasts produce surface antigen, are equally effective.

Combined passive–active prophylaxis using both hepatitis B immunoglobulin and hepatitis B vaccine improved the protective efficacy to > 90% in Taiwan (Beasley *et al.*, 1983b) and Hong Kong (Wong *et al.*, 1984), whereas > 70% of untreated babies became chronic carriers. Presumably, some babies still become chronic carriers despite prophylaxis, because of intrauterine transmission.

In the UK, babies of e-antibody-positive mothers are not routinely given prophylaxis. However, there have been occasional reports of babies of e-antibody-positive mothers developing severe acute hepatitis B (Shiraki *et al.*, 1980; Sinatra *et al.*, 1982) as well as babies whose mothers were e antigen and antibody negative but surface antigen positive (Tong *et al.*, 1984). In the USA it is recommended that all babies of women who are surface antigen positive be given 0.5 ml of hepatitis B immunoglobulin (HBIg) as soon as possible after birth and 10 µg hepatitis B vaccine at birth, 1 and 6 months (Brunell *et al.*, 1985).

Breast feeding is felt to be indicated in developing countries where the risks of bottle feeding outweigh the very small risk of transmitting hepatitis B, but is not advised in developed countries where the relative risks may be reversed.

Members of the medical and nursing staff should be immunized against hepatitis B.

Human immunodeficiency virus (HIV)

Structure

The virus that causes acquired immunodeficiency syndrome (AIDS), now called the human immunodeficiency virus (HIV), is a lentivirus, which is a

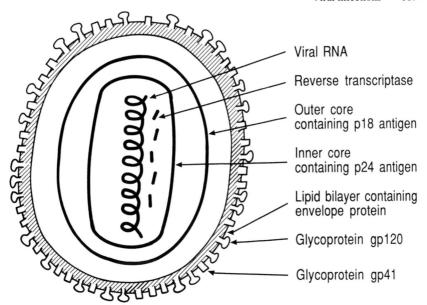

Viral RNA

Reverse transcriptase

Outer core
containing p18 antigen

Inner core
containing p24 antigen

Lipid bilayer containing
envelope protein

Glycoprotein gp120

Glycoprotein gp41

Figure 15.6 Diagrammatic representation of the human immunodeficiency virus
(HIV)

subfamily of the retroviruses. Although these are RNA viruses, they can
code for DNA synthesis directly by transcribing the RNA using an enzyme,
reverse transcriptase. The virus consists of a central core of RNA and
reverse transcriptase surrounded by two protein membranes (Figure 15.6).
The detection of circulating p24 antigen and of antibodies to p24 is often
used in serological tests. The outer lipid bilayer contains the envelope (env)
protein and from the bilayer protrude glycoproteins.

Epidemiology

HIV is important to neonatologists for a number of reasons. Infected babies
may sometimes present with symptoms in the neonatal period. There is an
unknown risk, however small, of staff and other babies acquiring infection
from an infected baby. There is also a risk of babies being infected by
receiving contaminated transfusions of blood or blood products and even by
contaminated human milk feeds. There are medical and ethical issues surrounding the early identification of infected or potentially infected babies
and their management (British Paediatric Association, 1989).

Approximately 1% of symptomatic HIV infections occur in children and,
of these cases, about 75% are perinatally acquired from a mother with HIV
infection with or without symptoms (Mok *et al.*, 1987; Centers for Disease
Control, 1988b; European Collaborative Study, 1988). Mothers with HIV
infection usually fall into one of the high-risk groups (Table 15.3), although
in some countries heterosexual spread is a growing problem, with increasing
numbers of infected women having no acknowledged risk factors.

Table 15.3 Risk groups for maternal HIV infection

Intravenous drug users
Prostitutes
Women from countries with a high prevalence of HIV infection (Haiti, Central Africa, Middle East)
Women with sexual partner in high-risk group (homosexual/bisexual, intravenous drug user, haemophiliac)
Women who received unscreened blood transfusions, particularly in countries with a high prevalence

Transmission

Vertical transmission could be transplacental or peripartum. Transplacental infection probably occurs, as virus has been detected in fetuses at 13–20 weeks and the incubation period for vertically acquired infection is shorter than that for other modes of infection (Falloon *et al.*, 1989). On the other hand, cases have been described in which only one monozygotic twin was infected so there are important unknown variables. Caesarean section has not been shown to protect against vertical transmission; nevertheless, peripartum infection from infected maternal secretions is probably also an important mode of transmission. The proportion of babies of HIV-positive mothers who become infected has varied in most studies between 25 and 50%, although Mok *et al.* (1989) reported that only 7% of such babies in Edinburgh became infected. It was originally thought that symptomatic mothers were more likely to have infected babies, although this was not confirmed in the European Collaborative Study (1988). This issue remains unresolved, although it seems likely that the stage of the mother's HIV infection, and hence the level of maternal viraemia, will affect transmission to the fetus or neonate.

Babies have been infected by receiving contaminated blood in the neonatal period. Screening of blood donors' HIV antibody status has made this an unlikely occurrence, but still a possibility as there may be a long latent period of 6 or more months between viraemia and seroconversion.

There have been a few reports of babies developing HIV infection when their mothers were only infected postnatally by blood transfusion (Ziegler *et al.*, 1985; Lepage *et al.*, 1987; Oxtoby, 1988). Because HIV can be isolated from cell-free breast milk of healthy HIV-infected mothers (Thiry *et al.*, 1985) it has been assumed that the babies were infected through their mother's breast milk. On the other hand, women recently infected by blood transfusion may be shedding far more virus than women who are asymptomatic or have had symptoms throughout pregnancy. The risk of a baby acquiring HIV infection through breast milk appears to be low, as studies have not shown any difference in the incidence of HIV infection in at-risk babies who were breast-fed or bottle-fed (European Collaborative Study, 1988; Italian Multicentre Study, 1988).

In developed countries it has generally been recommended that HIV positive mothers do not breast feed, although in developing countries breast-feeding is encouraged since the risks of bottle feeding outweigh those of transmitting HIV to the baby (DHSS, 1989).

Mothers of preterm babies without risk factors for HIV infection can express breast milk for their own babies. However, milk banks are under some threat. Eglin and Wilkinson (1987) have shown that milk spiked with high titres of HIV and pasteurized by the Holden method no longer contains detectable virus or reverse transcriptase. Nevertheless, the DHSS (1989) currently recommends that all donors to milk banks should be serologically screened for HIV infection, and that the milk should be pasteurized before it is given to other mother's babies.

Clincial features

Some babies born to mothers with HIV infection have been said to have a characteristic facial appearance including a prominent forehead and large, wide eyes (Marion et al., 1986, 1987; Iosub et al., 1987) but others have not confirmed these findings (Qazi et al., 1988). It is still not clear whether a true embryopathy exists or whether the features described reflect the babies' racial background.

Occasionally, babies have had lymphadenopathy and hepatomegaly at birth. It is rare for babies to present in the neonatal period, although there have been occasional reports of babies becoming symptomatic by 1 month of age with diarrhoea, failure to thrive and infections with opportunist organisms such as Pneumocystis carinii (Thomas et al., 1984b; Rubinstein, 1986). Infants who develop symptoms within a few weeks of birth may be co-infected with CMV.

Staff and HIV

Are staff and other babies at risk of infection from a baby with HIV infection? The risk to other babies, provided that normal precautions are followed, is negligible and no cases of cross-infection have yet been documented. The risk to staff is extremely low, but this is of little comfort to the few who have been infected. It appears that simple needlestick injuries rarely cause infection, but that staff occasionally have been infected by accidentally injecting infected blood or by pouring infected blood over bare hands with open sores and not washing it off immediately. The overall risk from needlestick injury with an infected needle is of the order of 0.4%.

Currently, women in the UK are not routinely screened for HIV infection in pregnancy. The Royal College of Obstetricians and Gynaecologists (RCOG Sub-Committee, 1987) has recommended a general improvement in standards of hygiene for delivery, and extra precautions for women known to be seropositive or from high-risk groups. For such deliveries the paediatrician should wear a mask, gown and apron, surgical gloves and safety spectacles. Mouth-to-endotracheal-tube suction to clear meconium should no longer be used for any delivery.

Lissauer (1989) has argued that paediatricians should not adopt a 'two tier' system of care for babies with possible HIV infection and those not thought to be at risk, but that paediatricians should treat every delivery and neonatal procedure as if the mother and baby were infected. This seems reasonable around delivery where there is a great deal of blood and liquor.

The implication for the neonatal unit, however, is that paediatricians and nurses should wear gloves and eye protection for every procedure in which blood or other potentially infected secretions might conceivably be spilt. Isaacs (1989) has argued that this is an over-reaction to a risk more theoretical than proven and that it should suffice for staff with open lesions (cuts or eczema) to cover them with waterproof tape and otherwise to wear gloves only when handling blood from known or suspected seropositive babies.

Diagnosis

Antibodies to HIV are detected by an ELISA screening test confirmed by Western blot. Because a newborn receives passive maternal antibody which persists, a definitive diagnosis of HIV infection can be made in a baby only by virus culture or detection of viral antigen or nucleic acid, although a symptomatic baby with antibodies is considered to be infected, for clinical and epidemiological purposes. Virus culture is not always readily available. Detection of p24 viral antigen in blood or tissue fluids indicates infection but many infected babies do not have detectable antigen. Viral nucleic acid (DNA) can be detected in white cells by the polymerase chain reaction, in which the concentration of nucleic acid is amplified, using enzymes, to a level at which it can be detected by probes. This method is exquisitely sensitive and may give false positives, so early reports of its use should be interpreted with caution (Laure et al., 1988). There is interest in the measurement of HIV-specific IgA to test for infection in infants.

In neonates the presence of serum (IgG) antibodies to HIV indicates only maternal infection and not whether the baby is infected. Maternal antibodies can persist for up to 15 months. IgM antibodies cannot yet be reliably tested. Testing a baby's HIV antibody status, therefore, is effectively testing the mother's status. The British Medical Association has stated that children can be tested without parental consent if it is essential to the child's care, even if this implictly tests the mother. Whenever possible, parental consent should be sought and obtained before testing a baby's HIV antibody status, and the family doctor should be informed if the test is positive. If the parents refuse to allow the baby to be tested or the diagnosis to be divulged to the family doctor, the parents' wishes should be respected, but the baby should be followed up closely (British Paediatric Association, 1989). Close follow-up of babies with suspected or proven infection is essential as the first symptom may be a life-threatening opportunist infection.

Treatment

Zidovudine (AZT) is of proven benefit in symptomatic HIV infection in children (Falloon et al., 1989). Prophylactic cotrimoxazole to prevent *Pneumocystis carinii* pneumonia (PCP) is usually well tolerated by children. Alternatives for PCP prophylaxis are dapsone and nebulized pentamidine. The roles of the treatment of asymptomatic HIV-positive children with AZT and of the treatment of symptomatic children with regular intravenous immunoglobulin infusions are still being evaluated.

Respiratory syncytial virus

Respiratory syncytial virus (RSV) occasionally causes neonatal unit outbreaks of infection, nearly always during the winter epidemic season, and
predominantly affecting babies > 3–4 weeks old. The clinical features of
neonatal RSV infection are non-specific and may include rhinitis, apnoeic
episodes, irritability, lethargy, poor feeding, fever, tachypnoea, pulmonary
infiltrates and increased requirements for respiratory support. Lower respiratory involvement is more often seen in older babies, but chest signs (rales,
rhonchi, intercostal recession) are not often present (Hall *et al.*, 1979; Mintz
et al., 1979; Rudd and Carrington, 1984). Younger babies may have merely
cough or coryza. Asymptomatic infection is not uncommon.

Hall *et al.* (1979) reported that 23 of 82 babies (28%) on a neonatal unit
studied during a community outbreak developed RSV infection. Four
babies died in association with RSV infection: one was already terminally ill;
one had bronchopulmonary dysplasia, which decompensated, and two died
suddenly and unexpectedly. This was an early report of babies studied in
1977. It seems likely that, with better intensive care and greater awareness of
RSV infection, the mortality from neonatal RSV infection would now be
considerably lower.

Certain groups of patients are at increased risk from RSV infection,
particularly babies with cyanotic congenital heart disease and bronchopulmonary dysplasia.

The American Academy of Paediatrics (1987) recommended that the
antiviral agent ribavirin should be considered for high-risk patients, including babies with congenital heart disease or bronchopulmonary dysplasia, 'certain premature infants' and severely ill infants. However, there
are considerable problems in delivering ribavirin to ventilated babies because it precipitates in ventilator tubing, the drug is expensive and there is no
evidence that it reduces mortality or obviates the need for mechanical
ventilation (Isaacs *et al.*, 1988b). We do not routinely use ribavirin for
preterm or high-risk babies infected with RSV but consider it for critically ill
babies and those with cyanotic congenital heart disease or bronchopulmonary dysplasia. Hand-washing is the most important way of preventing spread
in the neonatal unit, which occurs predominantly via infected nasal secretions, either carried from baby to baby on the hands of staff or via the
staff themselves becoming infected (Hall and Douglas, 1981).

Other respiratory viruses

Parainfluenza, influenza and rhinoviruses can cause sporadic infections or
neonatal unit outbreaks in which babies characteristically develop rhinitis,
cough, fever, apnoeic episodes, pulmonary infiltrates and feeding difficulties. These signs and symptoms are similar to those of RSV infection. In
simultaneous outbreaks of RSV and rhinovirus (Valenti *et al.*, 1982) and of
RSV and parainfluenza virus type 3 (Meissner *et al.*, 1984), babies infected
with RSV were clinically indistinguishable from those infected with the
other respiratory viruses. The clustering of cases in the second outbreak
strongly suggested patient-to-patient spread.

Most mothers have antibodies to measles. Measles is rare in pregnancy and does not cause a recognized syndrome of congenital infection, although there have been reports of sporadic fetal abnormalities in association with gestational measles. Gestational measles is associated with a high risk of spontaneous abortion. Neonatal unit outbreaks are extremely rare. Postnatal measles with rash occurring at 14–30 days, and usually resulting from postnatal maternal infection or from a sibling, is generally mild. However, congenital measles, in which the rash is present at birth or appears in the first ten days, may be severe, and dominated by pneumonia or pneumonitis. There is an obvious parallel with congenital chickenpox, although less is known about transfer of maternal antibody. The mortality appears to be the same, whether rash is present at birth or appears in the next ten days (Dyer, 1940; Kohn, 1933), and in one report, 7 of 16 preterm babies exposed to measles died from pneumonitis without developing a rash (Richardson, 1920). In Greenland, however, none of 13 babies whose mothers had measles at delivery developed congenital measles. The age of these reports should be emphasized and the mortality of 30–44% almost certainly no longer applies; there is no information on the current mortality from congenital measles. Given the potential severity, it would seem wise to give hyperimmune measles gamma-globulin to babies of mothers with peripartum measles and to neonates whose siblings have measles and whose mothers are non-immune.

First-trimester maternal mumps carries a modestly increased risk of abortion (Siegel et al., 1966). There is also a possible slightly increased long-term risk of the baby later developing diabetes (Fine et al., 1985). No consistent congenital syndrome has been described, although attempts have been made to link gestational mumps with endocardial fibroelastosis, Down's syndrome and other malformations. Even if the mother has mumps at the time of delivery, neonatal illness is rare, and parotitis exceedingly so. Jones et al. (1980) and Reman et al. (1986) reported babies aged 7 and 3 days respectively with mumps pneumonitis.

Chapter 16

Congenital infections

Introduction

Maternal infections during pregnancy can result in congenital infections which may be apparent at birth, or may be inapparent at birth but can result in late sequelae. In most, but not all, cases of infections by the 'TORCH' group of agents (*Toxoplasma gondii*, rubella, cytomegalovirus and herpes simplex virus), symptomatic congenital infection is most likely to result from maternal infections occurring in the first trimester at the time of maximum fetal organogenesis. Such infections are, of course, transmitted transplacentally and might better be called intrauterine infections. Babies may also be born with similar symptoms but resulting from peripartum maternal infection: examples are HSV and enterovirus infections (Chapter 15) and congenital listeriosis (Chapter 13). In the United States, although not in Britain, more babies have a rash in the first 24 h after birth caused by HSV than by any other agent. In cases of peripartum infection the origin may be mainly transplacental, as in listeriosis, or mainly attributable to ascending infection, as for HSV.

This chapter deals only with congenital intrauterine infections with *Toxoplasma*, rubella and CMV. A baby born with a rash does not necessarily have an infection caused by one of these three organisms. HSV is a very rare cause of first-trimester intrauterine infection but may sometimes cause an early rash. This, however, is usually vesicular and clinically distinctive from the purpuric rashes of the other TORCH agents. The rash of congenital listeriosis is also distinctive, the baby is usually sick, and there are other features of the mother's history and the baby's clinical state to suggest listeriosis (Chapter 13). In enterovirus infection the rash is only very rarely present at birth, although it may closely resemble the rashes of intrauterine infections. Autoimmune or isoimmune thrombocytopenia may result in a purpuric rash at birth and may be a difficult differential diagnosis.

In the John Radcliffe Hospital, Oxford, IgM antibodies to *Toxoplasma gondii*, rubella and CMV but not routinely to HSV are sought when there is clinical suspicion of intrauterine infection. This would, of course, include babies with rash and other classic features. If all babies who are small for gestational age are screened for congenital infection, the yield is extremely low and those babies identified have other suggestive signs. Therefore, we test babies who are small for gestational age only if they are without maternal risk factors such as hypertension.

Toxoplasmosis

Congenital infection with the protozoan parasite, *Toxoplasma gondii*, can result in clinical features surprisingly similar to those caused by CMV and rubella.

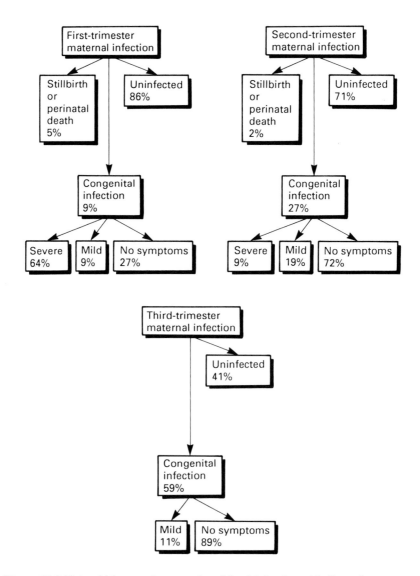

Figure 16.1 Natural history of maternal and fetal infection with *Toxoplasma gondii* (adapted from Remington and Desmonts, 1990). 'No symptoms', only serological evidence of infection; 'mild', retinal scars *or* intracerebral calcification, child neurologically normal; 'severe', chorioretinitis *and* intracerebral calcification or child neurologically abnormal

Transmission

Toxoplasmosis is a zoonosis. The parasite was first identified in 1908 in rabbits and rodents. It is commonly found in cats, dogs, pigs, sheep and cattle. Desmonts and Couvreur showed that 9% of children in a TB hospital in Paris seroconverted to *Toxoplasma* every month when fed undercooked mutton. They also showed that about 1% of young married women in Paris seroconverted each year at the time that they started keeping house and preparing food (Remington and Desmonts, 1990). Toxoplasmosis has been caused by eating undercooked meat from sheep, cows and pigs, including hamburgers. It also occurs in strict vegetarians. Ingestion of cysts from cat, dog or other animal faeces is a likely mode of transmission. Other possible modes such as milk, eggs, chicken and blood transfusion have not been confirmed.

Incidence

In the UK, congenital toxoplasmosis is diagnosed in ∼ 0.2 per 1000 pregnancies, probably an underestimate. Prospective studies in the USA and Europe have shown the incidence of maternal infection in pregnancy to vary from 2 to 12 per 1000 and the incidence of congenital infection, diagnosed by cord blood IgM, from 1 to 7 per 1000 live births. Most women who have an affected baby were asymptomatic in pregnancy but 10–20% report an episode of lymphadenopathy or a flu-like illness. It is controversial whether maternal toxoplasmosis can cause recurrent abortion.

Congenital infection can be demonstrated serologically, with increasing frequency the later in pregnancy that infection occurs (Figure 16.1). In contrast, the severity of fetal infection is greater the earlier in pregnancy that maternal infection occurs (Figure 16.1). Severe fetal infection will occur in about 6% of first-trimester infections, 2% of second-trimester infections and in no third-trimester infections.

Clinical features

Sabin (1942) described a tetrad of clinical features of congenital toxoplasmosis: internal hydrocephalus or microcephaly, chorioretinitis, convulsions or other signs of CNS involvement and intracerebral calcification. Since then, a wide range of other clinical manifestations have been described. Neonates may present early with features of generalized infection or with predominantly neurological manifestations. In generalized infection there may be hydrops fetalis from anaemia; rash due to thrombocytopenic purpura or to the 'blueberry muffin' appearance of dermal erythropoiesis (Figure 16.2), which occurs in 25% of such cases although in < 10% of all cases of congenital toxoplasmosis; jaundice, which may appear late; hepatosplenomegaly; lymphadenopathy, and pneumonitis. There may be systemic symptoms such as vomiting, diarrhoea, fever or hypothermia and neurological signs and symptoms, as described below.

Sometimes, neurological signs and symptoms are the only clue to neonatal infection. These include convulsions, bulging fontanelle, nystagmus, chorioretinitis (Figure 16.3), microphthalmia, cataracts and microcephaly or hydrocephalus. Alford *et al.* (1974) described 'CSF abnormalities' in all

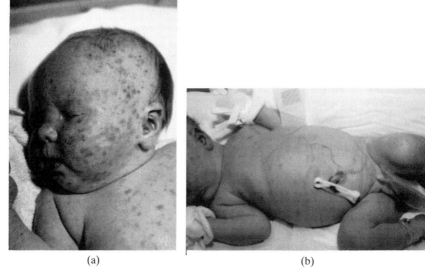

(a)   (b)

Figure 16.2 Congenital toxoplasmosis: (a) 'blueberry muffin' appearance of dermal erythropoiesis; (b) hepatosplenomegaly

eight subclinical cases examined, with 10–110 lymphocytes per ml (which might be considered normal) and protein levels of 1.5–10 g/l (150–1000 mg/100 ml). Thus, CSF abnormalities, of which elevated CSF protein is the commonest, may or may not be present and, if so, are presumably attributable to meningoencephalitis.

Infected babies may be normal at birth but develop problems, often severe, weeks or months later. These are usually caused by eye involvement (chorioretinitis) presenting as nystagmus, strabismus or blindness (Figure 16.4), but may also be due to CNS involvement (hydrocephalus) causing

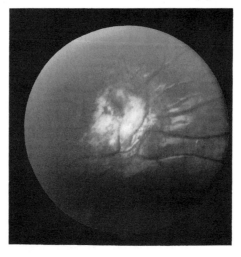

Figure 16.3 Congenital toxoplasmosis: optic fundus; area of chorioretinitis with surrounding pigmentation

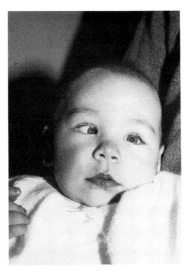

Figure 16.4 Congenital toxoplasmosis: presenting at 4 months of age with strabismus and blindness due to chorioretinitis

convulsions, bulging fontanelle or enlarging head circumference or to generalized infection causing late jaundice, hepatosplenomegaly or lymphadenopathy.

Choroidoretinitis may be delayed in onset until school age and ocular lesions may recur in childhood or adolescence. Occasionally, hydrocephalus may occur *de novo* in later childhood due to aqueduct stenosis.

Diagnosis

The diagnosis of congenital toxoplasmosis is confirmed by detecting specific IgM by immunofluorescence or ELISA in the cord or baby's blood. The organism can also be cultured from blood and placenta by inoculation into mice. Cerebral ultrasound scan may show hydrocephalus, and this and intracranial calcification may be seen on skull radiographs but is far better seen by CT scan. Calcification occurs classically as discrete foci (Figure 16.5)

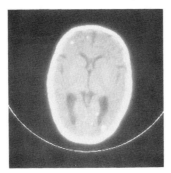

Figure 16.5 Congenital toxoplasmosis: punctate areas of cerebral calcification and mild ventricular dilatation

but very occasionally may be periventricular, as in congenital CMV infection.

Treatment

Three or four 21-day courses of pyrimethamine (1 mg/kg per day orally once daily) and sulphadiazine (50–100 mg/kg per day, orally 12-hourly), which act synergistically, alternating with 30- to 45-day courses of the erythromycin-like macrolide antibiotic spiramycin (100 mg/kg per day, orally 12-hourly) over the first year of life is recommended for overt congenital toxoplasmosis (Jacques Couvreur reported by Remington and Desmonts, 1990). More controversial are the authors' suggestions that steroids be added for severe infections with evidence of active inflammation, that a single 21-day course of pyrimethamine and sulphadiazine be given for subclinical congenital infection or possible infection, or that spiramycin alone be given to a healthy baby whose mother had a high *Toxoplasma* dye test in pregnancy but no confirmed infection. There is no controlled evidence for any of these suggestions for treatment of newborn babies and infants. Remington and Desmonts (1990) also state that, because pyrimethamine is a folic acid antagonist, folinic acid should be given. They recommend 3–10 mg i.m. or orally once daily to older children and adults, although there are no data on its use in newborns and infants.

Prevention

As only 10–20% of infected women will have symptoms, any screening programme depends on maternal serology. If infected women are identified, can the babies who are infected be identified antenatally, and is prenatal treatment effective or is termination the only option? It has been suggested that treating infected pregnant women with spiramycin may reduce the incidence and severity of congenital toxoplasmosis (Desmonts *et al.*, 1985; Daffos *et al.*, 1988; Hohlfeld *et al.*, 1989). Unfortunately, the studies performed to date have not been adequately controlled, so these claims have not been verified.

About two-thirds of severely affected fetuses have antenatal enlargement of the ventricles detectable by ultrasound scan (Desmonts *et al.*, 1985). Antenatal diagnosis is now possible by obtaining fetal blood samples for culture and IgM. Is screening of pregnant women a realistic proposal?

In France, serological screening to detect and treat women who acquire *Toxoplasma* infection during pregnancy is compulsory and the incidence of congenital toxoplasmosis is apparently falling (Daffos *et al.*, 1988; Hohlfeld *et al.*, 1989). Desmonts *et al.* (1985) studied 278 infected pregnant women: five requested immediate termination despite counselling; of the rest, information was available on 215 pregnancies. All women were treated with spiramycin 3 g daily until the end of pregnancy, and a fetal blood sample was performed at 20–24 weeks' gestation. Nine cases of continuing infection were diagnosed (six with hydrocephalus) and all were terminated. Four mothers requested termination although there was no evidence of continuing infection. Evidence of congenital toxoplasmosis could be found in only one of 199 babies thought antenatally to be free of infection. In an extension of this study, Daffos *et al.* (1988) reported 746 cases of maternal toxoplasmosis: there were 24 therapeutic terminations. Fifteen women with second-trimester infection elected to continue with pregnancy and were given spiramycin 3 g daily until delivery: six babies had mild infection but all were neurologically normal at follow-up.

It is arguable whether such intensive efforts to prevent congenital toxoplasmosis are justifiable in countries in which the incidence is apparently lower than in France. When the incidence is low, say 2 per 1000, a screening test with 99% specificity and 100% sensitivity might be expected to identify ten false-positive and two true-positive maternal infections in every 1000 pregnancies. In view of the level of anxiety that this will engender, as shown by requests for immediate termination in Desmont's study, and the risks of fetal blood sampling, the risks of screening may outweigh the benefits, particularly if the incidence is low.

McCabe and Remington (1988) called for prospective trials to evaluate maternal serological screening in the USA. They also state that providing information to women on how to avoid infection is the 'simplest, least expensive and ultimately the most efficient and effective means of preventing congenital infection'. Such instructions should be to eat only well-cooked meat, to wash fruit and vegetables before eating, and to wear gloves for gardening and handling cat (or dog) litters if the husband cannot be persuaded to do these tasks. Similarly, Jeannel *et al.* (1990) have questioned the validity of the French evidence that treatment of infected pregnant women with spiramycin prevents fetal infection, as no randomized placebo-controlled trial has ever been performed. They argue that the modes of transmission are linked to known living habits, and that health education to prevent maternal toxoplasmosis should be evaluated.

Rubella

In 1941 Sir Norman Gregg, an Australian ophthalmologist, described the association between congenital cataracts and a maternal history of rubella in early pregnancy. Children with congenital rubella syndrome are among the most distressing to care for: the combination of deafness and blindness means that it is virtually impossible to communicate with them – the so-called 'locked-in syndrome'. Rubella virus was first isolated in tissue culture in 1962 and this led to the development of vaccines which can, and should, effectively eliminate congenital rubella syndrome.

Epidemiology

In unimmunized populations, rubella virus circulates readily in young children, particularly those aged 5–9 years. Infection is commonest in the late winter and spring. In unimmunized populations, epidemics occur every 6–9 years but infections continue to occur at a lower rate in the interval between epidemics.

The attack rate for susceptible adults and children in closed situations, such as military camps or boarding schools, is 90–100%. However, in unimmunized populations 5–20% of women of child-bearing age are susceptible.

Intrauterine transmission of rubella virus via placental infection occurs in primary maternal rubella. Reinfections with rubella can occur and are usually clinically silent; they occur in 1–3% of the population in natural rubella and higher rates in immunized populations. Serum IgG rises and IgM sometimes appears. There is brief viral replication and there have been occasional reports of congenital rubella in association with reinfection (Strannegard *et al.*, 1970; Haukenes and Haram, 1972; Northrop *et al.*, 1972; Eilard and Strannegard, 1974; Forsgren *et al.*, 1979). In most of these cases the original rubella infection was not serologically confirmed, but very occasionally there have been convincing reports of documented reinfections causing congenital infection.

Clinical features

Maternal rubella

Maternal rubella is asymptomatic in about one-third of cases. In adults there is an incubation period of 14–21 days, and a prodromal period of 1–5 days. Prodromal signs and symptoms include fever, headache, sore eyes with conjunctivitis, sore throat, headache and anorexia. Lymphadenopathy, mainly posterior auricular, occipital and cervical, may precede the rash or appear at the same time. The rash, when it occurs, lasts about 3 days, and is fine, pink and maculopapular. It appears first on the face, spreading to the trunk and extremities and the lesions may coalesce to form a blush. There are many similar rashes caused by other viruses such as parvovirus B19 and enteroviruses, so serological proof of rubella infection should always be sought. Arthralgia and arthritis may occur before or after the rash. Reinfections are usually asymptomatic (Best *et al.*, 1989).

Congenital rubella

Congenital rubella is a chronic infection present from the time of prenatal infection to many months or years after birth. Most congenital infections result from primary maternal infections but occasional well-documented cases have followed maternal reinfection (Best *et al.*, 1989). The timing of maternal rubella infection is critical, in that infections before 11 weeks almost always cause multiple congenital abnormalities, infections from 11 to 16 weeks may cause deafness, while infections after 17 weeks rarely cause

Table 16.1 Estimated risk of congenital defect due to maternal rubella occurring at different times in gestation

Timing of maternal rubella in pregnancy (weeks)	Estimated risk of congenital defect (%)	Type of defect
< 11	90	Congenital rubella syndrome
11–12	33	Sensorineural deafness
10–14	20	Sensorineural deafness
15–16	10	Sensorineural deafness
17–18	0	—
> 18	0	—

After Miller *et al.* (1982)

Table 16.2 Some of the commoner manifestations of congenital rubella syndrome

Organ	Defect
Eye	Congenital cataracts Cloudy cornea Glaucoma Choroidoretinitis (salt and pepper) Microphthalmia
Ear	Sensorineural deafness
Heart	Pulmonary artery stenosis/hypoplasia Persistent ductus arteriosus
CNS	Microcephaly Active encephalitis
Growth	Intrauterine growth retardation
Reticulo-endothelial	Hepatosplenomegaly Lymphadenopathy
Lung	Interstitial pneumonitis
Skin	Thrombocytopenic purpura
Bone	Radiolucencies

problems (Miller *et al.*, 1982, Table 16.1). Almost any organ can be affected in the full congenital rubella syndrome, but some of the commoner manifestations are shown in Table 16.2. The eyes are often cloudy due to corneal opacification (Figure 16.6) with or without cataracts (Figure 16.7). If the retina can be seen there may be 'salt-and-pepper' chorioretinitis (Figure 16.8). The baby may have a purpuric rash due to thrombocytopenia or a

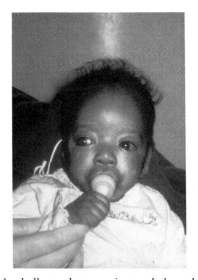

Figure 16.6 Congenital rubella syndrome: microcephaly and cloudy cornea

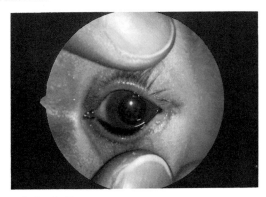

Figure 16.7 Congenital rubella: cataract

'blueberry muffin' appearance due to dermal erythropoiesis (also sometimes seen in congenital toxoplasmosis, as in Figure 16.2).

The CSF protein may be high, with or without lymphocyte pleocytosis, suggesting active encephalitis. Pulmonary artery stenosis is the commonest heart lesion, but patent ductus arteriosus is also common, while coarctation of the aorta may occur. The ECG may show an infarct pattern due to necrotic heart lesions. A skeletal survey may reveal bony translucencies. Pneumonitis usually presents postnatally with tachypnoea. Renal abnormalities (polycystic kidney, double ureter, hydronephrosis, renal artery stenosis) may very occasionally occur and babies with proven congenital rubella should have an abdominal ultrasound scan. Severely

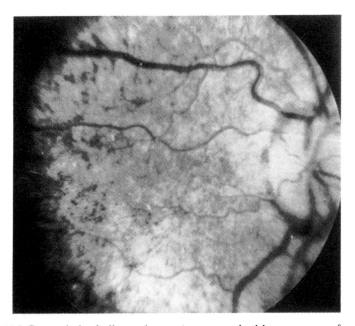

Figure 16.8 Congenital rubella syndrome: 'pepper and salt' appearance of chorioretinitis

affected babies may die from hepatitis, pneumonitis, cardiac lesions or prematurity.

Prognosis

Babies apparently normal at birth but with confirmed congenital infection following first- or second-trimester rubella should be closely followed up. Sensorineural deafness may occur in the absence of other clinical features and hearing should be tested regularly, because deafness may be progressive. Hearing loss is easily the commonest manifestation of congenital rubella infection. Other rarer long-term problems from congenital rubella syndrome include a subacute encephalitis resembling subacute sclerosing panencephalitis and usually occurring at 8–14 years, in which CSF and serum antibodies to rubella are raised. Endocrine problems may emerge, including diabetes mellitus, precocious puberty, hyper- and hypothyroidism and growth hormone deficiency. There may be visual deterioration from progressive neovascularization of the retina in babies with choroidoretinitis.

Diagnosis

Primary maternal infection is ideally diagnosed by showing seroconversion or a rising titre of IgG antibodies to rubella as measured by haemagglutination inhibition, single radial haemolysis, ELISA or radioimmunoassay. If IgG antibodies are detected within 10 days of contact the woman is immune, but if no antibodies are detected a second sample should be obtained 2 weeks later. If a woman presents some time after a contact and her previous rubella status is unknown, rubella infection can be diagnosed by looking for IgM antibodies, which appear 5–10 days after the rash and persist for 50–70 days. Antenatal diagnosis by measurement of specific IgM in fetal blood samples is possible in some centres (Daffos *et al.*, 1984). Reinfections are diagnosed by showing the appearance of specific IgM in a woman previously shown to have high-titre IgG antibody (Best *et al.*, 1989).

In congenital rubella the diagnosis can be made by detecting specific IgM in serum or cord blood, or alternatively by culturing rubella virus. The best specimens for virus isolation are nasopharyngeal aspirates, eye swabs, urine, faeces and CSF. Virus may persist in the eye and CSF for a year or more. Babies are infectious and should be isolated from pregnant women.

Prevention

In countries such as the USA and Canada, where rubella vaccine (alone or in the form of measles, mumps and rubella (MMR) vaccine) has been given for many years to all children at about 15 months, congenital rubella syndrome has virtually disappeared. In the United States only two cases were reported in 1984 and again in 1985 (Centers for Disease Control, 1987). This approach to prevention depends on uptake of the vaccine being adequate to prevent exposure of unimmunized non-immune women to the virus. In the USA, where rubella vaccines have been used in this way since 1969, most cases of rubella now occur in adults. It is recommended that non-pregnant susceptible women of childbearing age also be immunized.

In the UK a different strategy was initially adopted: selective immunization of schoolgirls aged 13–14 years and of non-immune primigravid
women after delivery. As rubella virus could then circulate in school-
children, this approach depended on an extremely high uptake in schoolgirls. In practice, ~ 2 per 1000 pregnancies were affected, even in
non-epidemic years, resulting in up to 800 terminations of pregnancy and
about 80 cases of congenital rubella infection each year. Despite universal
antenatal screening of rubella serology, an unacceptably high proportion of
cases occurred in second or subsequent pregnancies because, for various
reasons, non-immune primigravidas had not been immunized (Wild *et al.*,
1986). Since 1988, MMR vaccine has been given to British children at 13–15
months but selective vaccination will also continue indefinitely.

There is a small but definite risk of congenital rubella syndrome following
maternal reinfection and any woman, even if immune, in contact with
rubella in the first 16 weeks of pregnancy should be screened for IgM
antibodies to rubella.

A large number of terminations of pregnancy are performed each year
for inadvertent immunization with rubella vaccine during pregnancy. The
vaccine viruses used are live but attenuated. The situation is not entirely
clear because of changes in vaccine strains: in the USA the Cendehill and
HPV-77 strains have been completely replaced by RA 27/3 vaccine. There
is evidence that the vaccine virus can cross the placenta and infect the
fetus in up to 20% of cases, when products of conception have been cultured
(Modlin *et al.*, 1976; Preblud *et al.*, 1981). The vaccine virus has been
isolated from the kidney of an abortus (Vaheri *et al.*, 1972) and, most
worryingly, from the eye of an aborted fetus which had lens abnormalities
suggestive of congenital rubella (Fleet *et al.*, 1974). It is not advisable for
women to become pregnant for 3 months after rubella immunization, because virus has been cultured from an abortus when vaccine was given 7
weeks before pregnancy. On the other hand, 364 pregnant women accidentally immunized with rubella vaccine, of whom 112 were known to be
non-immune, have elected to proceed to term and there have been no
detectable malformations (Preblud *et al.*, 1981). Thus the risk of vaccine-
associated congenital infection appears to be extremely small, almost certainly < 3%, and pregnant women who are accidentally given the vaccine
should be counselled accordingly.

Cytomegalovirus

Cytomegalovirus (CMV) is the commonest cause of congenital infection in
developed countries and an important cause of mental retardation and
deafness world wide. Postnatal CMV infection may also cause significant
problems in preterm neonates and is dealt with here.

The organism

CMV is a herpesvirus and has the potential, like the other herpesviruses, to
cause persistent infection and to reactivate. There are at least two serotypes
of CMV. CMV infection of cells results in large intranuclear inclusions

and occasional intracytoplasmic inclusions in enlarged cells (hence the old name cytomegalic inclusion disease).

Transmission

CMV can be found in cervical secretions, semen and saliva and may be transmitted between adults by sexual activity or kissing. In developing countries most women of child-bearing age have already been infected in childhood, when transmission is probably by respiratory spread of droplets or secretions. The virus can cross the placenta, either during a primary maternal infection or during reactivation, and infect the fetus prenatally. It may also be acquired at delivery from cervical secretions, or postnatally from breast milk (Stagno *et al.*, 1980) or infected blood transfusion (Yeager, 1974). Postnatal infection can be devastating in preterm babies (Yeager, 1974), but in term babies, although symptoms (rash, pneumonitis, hepato-splenomegaly, lymphadenopathy) develop in up to one-third (Kumar *et al.*, 1984a), is rarely life-threatening or damaging. In contrast, prenatal infection can have major long-term sequelae.

Epidemiology

Congenital CMV infection, as determined by screening all babies by urine culture and/or cord blood IgM, occurs in ~ 3 per 1000 live births in Britain (Peckham *et al.*, 1983), and Sweden (Ahlfors *et al.*, 1979), but in 5 to 25 per 1000 live births in the USA (Birnbaum *et al.*, 1969; Stagno *et al.*, 1977). However, only 5–10% of infected infants are symptomatic at birth (Preece *et al.*, 1984).

The proportion of women of childbearing age who are seropositive to CMV varies in different populations. In Britain and the USA, ~ 50% of pregnant women are seropositive, but 80% of girls of low socio-economic status in Alabama were seropositive by puberty (Stagno *et al.*, 1977). In Japan 65% are seropositive by age 13 (Numazaki *et al.*, 1970) while in Africa > 90% have been infected by puberty (Schopfer *et al.*, 1978).

About 1% of non-immune women develop primary CMV infection during pregnancy and about one-half of their babies are infected (Griffiths *et al.*, 1980; Grant *et al.*, 1981; Stagno *et al.*, 1982; Peckham *et al.*, 1983).

Women who are seropositive at the start of pregnancy may reactivate. About 5% of pregnant women excrete CMV in the urine and CMV may be isolated from the cervix in up to 28% of pregnancies. Serological studies are unhelpful in diagnosing the rate of reactivation, because this may occur at any time during pregnancy and cultures of urine or cervical secretions suffer from a similar problem. In Figure 16.9, in which an estimate is made of the relative importance of primary and secondary infections, the rate of reactivation has been given as 10%, which is an approximation. About one-half of the babies will be infected perinatally, from cervical secretions or breast milk, while ~ 5% will develop intrauterine infections.

Congenital CMV infection can result from primary maternal CMV during pregnancy or from recurrence. The relative importance of these two modes of transmission varies according to the rate of seropositivity of women of childbearing age. Of 2698 pregnant women of middle or high income,

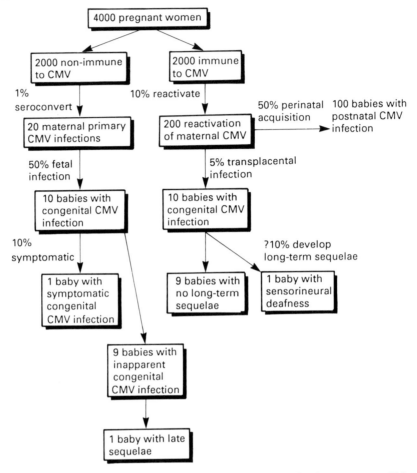

Figure 16.9 Theoretical scheme of outcome of CMV infection in pregnancy. This assumes a 'developed' country, where 50% of women of childbearing age are immune to cytomegalovirus (CMV) and the rate of congenital infection is 5 per 1000 live births

16 babies (0.6%) had congenital CMV infection, eight due to primary infections and eight due to recurrences, whereas of 1014 women of low income, 16 babies (1.6%) had congenital CMV but only three were due to primary infections and 13 to recurrences (Stagno *et al.*, 1982).

It was originally thought that congenital CMV infection with severe sequelae, like congenital infections with toxoplasma and rubella, was likely to follow primary maternal CMV only in the first trimester. Although it is clear that this is the major risk period, there is growing evidence that severe sequelae may result from primary infections in the second and third trimesters and from recurrent infections. Stagno *et al.* (1986) reported severe handicaps in five of 23 babies with congenital CMV resulting from primary maternal CMV occurring at up to 27 weeks' gestation, whereas the only abnormal baby out of 12 with congenital CMV from late primary infection (28–40 weeks) had only hypoplastic dental enamel. Other studies, however, have shown that at least some babies will have severe sequelae from primary maternal infection occurring in late pregnancy (Grant *et al.*, 1981; Ahlfors *et al.*, 1984; Griffiths and Baboonian, 1984; Preece *et al.*, 1984).

Although serious handicap is more likely in congenital CMV resulting from primary maternal infection (Stagno *et al.*, 1982; Ahlfors *et al.*, 1984), such handicap sometimes follows recurrent infection and these babies may rarely be symptomatic at birth (Ahlfors *et al.*, 1984; Preece *et al.*, 1984; Rutter *et al.*, 1985).

The interpretation of studies of babies with congenital CMV infection is complicated by the observations of Preece *et al.* (1986) that women in London with affected babies are more likely to be < 20 years old, Black and unmarried.

Clinical features

Only 5–10% of babies with congenital CMV infection are symptomatic at birth. Those with 'cytomegalic inclusion disease' (Figure 16.10) typically have a purpuric rash due to thrombocytopenia (usually with pinpoint petechiae), hepatosplenomegaly, jaundice, microcephaly, chorioretinitis and intracerebral calcification. Jaundice may appear within 24 h of birth and require exchange transfusion or appear at 2–5 days. The chorioretinitis of CMV resembles that of toxoplasmosis (Figure 16.3). Cataracts and microphthalmia are very rare in congenital CMV. Cerebral calcification is classically periventricular, and is found in the subependymal region (Figure 16.11). This appearance may rarely be seen in congenital toxoplasmosis. If the calcification is widespread it may cause obstructive hydrocephalus.

Pneumonitis may develop as a late manifestation of congenital CMV infection, usually occurring at 1–4 months of age. Preece *et al.* (1984) described 6 of 50 children with congenital CMV infection who developed an afebrile pneumonitis at this age, characterized by tachypnoea and hyperinflation. Two children also developed transient hepatosplenomegaly.

Deafness may be present from birth, usually in children who have other manifestations of disease, or may develop as a late sequel which can appear

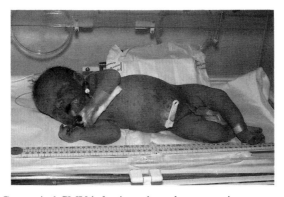

Figure 16.10 Congenital CMV infection: thrombocytopenic purpura

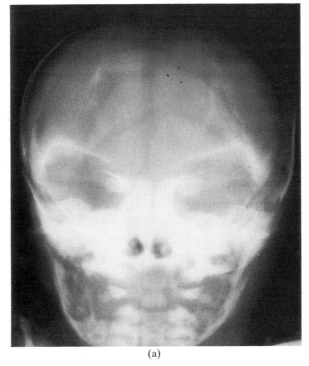

(a)

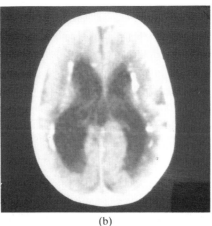

(b)

Figure 16.11 Congenital CMV infection: periventricular calcification and ventricular dilatation shown (a) on skull radiograph; (b) on computerized tomographic scan of brain

in the first five years of life. About 6% of babies with congenital CMV become deaf, making it one of the most important causes of hearing loss in children (Reynolds *et al.*, 1974; Hanshaw *et al.*, 1976; Saigal *et al.*, 1982; Kumar *et al.*, 1984b; Preece *et al.*, 1984). Hearing loss apparently results from viral replication in the inner ear (Davis *et al.*, 1979).

Yeager and colleagues (1981) took viral cultures from 51 preterm babies who were in a neonatal intensive care unit for over 28 days: 16 of these 51 infants began excreting the virus at 1–4 months of age (mean 55 days) and 14 of these babies developed respiratory deterioration with added pulmonary shadowing, grey pallor, hepatosplenomegaly and atypical lymphocytosis. These babies had apparently acquired CMV infections from blood transfusions. Such infections can be fatal, and are particularly severe in babies of seronegative mothers.

Diagnosis

No test has 100% sensitivity in diagnosing congenital CMV infection. The newer methods of detecting specific IgM, such as radioimmunoassays and ELISAs, have, however, greatly increased the sensitivity of testing cord or baby's blood. If urine, throat swab or nasopharyngeal aspirate are positive for CMV by culture in the first week of life, this indicates congenital infection. After a week of age the significance of such cultures is not clear, as infection may have been postnatally acquired and virus shedding may continue for months.

Outcome

It has already been implied that appropriate controls must be included in follow-up studies of babies with congenital CMV infection, because the babies often have a disadvantageous social background. Well-controlled studies now suggest that ∼ 10% of babies with congenital CMV identified by screening at birth will have major neurodevelopmental sequelae. The risk is highest in babies who are symptomatic at birth but sequelae may occur in babies with inapparent infection. Mental retardation, spastic quadriplegia and deafness are the main problems, but visual impairment may result from chorioretinitis or optic atrophy.

All babies with congenital CMV infection should be followed up until at least school entry and hearing tests performed regularly to detect late deafness.

Treatment

There are now two drugs available with confirmed efficacy against CMV, namely ganciclovir and foscarnet. Neither of these drugs has been evaluated in babies, and it would be hard to justify their use except perhaps in babies with life-threatening CMV pneumonitis.

Prevention

Screening of pregnant women will not prevent all congenital CMV infections, as cases occur in all trimesters and with recurrences as well as primary infections. Furthermore, the risk to an infected fetus is fairly low, so even if prenatal fetal infection could be reliably diagnosed, many terminations would be of healthy fetuses. It seems hard to justify screening pregnant women for CMV.

At present there is little prospect of a successful vaccine. Although attenuated CMV vaccines have been used in renal transplant patients, the vaccine strain may be able to remain latent and could be oncogenic. Genetically engineered vaccines using viral proteins but no viral DNA are a possibility, but it is not known which proteins will induce protective antibody and cell-mediated immune responses.

Yeager *et al.* (1981) showed that blood transfusion-acquired CMV infection could be prevented by using only blood from a panel of regularly tested donors who were known to be seronegative to CMV. An alternative approach is to use blood which has been filtered to remove leucocytes, because virus is mainly cell-associated, and this approach reduced acquired CMV infection from 21% to zero in one study of neonates (Gilbert *et al.*, 1989).

Staff and CMV

There are conflicting data on whether female staff working with babies are at increased risk of CMV infection, although the weight of evidence suggests that they probably are at moderately increased risk of primary infection. This is of obvious concern, as many such staff are of childbearing age. Ahlfors *et al.* (1981) found that Swedish nurses were not at increased risk for primary CMV or for having a baby with congenital infection. Dworsky *et al.* (1983) similarly found no added risk for health care professionals in Alabama. In contrast, in a small study Yeager (1975) found an annual seroconversion rate of 4.1% for Denver neonatal intensive care nurses and 7.7% for general paediatric nurses, but none of 27 staff without patient contact seroconverted. Haneberg *et al.* (1980) found that 9.4% of student nurses in Norway seroconverted after a 2-month paediatric rotation. Friedman *et al.* (1984) in Philadelphia found that 10.9% of intensive care nurses, 18.2% of the venesection/intravenous team, 3.7% of the medical and surgical ward nurses and 2.9% of staff without patient contact seroconverted in a year.

Haldane and colleagues (1968) collected data by questionnaire and found a higher rate of congenital anomalies in babies of nurses working with infants than those working with older patients or off work. However, Ahlfors *et al.* (1981) could find no such increased risk.

Should female nursing, medical and paramedical staff be screened for CMV antibody status? The objection to this is the same as that to screening all pregnant women; it is difficult to know what advice could usefully be given to seronegative pregnant women or what course of action to take, should such a woman seroconvert during pregnancy. A Manchester special care baby unit which adopted a policy of screening staff and advising that seronegative pregnant women should not care for babies with known or suspected CMV infection, abandoned the policy after 18 months. They felt that it was a disaster, having served little useful purpose and generated all sorts of public relation, psychological and management problems (Young *et al.*, 1983). One of the prerequisites of a screening programme is that there should be a clearly accepted course of action for managing those at risk, and screening staff for CMV antibody status does not fulfil these criteria.

Chapter 17

Surveillance in the neonatal unit

Introduction

'Surveillance' is a term frequently used in the neonatal unit. Resistant organisms are frequently selected by the extensive use of antibiotics and may be transmitted from baby to baby. Traditional practice has been to perform routine bacterial and fungal culture of various sites from most or all babies on the neonatal unit, so-called 'surveillance cultures'; these would be performed at least once a week.

The rationale for performing frequent surveillance cultures is really two-fold. One intention is to know which organisms are colonizing an individual baby so that, if the baby develops systemic sepsis, appropriate antibiotic therapy based on the colonizing organisms can be started. The second aim of surveillance cultures is to identify resistant organisms that have spread from baby to baby, so that infection control measures can be introduced or reinforced to prevent spread and so that antibiotic policies can, if necessary, be changed if colonization is widespread.

In many neonatal units a large number of surveillance cultures is performed at great expense in time and cost. The advisability of these cultures has been questioned (Fulginiti and Ray, 1988).

Do surveillance cultures predict the organisms causing systemic sepsis?

Early studies suggested that babies with abnormal pharyngeal colonization, defined as a heavy growth of Gram-negative bacilli, *Staphylococcus aureus*, *S. epidermidis* or other organisms (*Haemophilus*, enterococci, yeasts) from throat swabs were the only babies who developed late-onset or nosocomial sepsis (Sprunt *et al.*, 1978). Babies with 'normal flora' (defined as no growth, a light growth, or alpha-haemolytic streptococci as the predominant organism), did not develop sepsis. Most of the babies who developed sepsis had required endotracheal intubation for hyaline membrane disease; we are not told what proportion of the controls required intubation, so the authors may merely have been describing an epiphenomenon in a high-risk group.

It is, perhaps, not surprising that intubated babies develop septicaemia. Storm (1980) showed that a transient bacteraemia lasting < 10 min occurred in three of 10 intubated babies during routine suctioning of the endotracheal tube. We, among others, have shown that most babies who develop late-onset sepsis are preterm babies receiving mechanical ventilation (Isaacs *et al.*, 1987a).

Harris *et al.* (1976) and Sprunt *et al.* (1978) found a close correlation between the organisms colonizing the oropharynx or endotracheal tube and the organisms causing subsequent sepsis. However, recent papers have tended to show that surveillance cultures are poorly predictive of the organisms responsible for systemic sepsis. Slagle *et al.* (1989) found that routine endotracheal cultures were poorly predictive of the organisms causing septicaemia and often misleading. Evans *et al.* (1988) analysed > 24 000 cultures taken from 3000 babies over 3 years: they found that the maximum sensitivity of cultures from ear, nasopharynx, axilla, umbilicus, groin, rectum, stomach and endotracheal tube in predicting the organisms causing sepsis was only 56%, with a specificity of 82%; only one in 30 babies with suspected sepsis proved to have true sepsis. Webber *et al.* (1990) found that endotracheal and nasopharyngeal cultures predicted the organism or organisms obtained from blood cultures in only one of seven babies with late-onset pneumonia and septicaemia.

It is not clear why there has been an apparent change in the value of surveillance cultures for predicting the organisms causing sepsis. It may be a facet of the increasingly invasive procedures needed to care for very preterm babies, including the use of central venous catheters, which have altered the possible routes of entry of organisms and increased the likelihood of catheter-associated organisms such as *S. epidermidis*. Whatever the reason for the change, surveillance cultures have been described by Fulginiti and Ray (1988) as 'an exercise in futility, wastefulness and inappropriate practice'. This would certainly appear true for predicting sepsis in an individual baby and we have argued already (Chapter 5) that the choice of antibiotics for a baby should be based on a unit antibiotic policy, itself based on episodes of sepsis, rather than on the organisms colonizing that baby.

Do surveillance cultures help in managing outbreaks?

If surveillance of cultures from surface and deep sites is not predictive of sepsis in an individual baby, it may be important to know what organisms are circulating on the neonatal unit, their sensitivity patterns and whether there is a lot of spread from baby to baby. Organisms may be colonizing the upper respiratory tract, skin or bowel and enter the bloodstream via the respiratory tract, for which endotracheal intubation is the most obvious risk factor, through the skin through local trauma or intravascular cannulas, particularly longstanding cannulas, or through the bowel wall, particularly where there has been necrosis as in NEC. Full surveillance cultures might then include cultures of nasopharyngeal or endotracheal secretions, skin and faeces. One of the main problems is that multiple organisms of varying sensitivities are usually present in each of these sites.

We have found that surveillance cultures do have a limited value in telling us which organisms are prevalent. We would not change the unit antibiotic policy because of widespread colonization with resistant organisms without episodes of systemic sepsis (Chapter 5). We did, however, find at one time that six preterm babies requiring artificial ventilation were colonized with gentamicin-resistant *Klebsiella oxytoca*. We have shown previously that this is the highest risk group for developing late sepsis (Isaacs *et al.*, 1987a). When two of the six babies developed septicaemia with gentamicin-resistant *Klebsiella oxytoca*, we changed our antibiotic regimen for suspected late sepsis from flucloxacillin and gentamicin to flucloxacillin and netilmicin (Isaacs *et al.*, 1988a). It was certainly helpful, when making the decision to change the antibiotic policy, to know the colonization status of the other high-risk babies. On the other hand, the same information could rapidly have been obtained by culturing endotracheal secretions from intubated babies only when there was an apparent outbreak of systemic sepsis.

Cultures for early-onset sepsis

Although these are not strictly surveillance cultures, it has become routine to collect cultures from a number of different sites in babies with suspected early-onset sepsis. As the babies with systemic sepsis are usually those most heavily colonized, all these superficial and deep cultures tend to be positive when a baby has systemic sepsis (Webber *et al.*, 1990). Thus, it should be possible to cut down on the number of such cultures without increasing the risk of missing those babies with negative blood and CSF cultures who are colonized with a pathogen such as group B streptococcus or *Listeria* (Chapter 5).

Cultures for new admissions

In many neonatal units it is standard practice to take multiple cultures from babies admitted to the unit. This may be confined to babies transferred from other hospitals or may include all inborn babies admitted to the neonatal unit.

We certainly take cultures from babies transferred to the unit from another hospital, because the baby may be colonized with an organism such as MRSA, with important implications for its management. If this proves to be the case, we isolate the baby if possible or at least reinforce the importance of hand-washing after handling the baby. On the other hand, we do not routinely take cultures from inborn babies unless they are suspected of being septic.

Which cultures are useful?

After 4 years of carefully documented experience using multiple cultures for suspected early and late sepsis, and only moderately restricted surveillance cultures, we came to a similar, if slightly less extreme, conclusion to that of Fulginiti and Ray (1988). We decreased the number of cultures for suspected early and late sepsis (Table 17.1). We also decreased surveillance cultures, from thrice-weekly endotracheal and nasopharyngeal cultures

Table 17.1 Investigations for suspected sepsis: cultures performed

Before 1988	After 1988	
Early and late onset	Early onset	Late onset
Throat		
Nose		
Ear		
Umbilicus	Ear	Endotracheal/nasopharyngeal
Endotracheal	Throat	Urine
Rectum	CSF	CSF
Urine	Blood	Blood
CSF		
Blood		

from all preterm babies who were being or had been artificially ventilated, to once-weekly endotracheal tube cultures from babies on mechanical ventilation. After 2 years we have not experienced any increased problems in monitoring or treating sepsis, nor have we had any babies who relapsed after stopping antibiotics after 48 h (S. Dobson, submitted for publication). We have estimated the annual saving by reducing these cultures to be > £24 000.

Surveillance of systemic sepsis and antibiotic use

Although we have found surveillance cultures to be of limited use in managing infections, on the other hand we have found it extremely helpful to monitor episodes of systemic sepsis and antibiotic use.

The system that has been devised in the John Radcliffe Hospital, Oxford, in conjunction with Dr Andrew Wilkinson, the senior neonatologist, is for one infectious disease specialist to perform a weekly ward round with the junior staff, which lasts ~ 2 h. All microbiology reports are seen by a junior doctor, signed and filed in alphabetical order of the baby's name in a box file (Figure 17.1). They are not filed in the babies' case notes until they have been seen and signed by the infectious disease specialist on the weekly ward round, who therefore has immediate access to the whole week's results.

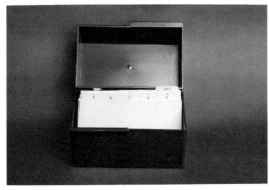

Figure 17.1 Box used for culture results

On the weekly ward round, and by reviewing after the ward round the case notes of babies discharged from the unit during the week, the infectious disease doctor records episodes of systemic sepsis and other infections, contaminants of blood or CSF and antibiotic use on a standard proforma (Figure 17.2). Infections and contaminants are defined as in Appendix 1. The number of baby-days and antibiotic baby-days are recorded, as well as the level of intensive care, as defined by the British Paediatric Association (1984) and shown in Appendix 2; we have used this as a marker of workload and found it to correlate with the spread of organisms (Isaacs

Week ending ....

NAME	DAYS	MAX CARE	ET TUBE CULTURES				CULTURES FROM OTHER SITES			CONTAMINANTS			INFECTION			ANTIBIOTICS	
		3 Int; 2 Spe 1 Ord	Organism	Sens	Pus cells		Organism	Sens	Site*	Organism	Site*	D:Def; P:Prob	Age at onset (full days)	Infection + organism (line-assoc or not)	Individual antibiotics x no of days	Antibiotic days

| | | | | | | | | | | | | | | | | |

| TOTAL BABY DAYS | | | | | | | |
| NO OF BABIES REQUIR-ING LEVEL 3 CARE | | | Int = Intensive / Spec = Special / Ord = Ordinary | | | *Site U = Urine O = Umbilicus NP = Nasopharynx S = Skin E = Ear I = Eye R = Rectum B = Blood C = CSF | |

Figure 17.2 Standard proforma for recording information on infections and antibiotic use

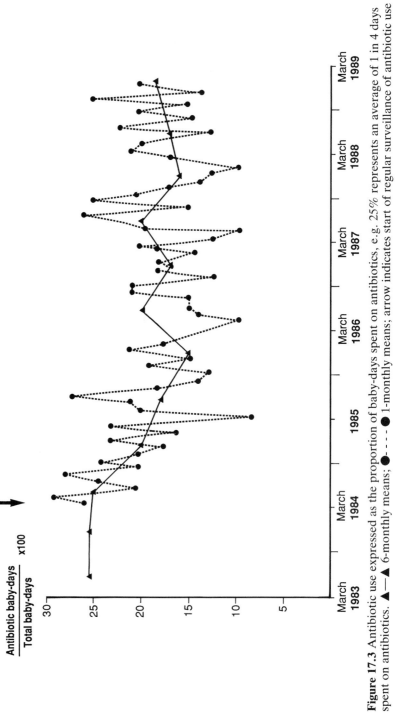

Figure 17.3 Antibiotic use expressed as the proportion of baby-days spent on antibiotics, e.g. 25% represents an average of 1 in 4 days spent on antibiotics. ▲——▲ 6-monthly means; ●- - - ● 1-monthly means; arrow indicates start of regular surveillance of antibiotic use

et al., 1988a). The ward round acts as a teaching round on neonatal infections and as an opportunity to collect data. It also reminds junior staff to consider stopping antibiotics after 2–3 days when cultures are negative. When the ward rounds were started in April 1984, the unit antibiotic policy was, as it is now, to stop antibiotics if systemic cultures were negative unless there was either pneumonia or suspected early sepsis associated with heavy colonization with group B streptococcus, *listeria* or another likely pathogen. In practice, however, antibiotics were often continued and at the start of surveillance the median duration of antibiotic courses was 5 days and on average a baby spent 1 in 4 days on antibiotics (Figure 17.3). The same average antibiotic use had occurred in the previous year. Within 2 years of starting infectious disease ward rounds, the median duration of antibiotic courses was 2 days, as it has remained (Isaacs *et al.*, 1987c). The proportion of baby-days spent on antibiotics had fallen from the previous level of 25% and, although there was great fluctuation in antibiotic use from month to month, when examined over 6-month intervals antibiotic use has remained constant at 15–20% of baby-days (Figure 17.3). This represents a substantial saving in antibiotic costs and in not having to perform serum aminoglycoside assays, which are generally done only if antibiotics are continued for > 3 days. The infectious disease doctor maintains a close liaison with the microbiology department on the significance of blood culture isolates, antibiotic treatment and general policy.

We regularly review the organisms using sepsis and the outcome of episodes of sepsis at a 6-monthly meeting. This allows us to be aware rapidly of changing patterns of sepsis (Chapter 1) and of whether our antibiotic policy is appropriate or is resulting in increased morbidity or mortality.

We would recommend this system of monitoring or 'surveillance' of infections and antibiotic use as being simple, cheap, economical of time and highly educational for the infectious disease doctors as well, it is hoped, as for the junior staff.

Chapter 18

Prevention

Introduction

In view of the high mortality and morbidity of neonatal infections, prevention of such infections should have a high priority. Reference to this has been made in many of the chapters on specific infections, but this chapter examines more general aspects of prevention.

Congenital intrauterine infections

Immunization is arguably the single most effective preventative measure available to doctors. Immunization of mothers against rubella has the potential to eliminate congenital rubella syndrome, while maternal immunization against tetanus could prevent neonatal tetanus. When immunizations are not available, as for toxoplasmosis and CMV infection, other strategies of prevention need to be considered. Serological screening programmes for pregnant women for toxoplasmosis have been introduced in France and their possible use in other countries may be considered in future.

Any maternal illness in the first trimester of pregnancy should be taken seriously, and serological tests for toxoplasma, rubella and CMV, if clinically indicated, may help to identify at-risk pregnancies. Antenatal diagnosis of fetal infections using fetal blood samples or cordocentesis is increasingly possible, and counselling based on the state of knowledge can then be offered.

Early-onset infections

We have discussed under the relevant headings the prevention of infections due to group B streptococci (GBS) and *Listeria*. Screening of pregnant women for GBS carriage, by culturing either cervical secretions or urine, can identify high-risk pregnancies. Maternal *Listeria* infection is often undiagnosed clinically, but dietary advice may allow women to reduce their risk of contracting *Listeria* infection during pregnancy.

When women in labour have risk factors for neonatal infection (fever, prolonged membrane rupture, premature onset of labour) it may be decided to start them on antibiotic therapy. Although this is the obstetrician's decision, paediatricians should not be slow in pointing out that there is sound evidence that intrapartum ampicillin (2 g i.v. at once and 1 g i.v. 4-hourly until delivery) reduces maternal and neonatal GBS infection

(Boyer and Gotoff, 1986) and it may also reduce the severity of neonatal listeriosis. Ampicillin is probably effective cover against *H. influenzae* and pneumococcus as well as some Gram-negative organisms, so it seems the antibiotic of choice for intrapartum therapy.

Women who have had a baby with congenital listeriosis are at low risk for their subsequent babies to be infected. This is not true for women who have had a baby with early-onset GBS sepsis, and they should be given intrapartum ampicillin at the above dose from the onset of labour in all subsequent pregnancies.

Late-onset infections

Breast feeding

Human breast milk is protective against gastroenteritis, many respiratory infections including RSV infection and otitis media (Fallot *et al.*, 1980), and necrotizing enterocolitis. Although the advent of HIV infection has complicated the use of milk banks of donated human breast milk, it appears that most donors will agree to being tested for HIV infection as recommended by the DHSS (1989). Women should be strongly encouraged to breast-feed their babies. If the baby is preterm and not sucking, the mother should be given encouragement and assistance in expressing her milk. If she is unable to provide sufficient milk, the use of pasteurized donor breast milk from an HIV-seronegative donor has advantages over artificial milks in protecting against infections.

Early enteral feeding

In our unit at Oxford, enteral feeding has traditionally been introduced very early, even for very preterm babies requiring ventilatory support, because of its importance in stimulating gut hormonal development. This has meant that it has often been possible to maintain babies' nutritional status without resort to central venous catheters and parenteral nutrition, both of which carry an inherent risk of sepsis.

Skin care

There have been worries about systemic absorption of disinfectants, such as hexachlorophane, leading to neurotoxicity; babies are now cleaned at birth by washing with soap and water.

Umbilical cord care

There is little doubt that attention to umbilical cord care was highly important in reducing the incidence of local and systemic staphylococcal infections in the 1950s and 1960s. There is some debate as to the relative merits of various topical antibiotics and antimicrobials including triple dye, gentian violet, bacitracin ointment or powder, and of alcohol to sterilize the cord. What is clear is that, if no cord care is given, we can expect to see a return of serious infections due to *Staphylococcus aureus* and, in the neonatal unit, necrotizing fasciitis due to Gram-positive and Gram-negative organisms (Mason *et al.*, 1989).

Eye care

The use of prophylactic antibiotics to prevent gonococcal and chlamydial conjunctivitis is discussed in Chapter 11. In the UK, prophylactic antibiotics are not given, the occurrence of gonococcal conjunctivitis being used as a marker to treat the baby, the mother and her sexual contacts. Chlamydial conjunctivitis is under-diagnosed, but it may be important to attempt to diagnose it rather than to prevent it, because without systemic erythromycin about one-half of the babies with chlamydial conjunctivitis will develop chlamydial pneumonitis. As the latter presumably follows nasopharyngeal colonization, eye prophylaxis would not prevent pneumonitis but would prevent recognition of at-risk babies.

Invasive procedures

Invasive procedures for monitoring and treating the fetus and newborn baby have become an integral part of obstetric and neonatal care. To a large extent these have been inextricably linked with falling perinatal mortality, but they carry a price in terms of infection.

Fetal scalp monitors should be used with circumspection and care because they may result in scalp abscesses and, very occasionally, osteomyelitis of the skull. They should not be used when there is active herpes simplex virus infection of the cervix or a history of maternal HSV, because neonatal HSV infection has been introduced through fetal scalp monitors.

Umbilical vessel catheterization carries a modest risk of infection, but this is far higher for umbilical venous than for arterial catheters. If umbilical venous catheters are to be used it should be for as short a time as possible. Although infection of umbilical artery catheters is fairly uncommon, infection of peripheral artery catheters is even rarer (Adams *et al.*, 1980) and they may be safer as regards infection.

Bacteraemia or fungaemia complicate the use of central venous catheters in ~10% of patients (Nelson, 1983). Indwelling peripheral venous polyethylene catheters used for prolonged intravenous therapy may become infected in up to 8% of cases (Nelson, 1983). The use of topical antibiotics at the site of catheter entry and the use of prophylactic parenteral antibiotics have no effect on the incidence of bacteraemia (Nelson, 1983).

Heat is generally a more effective disinfectant than solutions and, whenever possible, equipment should be autoclaved rather than using liquid disinfectants. This applies particularly to ventilator tubing, humidifiers and suction equipment, which should be changed and autoclaved regularly. Nebulizer equipment and humidifiers are particularly prone to contamination with water-loving organisms. Closed incubators must be cleaned with disinfectant if they cannot be autoclaved, and an iodophor or quaternary disinfectant is preferable.

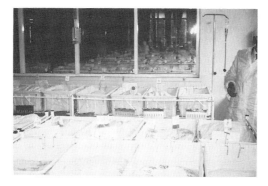

Figure 18.1 Overcrowding in a neonatal unit in China (photograph courtesy of Professor Peter Rolfe). There was an exceptionally high incidence of staphylococcal skin infections

Staffing arrangements

Understaffing and overcrowding (Figure 18.1) have been associated with an increased risk of all nosocomial infections (Goldmann *et al.*, 1981), with spread of gentamicin-resistant Gram-negative bacilli (Isaacs *et al.*, 1988a) and with outbreaks of staphylococcal infection (Haley and Bregman, 1982). The most likely explanation for this is that normal infection control measures such as hand-washing are compromised by increased workload, but whether this is because staff are busy and forget to wash their hands between handling different babies, or whether they do wash their hands but are looking after more babies, is not clear. It seems unlikely that droplet spread is a major mechanism of baby-to-baby transmission.

Spread from sinks seems to be less important than was once thought. Although swabbing sinks will often yield water-loving organisms such as *Pseudomonas* species, in outbreaks of *Pseudomonas* species infection in adult intensive care units the patients are usually infected with different strains from those found in the sink (Morrison and Wenzel, 1984).

Hand-washing

Hand-washing is the single most effective infection-control measure available in the neonatal intensive care unit. Despite this, countless studies have shown that medical staff are extremely poor at washing their hands before handling babies, and that doctors are consistently the worst offenders. Semmelweis, working in Vienna in 1861, noted that women delivered by doctors had an incidence of puerperal fever three times greater than that in women delivered by midwives. When a colleague died from sepsis after cutting his hand performing an autopsy, Semmelweis realized that the doctors were probably transmitting organisms acquired when performing autopsies. He introduced strict hand-washing with chlorine water, and maternal mortality dropped from 12% to 3% within weeks.

Larson (1988) reviewed > 400 articles on hand-washing published from 1879 to 1986 and concluded that there was strong evidence that hand-washing prevents infection. The use of soap and water for 15 s removes most superficial bacteria from hands, while chlorhexidine or iodine-based soaps increase the effectiveness (Sprunt *et al.*, 1973). Alcohol rubs are very effective in preventing spread of viruses (Isaacs *et al.*, 1989). Constant reminders on ward rounds about not leaning on incubators and about washing hands before and after handling babies can help to reduce the spread of organisms.

Management of outbreaks

There are many reports of outbreaks of neonatal infection, often with resistant Gram-negative bacilli, other bacteria, fungi or enteroviruses. In some reports it is clear that a new organism has entered the neonatal unit and spread to many babies, colonizing many and infecting some. In other cases the evidence of a true outbreak is less clear-cut. We have reported previously (Isaacs *et al.*, 1987a) that, when we started surveillance of infections in Oxford, ~ 30% of all babies cultured were colonized with *Pseudomonas aeruginosa*, which was the commonest cause of late-onset sepsis. Nine months later, and without introducing any special infection control measures, we were very rarely able to culture *Pseudomonas* from any of the babies (Figure 18.2). In our opinion, this casts doubt on the validity of expensive infection-control measures, such as bacterial surveillance cultures on all babies and swabbing possible environmental sources such as sinks, unless there is clear evidence of a true outbreak. Babies will inevitably become colonized with one or more organisms, and systemic sepsis with those organisms is likely to occur in babies with multiple risk factors for infection. Our observations (Table 1.5) suggest that approximately the same total number of late-onset infections occur each year, but with different organisms, depending on which are colonizing babies. Thus, the particular virulence of organisms does not appear to be a major factor in determining the incidence of late-onset infection.

We have found a low mortality from late-onset infections. Unless an organism colonizing babies was causing particularly frequent, severe

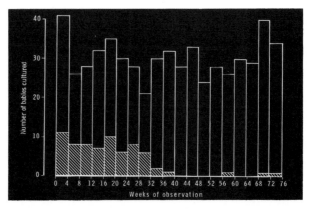

Figure 18.2 Sequential observations on colonization of babies with *Pseudomonas aeruginosa*. Neonatal unit, John Radcliffe Hospital, Oxford, starting May 1984. Shaded areas represent babies colonized with *P. aeruginosa*

infections, we would argue that infection-control measures, other than to reinforce the importance of hand-washing, are of unconfirmed benefit, often expensive and probably unnecessary.

Cohorting

'Cohorting' of staff and babies may be an effective measure if there is documented spread of an organism. Babies known to be colonized or infected are segregated from non-infected babies and cared for only by the same staff, who do not handle non-infected babies, including new admissions. If the staff are ill but still working, they handle only infected babies. In busy neonatal units, where infected babies require varying levels of intensive care, this is rarely a practical proposition.

Isolation

Isolation of babies who are colonized or infected is rarely necessary. The indications for isolation include suspected or confirmed infections with diarrhoeal organisms, rubella, chickenpox, herpes simplex virus, enteroviruses (particularly Coxsackievirus), syphilis and gonorrhoea. *Listeria* has occasionally caused serious nosocomial infections and we routinely isolate mother and baby. Group B streptococci occasionally cause outbreaks but this is rare and, as most colonized babies are not detected because they are never swabbed, we do not isolate babies with GBS colonization or sepsis.

Gloves, gowns and masks

Gloves, gowns and masks need be worn by staff only to prevent neonatal infections during surgical procedures. We do recommend that staff with colds wear masks and that staff feeding babies wear gowns to limit the spread of secretions on clothes.

There is controversy over whether staff need to wear such protective clothing to lessen their own risk of contracting HIV infection (Chapter 15).

Visitors

There are many reasons for allowing free access to relatives and friends to visit babies on the neonatal unit and, fortunately, nosocomial viral infections are fairly uncommon, even in winter (Rudd and Carrington, 1984). We ask visitors to wash their hands to the elbow and to handle their own baby only. We ask family and friends not to visit if they have a respiratory or gastrointestinal infection.

Antibiotic use

We have argued in detail (Chapter 5) that antibiotic use can be, and should be, kept to a minimum. Prolonged use of antibiotics creates 'antibiotic pressure' which selects for resistant organisms and is associated with an increased risk of systemic candidiasis (Weese-Mayer *et al.*, 1987). Antibiotics should not be continued for longer than 2–3 days just because the baby is 'still sick' or has 'lots of lines'. We have shown that, in most instances, antibiotics can safely be stopped after 48–72 h without risk of missing occult infection (Isaacs *et al.*, 1987b). Exceptions are babies with pneumonia and those babies with probable early-onset sepsis who have negative blood, urine and CSF cultures but heavy colonization with a probable pathogen.

Blood products

All human blood products used in the neonatal unit should come from donors who have been screened for antibodies to HIV and hepatitis B virus. Furthermore, the risk of transmitting CMV to babies should be minimized, either by using only blood products from known CMV seronegative donors (Yeager *et al.*, 1981) or by using filtered blood (Gilbert *et al.*, 1989).

Immunoglobulins

The potential ability of oral immunoglobulin preparations rich in IgG and IgA to prevent necrotizing enterocolitis is discussed in Chapter 12.

It has been proved that i.m. immunoglobulin preparations rich in specific antibody are effective in decreasing the severity of neonatal chickenpox (Chapter 15) and can protect against severe measles in older immune-compromised children. Specific immunoglobulin preparations have also been used, with less convincing evidence of efficacy, in attempting to ameliorate infections with group B streptococci (Christensen and Christensen, 1986) and RSV (Prince *et al.*, 1986).

Intravenous immunoglobulin preparations have been given prophylactically to low-birth-weight preterm babies who are at high risk of late infection and have relatively low levels of transplacental antibodies. In a controlled study in Saudi Arabia, a single dose of i.v. immunoglobulin 120 mg/kg given to preterm babies (< 37 weeks' gestation) within 4 h of delivery significantly reduced late-onset infections with Gram-negative organisms (Haque *et al.*, 1986). Chirico *et al.* (1987) in Italy found that weekly infusions of gammaglobulin to babies of < 34 weeks' gestation and babies weighing < 1500 g significantly reduced the incidence of, and mortality from, infection. Both these studies were conducted in countries with a high incidence of late-onset infections and with a high mortality. On the other hand, Stabile *et al.* (1988) found no benefit from giving multiple large doses of an Italian immunoglobulin preparation to preterm babies selected by the same procedure as that of Chirico *et al.* (1987). Studies are in progress in the USA and UK to determine whether improvement in incidence and outcome of late-onset infections is found. Until the results of such studies are known we are not routinely giving immunoglobulins to preterm babies.

Chapter 19

Clinical pharmacology

Introduction

Neonates have been called 'therapeutic orphans' by Shirkey (1970) because of the paucity of data on which their treatment is usually based. In the 1950s they were poisoned with chloramphenicol, which resulted in cardiovascular collapse – the 'grey baby syndrome' (Burns *et al.*, 1959) – and with sulphonamides, which displaced albumin-bound bilirubin and resulted in kernicterus (Silverman *et al.*, 1956). Although neonates are no longer treated therapeutically as miniaturized adults, nevertheless new drugs, including antibiotics, are introduced too often without adequate clinical trials. We believe that new antibiotics should be subjected to large-scale comparative trials in neonates before widespread use. Until such data on safety and efficacy are available, it is generally wise to be conservative. We, therefore, prefer to use antibiotics for which there is considerable experience, even if these drugs have known dose-related toxicity, as is the case for aminoglycosides.

Maternal antibiotics

If the pregnant mother is treated with antibiotics which cross the placenta, the fetus is given antibiotics antenatally. This can be used therapeutically: passage of the drug across the placenta can treat the fetus, as in the treatment of maternal syphilis to treat congenital syphilis. Treatment of the mother may prevent neonatal infection, as in intrapartum administration of ampicillin to prevent early-onset GBS sepsis (Boyer and Gotoff, 1986). However, drugs administered to the pregnant woman can also cause untoward effects to the fetus. Tetracyclines readily cross the placenta and are deposited in fetal bone (Totterman and Saxen, 1969), resulting in impaired bone growth (Cohlan *et al.*, 1963). They are also deposited in the deciduous teeth of the fetus, resulting in later discoloration, enamel hypoplasia and malformation (Kline *et al.*, 1964). Nitrofurantoin and sulphonamides can cause haemolysis if the fetus has glucose-6-phosphate dehydrogenase (G6PD) deficiency and sulphonamides may displace bilirubin, causing hyperbilirubinaemia and possibly kernicterus (Silverman *et al.*, 1956). Chloramphenicol given to the mother near parturition may cause neonatal circulatory collapse (Burns *et al.*, 1959). Aminoglycosides can be ototoxic to the developing fetus: streptomycin can definitely damage the eighth nerve

(Robinson and Cambon, 1964; Conway and Birt, 1965), while kanamycin (Yow *et al.*, 1962; Jones, 1973) and gentamicin (McCracken *et al.*, 1980) are potentially ototoxic.

Most antibiotics do not attain sufficient concentrations in breast milk to be toxic to the breast-fed baby. However, tetracyclines should be avoided for lactating mothers because they may stain the baby's teeth, and sulphonamides (Harley and Robin, 1962) and nalidixic acid (Belton and Jones, 1965) have caused haemolysis in breast-fed babies with G6PD deficiency.

Absorption

Enteral administration of antibiotics is not generally recommended in the newborn period because of poor absorption. For example, serum levels of ampicillin 1 h after oral administration of a 25 mg/kg dose to full-term infants were 2.6–7.2 µg/ml (McCracken *et al.*, 1978) compared with ~ 60 µg/ml 1 h after the same dose given i.v. (Axline *et al.*, 1967; Boe *et al.*, 1967), while oral nafcillin achieves blood levels about one-third of those with i.m. injection (Grossman and Ticknor, 1965). However, if the oral antibiotic achieves levels greatly in excess of the minimum inhibitory concentration (MIC) of the organism, and the response to treatment can be closely monitored, then enteral administration is a reasonable option. Infants of very low birth-weight have erratic absorption of enteral drugs and poor muscle bulk for i.m. injection, so i.v. administration of antibiotics is almost always indicated (Prober *et al.*, 1990).

Administration

Although relatively small doses of antibiotics are appropriate for neonates, antibiotics are often available only in vials for adult use, which require diluting. This can result in critical errors: in the study by Mulhall *et al.* (1983b) severe toxicity from chloramphenicol occurred due to errors in calculating the dilution factor. Even when the manufacturers produce a neonatal formulation, this is calculated as an appropriate dose for a full-term infant, but the dose for an infant of very low birth-weight may be considerably lower; either a very small volume has to be given or the antibiotic must be diluted further.

Antibiotics are usually administered to neonates i.v. in small volumes and cannot be diluted too much, or flushed through too vigorously, because of the low total feed volume, the need for calories and the danger of over-hydration; delivery systems must therefore minimize dead space in syringes and tubing (Rajchgot *et al.*, 1983).

Distribution

Antibiotics will become distributed in body tissues; the body can be considered as compartments comprising water, fat and protein. Hydrophilic drugs will distribute preferentially to the water compartment, hydrophobic drugs to fat and heavily protein-bound drugs to protein. In the full-term newborn, water comprises $\sim 75\%$ of body-weight, with extracellular water $\sim 40\%$ of body-weight. At 28 weeks' gestation, however, total water is $\sim 85\%$ and extracellular water $\sim 65\%$ of body-weight. After birth, total body water falls by up to 15% within 5 days (Prober *et al.*, 1990).

Body fat is $\sim 13\%$ by weight of a full-term infant but only 4% of a 1500 g baby and 1% of a 500 g baby. However, feeding leads to a rapid accretion of fat which comprises up to 30% of the baby's weight gain.

These variations in body composition indicate the difficulty in predicting drug disposition and the need for repeated assessments of serum levels of toxic drugs such as aminoglycosides.

Protein binding

Many drugs are bound to serum proteins such as albumin, but the biological significance of this is uncertain. For example, although it is often stated that protein-bound antibiotics have little or no antibacterial activity, dicloxacillin is 98% protein bound yet is no less effective than methicillin, which is 37% bound (McCracken and Freij, 1990). Sulphonamides (Silverman *et al.*, 1956) and some of the third-generation cephalosporins (Robertson *et al.*, 1988) bind avidly to albumin, will displace bilirubin from binding sites and potentially can cause hyperbilirubinaemia.

The serum albumin is lower in full-term infants than later in childhood, and lower still in preterm infants. The resulting increase in unbound drug may result in greater therapeutic efficacy and toxicity. Serum proteins rise with nutrition and with transfusions of blood or plasma.

Metabolism

The liver is the main organ involved in metabolism of antibiotics, by way of microsomal enzyme systems. Non-synthetic hepatic biotransformation reactions, hydrolysis, hydroxylation, oxidation and reduction, are all diminished in newborn compared with older children (Prober *et al.*, 1990). Of the synthetic biotransformation reactions, conjugation to glucuronide which is the commonest conjugation pathway, is poor in neonates, whereas conjugation to sulphate and glycine is 'normal'. Oxidation and glucuronidation are the two metabolic pathways in which neonatal function is lowest compared with older children and adults. After 2–12 weeks, hepatic metabolism becomes more efficient. Lower doses of chloramphenicol are needed in neonates because of slow maturation in glucuronidation: the glucuronide form is inactive.

Excretion

Drugs are excreted mainly by the kidneys or in the bile; the former is the most important route of excretion and the better studied. Renal excretion of drugs is mediated by filtration by the glomeruli and by reabsorption and secretion by the renal tubules. The glomerular filtration rate (GFR) at term is ~ 25% of the adult value, and at 28 weeks' gestation is ~ 15% (Aperia and Zetterstrom, 1982; Guignard and John, 1986). The GFR increases rapidly within 3 days of birth, but remains relatively low in preterm infants; it increases over several weeks and is directly related to postconceptional age (Oh, 1981). Drugs such as the aminoglycosides and vancomycin, which are excreted by glomerular filtration, should therefore be given less frequently the more immature is the baby. The GFR doubles by 2 weeks of age in term infants and dose intervals can be reduced, but this may not be appropriate for babies of very low birth-weight (Prober et al., 1990).

Tubular reabsorption and secretion have been less well studied than GFR. Penicillins may be cleared slowly because their excretion depends on tubular secretion, which matures slower than GFR (Besunder et al., 1988). However, tubular reabsorption is also low in neonates and some antibiotics may be excreted more rapidly. Weak bases are likely to be excreted more quickly, particularly by preterm infants, because acidification of the urine is relatively poor. Biliary excretion has not been intensively studied in neonates. Bile stasis is a recognized complication of total parenteral nutrition and also occurs in babies of very low birth-weight. Drugs or metabolites excreted through bile might be expected to accumulate in babies with bile stasis.

Specific drugs

For dosage schedules refer to Appendix 3.

Penicillins

Penicillins interfere with bacterial cell-wall mucopeptide synthesis, and block the cross-linking reaction which gives the bacterial peptidoglycan its rigidity. They bind to bacteria through penicillin-binding proteins in the cell wall. Gram-positive organisms exposed to beta-lactam antibiotics (penicillins and cephalosporins) release lipoteichoic acid from the cell wall and this apparently contributes to cell lysis. If the concentration of antibiotic is increased above a critical level there is a reduced bactericidal effect *in vitro* on Gram-positive organisms (the Eagle phenomenon); the relevance of this *in vivo* is unknown.

Organisms are inherently resistant to penicillins if the structure of their cell wall differs from the classic structure, as in the case of mycobacteria. Staphylococci, many Gram-negative bacilli and gonococci can produce beta-lactamases which degrade the beta-lactam ring common to all penicillins, which Greenwood (1989) has called their Achilles' heel. Coliforms may also produce acylases, which have variable action against penicillins and cephalosporins. Both Gram-positive and Gram-negative bacteria may be inhibited but not killed by beta-lactam antibiotics: these *persisters* will multiply when the antibiotic is stopped. *Tolerance* to penicillins, the phenomenon of inhibition greatly exceeding killing, is exhibited by some strains of staphylococci and streptococci. However these phenomena occurring *in vitro* are of uncertain clinical significance.

Penicillin is the antibiotic of choice for infections attributable to group B streptococcus, pneumococcus and most other streptococci, with the important exception of the faecal streptococci. It is the only effective treatment for congenital syphilis. Penicillin G is active also against *Listeria*, although there is more experience with ampicillin. It is active against most anaerobes except *Bacteroides fragilis*.

Penicillin G is poorly absorbed when given orally. After parenteral administration the half-life is inversely correlated with birth-weight and postnatal age: in the first week after birth the half-life of aqueous (crystalline) penicillin G is 1.5 h at term but 10 h in babies weighing <1500 g (McCracken and Freij, 1990). Procaine penicillin G produces serum levels > 25 times the MIC of group B streptococci, 24 h after a dose of 50 000 units/kg has been given to a full-term infant < 1 week old (McCracken *et al.*, 1973). The clearance of penicillin increases with increasing postnatal age. Benzathine penicillin G gives peak concentrations 12–24 h after a single dose and serum levels equal to the MIC of group B streptococcus at 12 days (McCracken and Freij, 1990). There is evidence *in vitro*, but none *in vivo*, of synergy between penicillin and aminoglycosides.

Penicillin G does not penetrate well into the CSF, even if the baby has bacterial meningitis. Peak CSF levels are 2–5% of serum levels but still exceed the MIC of group B streptococci by a factor of 50. The recommended daily dose for group B streptococcal meningitis is 150 000–250 000 units/kg (see Appendix 3).

Ampicillin

Ampicillin is more active *in vitro* than penicillin G against enterococci (faecal streptococci), *Listeria monocytogenes* and some Gram-negative organisms, e.g. *E. coli*, *Proteus*, *Salmonella*. On the other hand, penicillin G is more active than ampicillin against group B streptococcus and other streptococci (pneumococcus, group A streptococcus).

Oral absorption of ampicillin is fairly good in well, full-term babies, achieving serum levels 2–24 times lower than after parenteral administration (Grossman and Ticknor, 1965; McCracken *et al.*, 1978). There is little information on oral absorption of ampicillin by sick and pre-term babies, to whom oral ampicillin should not be given. CSF penetration of ampicillin is slightly better than that of penicillin G, particularly if the meninges are inflamed.

The advantage of ampicillin over penicillin G for empirical therapy of suspected early-onset sepsis is its somewhat broader spectrum. This is also a disadvantage, as ampicillin is more likely to select for colonization with *Candida* and Gram-negative enteric organisms (Tullus and Burman, 1989). Oral ampicillin can cause diarrhoea, which is less commonly seen following parenteral administration. Ampicillin very occasionally causes rashes in neonates. Mild blood eosinophilia may develop.

Antistaphylococcal penicillins

The antistaphylococcal penicillins are semi-synthetic penicillins with a side chain that protects against binding of beta-lactamases. Flucloxacillin and cloxacillin have been widely used in the United Kingdom but there are no pharmacokinetic data for their use in neonates. Flucloxacillin is better absorbed enterally than cloxacillin by older children and adults. Oral naf-cillin gives serum levels about one-third of those after intramuscular use (Grossman and Ticknor, 1965). Clinical experience suggests that oral flu-cloxacillin may be used successfully to complete a course of treatment, as for example when treating bullous impetigo in term babies without bacterae-mia: we give 2–3 days of parenteral flucloxacillin followed by 4–5 days of oral flucloxacillin. However, this is done in the absence of sound pharmaco-logical or epidemiological data.

Oxacillin and methicillin are very poorly absorbed enterally and are only given parenterally. The pharmacokinetics of methicillin, oxacillin and naf-cillin are similar to those of penicillin G in terms of half-life, increased clearance after the first postnatal week and with increasing postnatal age, and decreased clearance with lower birth-weight (McCracken and Siegel, 1983). The antistaphylococcal agents all achieve CSF levels about 1.4–2% of serum levels when administered parenterally to rabbits with experimental meningitis (Strasbaugh *et al.*, 1980). There are no data on CSF penetration in neonates.

The antistaphylococcal penicillins are active against sensitive *Staphylo-coccus aureus* and coagulase-negative staphylococci. They also have good activity against most penicillin-sensitive organisms such as streptococci, so it is not usually necessary to prescribe penicillin and flucloxacillin simul-taneously. They have poor activity against *Treponema pallidum* and against anaerobes. Some strains of staphylococci are found to be 'tolerant' *in vitro*, in that the MBC greatly exceeds the MIC. Although this might suggest that organisms could be inhibited but not killed by flucloxacillin, there is little evidence to suggest that resistance attributable to tolerance is a signifi-cant clinical problem, except perhaps in endocarditis. On the other hand, multiply-resistant strains of *S. aureus* and *S. epidermidis* that are resistant to antistaphylococcal penicillins are an increasing problem (Chapter 13). Stud-ies *in vitro* suggest synergy between antistaphylococcal penicillins and ami-noglycosides, but the only clinical evidence is that *S. aureus* bacteraemia due to endocarditis in adult drug addicts resolves more quickly with nafcillin and gentamicin than with nafcillin alone (Korzeniowski and Sande, 1982).

There is very little toxicity with these drugs. Very occasionally they may cause neutropenia and drug eruptions.

Other penicillins

Ticarcillin, the thienyl variant of carbenicillin, and the ureidopenicillins, azlocillin, mezlocillin and piperacillin, are the only penicillins with signifi-cant antipseudomonal activity.

Cephalosporins

The cephalosporins are antibiotics derived from cephalosporin C, which itself is a natural product of the *Cephalosporium* mould. Although they contain a beta-lactam ring, they are relatively resistant to the action of beta-lactamases. Their main mode of action is by interfering with bacterial cell-wall synthesis.

Cephalosporin C was never marketed. The 'first generation' of cephalosporins, cephalothin and cephaloridine, were susceptible to Gram-negative beta-lactamases, had variable nephrotoxicity and have been superseded for the treatment of systemic infections. The 'second generation' cephalosporins include cefuroxime and cefoxitin, which are still used in neonatal infections. They are more stable to beta-lactamases and have a broad spectrum of activity against staphylococci, streptococci and some Gram-negative organisms. The 'third generation' cephalosporins, however, are almost completely stable to beta-lactamases. They have a broad spectrum of activity, although they are not the antibiotics of choice for staphylococcal or streptococcal infections. Cefotaxime is widely used in neonatal infections, but has little activity against *Pseudomonas*. Ceftazidime has by far the best antipseudomonal activity. Ceftriaxone has the longest half-life, but can displace bilirubin from albumin *in vitro* (Robertson *et al.*, 1988). Moxalactam is strictly an oxacephem, having an oxygen instead of a sulphur in its ring. It has more activity against anaerobes. It, too, can displace albumin-bound bilirubin, but also interferes with vitamin K metabolism and can cause bleeding, which is a major drawback for preterm babies who are at risk of intraventricular haemorrhage. Ceftizoxime and cefmenoxime are similar to cefotaxime. Cefoperazone has antipseudomonal activity but its activity against other organisms is otherwise less than that of cefotaxime. The cephalosporins have no activity against *Listeria* or enterococci (faecal streptococci).

The third-generation cephalosporins have excellent CSF penetration, even in the absence of meningeal inflammation (McCracken and Nelson, 1983); when meningitis is present, the CSF level is 10–30% of serum levels for moxalactam (Schaad *et al.*, 1981) and 27–63% for cefotaxime (Kafetzis *et al.*, 1982). However, they have not had the anticipated dramatic effect on morbidity and mortality of bacterial meningitis (McCracken *et al.*, 1984) and a recent report has suggested that cefotaxime therapy may be associated with a high rate of relapse (Anderson and Gilbert, 1990).

The second- and third-generation cephalosporins are safe and generally well tolerated by neonates, with the exceptions already outlined regarding bilirubin displacement and interference with vitamin K metabolism leading to hypoprothrombinaemia. Renal toxicity has not been a significant problem for neonates. Drug levels do not need to be monitored, which is a significant advantage. Some workers have found that rapid selection of resistant organisms occurs after the introduction of third-generation cephalosporins (Modi *et al.*, 1987) whereas others have used them for years without selection for resistant strains (Spritzer *et al.*, 1990): the difference may be in the duration of antibiotic 'courses' used in the institutions.

Vancomycin

Vancomycin is a complex heterocyclic molecule classified as a glycopeptide antibiotic, and unrelated to the aminoglycosides. The molecule is too large to penetrate Gram-negative bacteria and vancomycin is active only against Gram-positive bacteria. Teichoplanin, a related glycopeptide, is an experimental antibiotic with similar activity. Vancomycin was originally used in the 1950s to treat penicillin-resistant staphylococci and gained a reputation for toxicity. This was largely attributable to impurities, which have now been removed. It was reintroduced in 1978 because of MRSA. It acts by interfering with cell-wall synthesis and inhibiting RNA synthesis. It is excreted renally and is not metabolized.

Vancomycin is active against *Staphylococcus aureus* and coagulase-negative staphylococci, streptococci and Gram-positive anaerobes, including *Clostridium difficile*, but not Gram-negative organisms. It is currently the treatment of choice for infections with methicillin-resistant strains of *S. aureus* and *S. epidermidis*. It is not absorbed orally but can be given enterally to treat staphylococcal enterocolitis and *C. difficile* diarrhoea. When given parenterally it must be infused slowly over at least 30 min, because faster infusions can cause an erythematous rash over the head and upper trunk, the 'red man syndrome'. If this rash does develop it can be abolished by slowing the infusion rate. Vancomycin is potentially nephrotoxic and ototoxic, and drug levels must be monitored. CSF levels are 10–15% of serum levels in shunt infections with mild inflammation (Schaad *et al.*, 1980). Vancomycin can be given into a ventricular reservoir (such as a Rickham reservoir) in severe or persistent shunt infections, but may itself cause a chemical ventriculitis.

Aminoglycosides

The first aminoglycoside, streptomycin, was discovered in 1943. Since then, various related antibiotics have been described: the aminoglycosides with 'mycin' (e.g. kanamycin) come from the mould *Streptomyces* while those with 'micin' (e.g. gentamicin) come from *Micromonospora* species. The exact mode of action is uncertain: streptomycin acts by binding to a ribosomal protein, whereas the other aminoglycosides appear to alter the bacterial mRNA, causing production of defective proteins (Greenwood, 1989).

The main activity of aminoglycosides is against Gram-negative organisms. However, their weak activity against staphylococci and streptococci may be clinically important because they act synergistically, at least *in vitro*, with penicillins.

Resistance to aminoglycosides is mainly attributable to plasmid-mediated enzymes which interfere with drug transport into the bacteria. Bacteria with resistance to one aminoglycoside due to a plasmid may be resistant also to one or more of the other aminoglycosides. If an organism resistant to only one aminoglycoside is selected by antibiotic pressure and is causing sepsis, the resistant organism can often be eradicated by changing the antibiotic policy to use a different aminoglycoside (Raz *et al.*, 1987; Isaacs *et al.*, 1988a).

There is relatively little evidence of significant nephrotoxicity and ototoxicity in neonates (Buchanan, 1985), even in babies accidentally overdosed with gentamicin (Fuquay *et al.*, 1981) and neonates may be relatively resistant to toxic effects of aminoglycosides. Combinations of aminoglycosides, e.g. tobramycin and gentamicin, or amikacin and gentamicin, are more toxic to the vestibular nerve than is single-drug therapy (Eviatar and Eviatar, 1982). Gentamicin accumulates in the body of neonates (probably in the kidneys) even if serum levels are kept within the recommended ranges, as it does in adults, particularly when treatment is for > 7 days (Assael *et al.*, 1980). Thus it is advisable to stop aminoglycosides as early as possible. For example, if an aminoglycoside is being used for its synergistic activity with penicillin to treat babies with GBS sepsis, the aminoglycoside should be stopped when the baby shows sustained improvement, and certainly by 7 days. Frusemide can potentiate aminoglycoside toxicity and other drugs should be used in preference to aminoglycosides if frusemide is prescribed.

Monitoring of serum aminoglycoside levels has been strongly recommended for all babies receiving these antibiotics. Buchanan (1985) has advocated a more selective approach because of their low toxicity to neonates. He suggests measuring levels only in certain high-risk situations: these include babies with renal dysfunction, babies responding poorly to therapy for a sensitive organism, babies on prolonged therapy, babies receiving two aminoglycosides simultaneously, and babies also receiving frusemide. Babies weighing < 1500 g should also be included because their renal immaturity and variable fluid balance result in unpredictable aminoglycoside pharmacokinetics (McCracken and Siegel, 1983). Indeed, most paediatricians would routinely monitor aminoglycoside levels in all babies requiring > 48 h therapy.

Gentamicin, netilmicin, amikacin and tobramycin are widely used in neonates. There is relatively little to choose between them: tobramycin has more activity against *Pseudomonas*, whereas amikacin is preferred for *Serratia* infections. They are poorly absorbed enterally and are administered i.m., by slow i.v. injection or by i.v. infusion. Intravenous boluses are not recommended because of the possibility of very high levels being toxic. CSF penetration is poor, even in meningitis, yet the combination of ampicillin and an aminoglycoside has proved as effective as any other drug regimen so far tested in treating Gram-negative enteric meningitis. Aminoglycosides given by lumbar or intraventricular injection do not improve the outcome in bacterial meningitis, but aminoglycosides are often given into intraventricular reservoirs in persistent shunt infections, a practice that has not been critically evaluated. Aminoglycosides have been given orally as prophylaxis against necrotizing enterocolitis but their apparent efficacy has been based on longitudinal studies only (see Chapter 12) and there is heavy selection for resistant organisms.

Chloramphenicol

Chloramphenicol is a naturally occurring antibiotic produced by a *Streptomyces* strain, but can also readily be synthesized. Pro-drugs, inactive in themselves but metabolized to chloramphenicol, are used to overcome problems with pure chloramphenicol: the succinate is soluble, unlike the pure drug, and can be used for injection, while the palmitate and stearate are less bitter for oral use.

Chloramphenicol acts by peptidyl transferase on 70S ribosomes. Its spectrum includes most Gram-positive and Gram-negative bacteria. Although it is bacteriostatic for most enterobacteria, it is bactericidal for many other organisms. It has excellent CSF penetration and has been used extensively to treat bacterial meningitis. There are three main drawbacks to its use in the neonatal period. The first is its propensity to cause the 'grey baby syndrome' (Burns *et al.*, 1959). This condition, which can affect full-term as well as preterm babies, presents as vomiting, respiratory distress, poor feeding, abdominal distension and loose green stools. If chloramphenicol is continued, the babies develop circulatory collapse, becoming grey, poorly perfused and hypothermic, followed by death (McCracken and Nelson, 1983). The second problem is that chloramphenicol levels are very unpredictable at standard doses and are greatly affected by concomitant use of phenytoin, which increases serum levels of chloramphenicol, and phenobarbitone, which reduces them. This is because chloramphenicol is metabolized by glucuronidation, and glucuronyl transferase is affected by these drugs. The third problem is that most coliforms are inhibited but not killed by chloramphenicol. Additional problems are dose-related marrow suppression, mainly causing anaemia. Drug levels should be closely monitored if chloramphenicol is used in the neonatal period.

The reality of chloramphenicol use is that significant toxicity still occurs, despite wide recognition of the possible adverse effects (Mulhall *et al.*, 1983b). There are far safer and probably more effective antibiotics than chloramphenicol for treating neonatal meningitis, and chloramphenicol should now be used only in exceptional circumstances.

Erythromycin

Erythromycin is one of the macrolide antibiotics (named for their macrocyclic lactone ring) produced by a strain of *Streptomyces*. Erythromycin base is degraded by stomach acid and oral preparations are either enteric-coated (stearate) or are esters (erythromycin ethylsuccinate and estolate) which act as pro-drugs metabolized to active erythromycin. Erythromycin lactobionate and gluceptate are the intravenous preparations.

Erythromycin interferes with bacterial protein synthesis. It is active against Gram-positive organisms, including many penicillinase-producing staphylococci, and against mycoplasmas and ureaplasmas. It is also the drug of choice for chlamydial infections and for prophylaxis and treatment of *Bordetella pertussis* infections. Most Gram-negative organisms, with the exception of *Haemophilus influenzae* and *Neisseria*, are not susceptible to erythromycin.

Erythromycin esters, particularly the estolate, can cause cholestatic jaundice. The pharmacokinetics of the oral preparations have been studied in neonates, but there are little or no data on intravenous use.

Clindamycin

Clindamycin is a lincosamide, related to lincomycin, and both are produced by *Streptomyces lincolnensis*. They interfere with bacterial protein synthesis. Clindamycin has somewhat better antibacterial activity and causes less marrow toxicity than lincomycin. It is active against staphylococci, streptococci and *Bacteroides fragilis*, as well as some other anaerobes. It has been used in the treatment of neonatal infections caused by anaerobes and by staphylococci, and in necrotizing enterocolitis (Faix *et al.*, 1988). There are no good pharmacokinetic data and although there have been few reports of toxicity, this may be because there are so few trials of its use.

Trimethoprim–sulphamethoxazole (cotrimoxazole)

Trimethoprim is a selective bacterial dihydrofolate reductase inhibitor. It acts synergistically with sulphonamides, which block an earlier stage in folate synthesis, so that lower concentrations of the two drugs can be used. As sulphonamides can displace bilirubin bound to albumin it should always be considered, when prescribing for a neonate, whether trimethroprim alone might not be equally effective to cotrimoxazole (trimethoprim–sulphamethoxazole).

Trimethoprim is active against staphylococci, enterococci, *E. coli*, *Proteus*, many coliforms but not *Pseudomonas*. It diffuses well into the CSF and brain. Sulphamethoxazole has a spectrum of antibacterial activity similar to that of trimethoprim. Cotrimoxazole, but not trimethoprim alone, has occasionally been used in treating neonatal Gram-negative enteric bacillary meningitis (Sabel and Brandberg, 1975; Ardati *et al.*, 1979) but there have been treatment failures. High-dose i.v. cotrimoxazole (20 mg/kg per day of trimethoprim) is the treatment of choice for *Pneumocystis carinii* pneumonia. Cotrimoxazole has been given p.o. and i.v. and, although few adverse reactions have been reported, even with high-dose i.v. use, the use of the drug has not been studied systematically. Trimethoprim given to the mother will cross the placenta and diffuse into breast milk at high concentrations (McCracken and Siegel, 1983).

Metronidazole

Metronidazole is a nitroamidazole antibiotic with excellent activity against anaerobes, including *Bacteroides fragilis*. It is active against *Entamoeba histolytica*, but has no important action against aerobes. The half-life is 23–25 h in full-term infants but is prolonged to 59–109 h in preterm infants (Jager-Roman *et al.*, 1982; Hall *et al.*, 1983). Peak levels decrease with duration of treatment and there is controversy as to whether or not the half-life becomes shorter with treatment. CSF penetration is excellent and metronidazole has been used successfully to treat *B. fragilis* meningitis (Feldman, 1976). It is commonly used in the UK in combination with antibacterial agents to treat necrotizing enterocolitis. Toxicity has not been described although high doses can cause reversible neuropathy in adults.

Aztreonam

As multiply-resistant Gram-negative organisms become an increasing problem, newer antibiotics are being developed. Aztreonam is a beta-lactam antibiotic with activity against Gram-negative enteric bacilli, including *Pseudomonas aeruginosa*. The pharmacokinetics of aztreonam have been studied in neonates (Likitnukul *et al.*, 1987; Umana *et al.*, 1990) and it appears to be of low toxicity. It will penetrate inflamed meninges.

Ciprofloxacin

Ciprofloxacin, a nalidixic acid derivative with a spectrum similar to that of aztreonam, has been used with limited success to treat infections with resistant *Enterobacter cloacae* (Bannon *et al.*, 1989) and has been used successfully to treat a baby with a CSF shunt infection caused by a multi-resistant *Pseudomonas aeruginosa* (Isaacs *et al.*, 1986b), although CSF penetration is only moderate (Isaacs *et al.*, 1986b; Bannon *et al.*, 1989). Ciprofloxacin can damage cartilage in laboratory animals and is not generally recommended in childhood.

Imipenem–cilastatin

Imipenem is a carbapenem produced by a strain of *Streptomyces*, and is used in combination with cilastatin, a renal dipeptidase inhibitor with no intrinsic antibacterial activity. It is active *in vitro* against *Staphylococcus aureus*, *S. epidermidis*, streptococci excluding *S. faecium*, and a wide range of Gram-negative organisms. It will penetrate inflamed but not uninflamed meninges. Because of CNS toxicity it is not recommended for the treatment of meningitis. It has been evaluated in children (Ahonkhai *et al.*, 1989) but not to our knowledge in newborns.

The drug is a very powerful inducer of beta-lactamases and although these do not act on imipenem they can result in resistance to penicillins and cephalosporins.

Appendix 1

Definitions of neonatal infections

Table A1.1 Definitions of neonatal infections

Dubious	Probable	Definite
A Pneumonia	Clinical picture of respiratory distress consistent with pneumonia and radiographic appearance of streaky densities or confluent lobar opacification persisting for > 24 h. Possible organisms: grown from endotracheal aspirate.	As for probable pneumonia but with positive blood cultures for a respiratory pathogen or post-mortem confirmation of the diagnosis.
B Necrotizing enterocolitis (NEC) I: Blood in stools; normal clotting screen. II: Abdominal distension, suspicious abdominal X-ray but no blood and no intramural gas. I and II tolerate early reintroduction of enteral feeds.	III: Bloody stools, abdominal distension and suspicious abdominal X-ray without intramural gas.	IV: As for III but with pneumatosis intestinalis. V: Per-operative or post-mortem diagnosis.
C Bacteraemia/septicaemia Contaminant: growth of *Staphylococcus epidermidis*, fastidious streptococcus or other aerobic or anaerobic organism from blood cultures taken from a neonate with possible sepis, but in whom the clinical picture subsequently suggests the organism was a contaminant.	Group B streptococcus: Early RDS or persistent fetal circulation and colonization with group B streptococcus but no positive systemic cultures. *Pneumococcus, Haemophilus, Listeria*, etc.: Clinical sepsis with colonization at birth but no positive systemic cultures.	Pure growth of pathogen from one or more blood culture bottles or antigen detection associated with clinical picture of sepsis. Includes *S. epidermidis*, etc., when risk of infection high (e.g. when a long line is *in situ*) or strong clinical evidence of sepsis.
D. Meningitis Contaminant: growth of possible CSF pathogen from CSF, only on enrichment culture, and without CSF pleocytosis, with subsequent clinical picture not truly suggestive of meningitis.		Pure growth of pathogen from CSF; or CSF pleocytosis and positive blood cultures; or virus isolated from CSF or other site with aseptic meningitis

Dubious	Probable	Definite
E **Conjunctivitis**		Purulent discharge from one or both eyes with presence of pus cells and pure growth of bacterial pathogen, virus or *C. trachomatis* (or antigen detection of the latter).
F **Skin: septic spots (Micro-abscess)**		Discrete pustules containing pus cells and a pure growth of *Staphylococcus aureus* or other pathogens.

	Probable	Definite
G **Cellulitis**		Spreading area of skin inflammation with positive bacteriology on needle aspiration or blood cultures.
H **Skin abscess**		Raised, often fluctuant, swelling yielding pure growth of a bacterial or fungal pathogen.
I **Omphalitis**		Inflammation around umbilicus with pure growth of an organism from the umbilicus
J **Wound infection**		Inflammation of skin incision with discharge of pus from wound.
K **Urinary tract infection**	Pure growth $\geq 10^5$ organisms/ml of urine from bag specimen (needs SPA).	Pure growth of pathogen from SPA or clean catch of urine. (Pyelonephritis may be diagnosed *post-mortem*.)
L **Osteomyelitis**		Clinical evidence and/or radiographic changes (lytic lesions, bone scan, etc.) with or without microbiological confirmation.
M **Gastroenteritis**		Loose or watery stools persisting for > 24 h associated with presence of an intestinal pathogen.
N **Bacterial endocarditis**		Characteristic clinical picture, usually in association with persistently positive blood cultures and vegetations on echocardiogram.

	Probable	Definite
O Systemic fungal infection		CSF, SPA urine and/or positive blood cultures. Culture from SPA urine alone may merely be renal candidiasis.
P Congenital infections		Laboratory evidence (specific IgM or culture of organism), often supported by clinical picture.
Q Peritonitis		Growth of organism(s) from peritoneal fluid.
R Upper respiratory tract infection		Rhinorrhoea, cough, increased ventilatory requirements, apnoea, fever associated with respiratory virus identification.
S Asymptomatic virus shedding		Positive virus identification but no attributable symptoms.
T Systemic viral infections		Hepatitis, myocarditis, meningitis, encephalitis and virus identification.
U Localized viral infections		Skin (HSV, enterovirus), eye or other site not previously covered.
V Deep abscess		Abscess in lung, liver, spleen, etc.
W Empyema		Purulent pleural exudate.
X Fungal dermatitis		Skin rash with isolation of fungus.

Categories of neonatal care

Categories of neonatal care
(British Paediatric Association, 1984)

Intensive care

Care is given in a special or intensive care nursery which provides continuous skilled supervision by nursing and medical staff.

Special care

Care is given in a special care nursery or on a postnatal ward which provides observation and treatment falling short of intensive care but exceeding normal routine care.

Normal care

Care given, usually, by the mother in a postnatal ward, supervised by a midwife and doctor but requiring minimal medical or nursing advice.

The use of categories of neonatal care in hospital

Intensive care

1 Babies receiving assisted ventilation [Intermittent Positive Pressure Ventilation (IPPV), Intermittent Mandatory Ventilation (IMV), Constant Positive Airway Pressure (CPAP)] and in the first 24 h following its withdrawal.
2 Babies receiving total parenteral nutrition.
3 Cardiorespiratory disease which is unstable, including recurrent apnoea requiring constant attention.
4 Babies who have major surgery, particularly in the first 24 h postoperatively.
5 Babies of < 30 weeks' gestation during the first 48 h after birth.
6 Babies who have convulsions.
7 Babies transported by the staff of the unit concerned. This would usually be between hospitals, or for special investigation or treatment.
8 Babies undergoing major medical procedures, such as arterial catheterization, peritoneal dialysis or exchange transfusion.

Special care

1 Babies who require continuous monitoring of respiration or heart rate, or by transcutaneous transducers.
2 Babies who are receiving additional oxygen.
3 Babies who are receiving intravenous glucose and electrolyte solutions.
4 Babies who are being tube fed.
5 Babies who have had minor surgery.
6 Babies with a tracheostomy.
7 Dying babies.
8 Babies who are being barrier nursed.
9 Babies receiving phototherapy.
10 Babies who receive constant supervision (for example, babies whose mothers are drug-addicts).
11 Babies who receive special monitoring (for example, frequent glucose or bilirubin estimations).
12 Babies receiving antibiotics.
13 Babies with conditions requiring radiological examination or other methods of imaging.

Normal care

Babies other than those above.

Appendix 3

Suggested schedules for antimicrobial agents in neonatal sepsis

Table A3.1 Penicillins

Approved name	Total daily dose (mg/kg)	Daily doses (n)
Penicillin G	120 (200,000U)	2–4
(Benzylpenicillin)	240 (400,000U) for meningitis	2–4
Ampicillin	150–200	3
	300–400 for meningitis	3
Flucloxacillin	100–400	2–3

Table A3.2 Aminoglycosides

	Dose[a]	Therapeutic range	
Approved name	(mg/kg per dose)	Trough	Peak (mg/l)
Amikacin	7.5	< 8	20–30
Gentamicin	2.5	0.5–1.5	6–8
Netilmicin	3.5	< 2	10–12

[a] N.B. NOT daily

Table A3.3 Frequency of administration of aminoglycosides

Age	Birth-weight (g)		
	< 1500	1500–2500	> 2500
First week of life	18-hourly	12-hourly	12-hourly
Older than 7 days	12-hourly	12-hourly	8-hourly

Table A3.4 Cephalosporins

Approved name	Dose[a] (mg/kg)	Daily doses
Cefuroxime	50 per dose	2
Cefotaxime	50 per dose	2 (3 for meningitis)
Ceftazidime	50 per dose	2 (3 for meningitis)
Ceftriaxone	50 per dose	1

[a] N.B. NOT daily

Table A3.5 Other commonly used antimicrobials

Approved name	Dose[a] (mg/kg)	Daily doses (n)
Erythromycin	10 (orally or by i.v. infusion at 5 mg/ml in 5% dextrose)	2–3
Metronidazole	7.5	1–3
Vancomycin	25 (i.v. infusion over 20–30 minutes)	36-hourly at < 800 g 24-hourly at 800–1200 g 12-hourly at > 1200 g

[a] N.B. NOT daily dose

Table A3.6 Antimicrobials less commonly used

Approved name	Dose[a] (mg/kg)	Daily doses (n)
Chloramphenicol	25	1 (2 for full-term babies over 7 days). Monitor levels
Methicillin	25 50 for meningitis	2–4 2–4
Oxacillin	25	2–4
Piperacillin	100	2
Ticarcillin	75	2–4
Tobramycin	2	2–3

[a] N.B. NOT daily dose

Table A3.7 Oral regimens (for well full-term babies completing a course of antibiotics)

Approved name	Oral regimen
Ampicillin	62.5 mg 6-hourly[a]
Flucloxacillin	30 mg/kg per dose 8-hourly
Penicillin V	62.5 mg 6-hourly[a]

[a] NOT per kg

Table A3.8 Antifungal agents

Approved name	Dose (mg/kg)	Daily doses (n)
Amphotericin B	0.25[a]	2–4
5-Fluorocytosine (flucytosine)	75	2 (Monitor levels)

[a] Infusion in 5% dextrose over 4–6 h. Giving bottle and tubing wrapped in aluminium foil.
   Total dose should not exceed 20–30 mg per kg (see Chapter 14).

Oxford guidelines on investigations for suspected bacterial and viral infection

Guidelines on bacteriological investigations for sepsis or surveillance

Early-onset sepsis (in first 48 h after birth)

'Surface' cultures: Nasopharyngeal aspirate for bacteria
External ear swab

Systemic cultures: Blood
CSF (unless severe respiratory compromise)
    Gastric aspirates are potentially misleading and should *not* be sent from delivery suite or the nursery.
    The above 'surface' cultures also apply to babies with maternal risk factors (e.g. prolonged rupture of membranes) in delivery suite.

Late-onset sepsis (after 48 h)

'Surface' cultures: Nasopharyngeal or endotracheal aspirate for bacteria.
No surface swabs, unless clinically indicated (e.g. pus from septic spot, umbilical swab if omphalitis, etc.)

Systemic cultures: Blood
CSF
Urine (bag specimen unless strong clinical suspicion of urinary tract infection in which case an SPA).

Endotracheal tube aspirates

Babies receiving artificial ventilation currently have endotracheal cultures sent routinely once a week on a Monday.
    Suspected pneumonia in a baby on artificial ventilation is an indication for culture of endotracheal secretions.

Guidelines on viral studies

Suspected intrauterine infection: 1 ml clotted blood for TORCH
                                                   antibodies

	Bag urine and nasopharyngeal aspirate to be cultured for CMV (do not need to put in viral transport medium)
Gastroenteritis	Stool specimens in separate pots to Virology and Bacteriology.
Suspected viral respiratory infection	Nasopharyngeal aspirate for viral culture (and immunofluorescence for RSV if suspected).
Suspected viral meningitis	CSF to Virology as well as Bacteriology. Stool to Virology. Throat swab in viral transport medium.
Suspected herpes simplex skin lesion	Urgent electron microscopy or immunofluorescence on vesicle fluid.

If in doubt about viral cultures, please discuss this with one of the paediatric infectious diseases team.

Oxford guidelines on immunizations

Immunization with DPT

Babies should receive their first DPT immunization at 2 months of age, without correcting for prematurity. If there is a worry over whether the pertussis component of the vaccine should be given, this should be discussed with one of the consultants.

Oral polio vaccine should not be given to babies still in the nursery as it can spread to other babies.

At discharge, recommendations on immunization should be included in the discharge summary. These would generally be that the baby should receive all his or her immunizations at the normal postnatal age. Any queries about individual babies should be discussed with the consultant.

BCG immunization of the newborn

Babies at risk of TB should be anticipated at booking or antenatal visits and the blue infant sheet marked at the appropriate place. This should be brought to the notice of the SHO doing the initial examination.

BCG immunization of infants is recommended where:

1 The infant is known to be a contact of a case of active respiratory TB.
2 The infant belongs to an immigrant community characterized by a high incidence of TB (for example from the Indian subcontinent). The reason for this is not only the possibility that the parents may carry TB: other friends and relatives from the high-risk country frequently visit these families and the children are often taken back to their ancestral home. BCG is also advisable for babies who will be in close contact with 'old' cases of respiratory TB.
3 The infant will reside in, or travel to, any area where the risk of TB is high or where crowded living conditions exist.

Immunization should be carried out soon after birth. Newborn babies need not be tested for sensitivity beforehand.

Bacillus Calmette-Guérin (BCG) vaccine (intradermal)

BCG vaccine (intradermal) contains a live, attenuated strain derived from *Mycobacterium bovis*. It is supplied freeze dried and should be stored at

2–8°C and protected from light. It should not be used after the expiry date stated on the label. The ampoule currently supplied should be diluted with 1 ml 0.9% saline or water for injections, and should be used within 1 h of reconstitution.

The dose for infants < 3 months of age is 0.05 ml; one vial therefore contains sufficient for up to 20 babies.

Method

The site of inoculation should be at the insertion of the deltoid muscle, as sites higher on the arm are more likely to lead to cheloid formation. The tip of the shoulder should be avoided. Before giving the intradermal injection, the skin should be swabbed with spirit and allowed to dry. When giving an intradermal injection the operator should stretch the skin between thumb and forefinger of one hand and with the other slowly insert the needle (25G, orange) with the bevel upwards for ~ 2 mm into the superficial layers of the dermis almost parallel with the surface. A raised, blanched bleb is a sign that the injection has been made correctly. Considerable resistance is felt from a correctly given intradermal injection. If this is not felt, and it is suspected that the needle is too deep, it should be removed and reinserted before more vaccine is given. For a struggling baby, an assistant is helpful.

Side effects and adverse reactions

A local reaction may develop at the site of the vaccination within 2–6 weeks. It begins as a small papule which slowly increases in size for 2–3 weeks; occasionally a shallow ulcer up to 10 mm in diameter develops. If this discharges, a temporary dry dressing may be used until a scab forms but it is essential that air should not be excluded. The lesion slowly subsides over about 2 months and heals leaving only a small scar. Faulty injection technique is the most frequent cause of severe injection site reactions (large ulcers and abscesses).

Contraindications

BCG vaccine should not be given to infants with pyrexia or a generalized skin condition. No further immunizations should be given in that arm for at least 3 months because of the risks of regional lymphadenitis.

Immunization programme for babies born to mothers who are Hepatitis B antigen positive

1 The Blood Transfusion Service screens all mothers for HBsAG (Hepatitis B Surface Antigen).
2 Blood samples from all HBsAG positive mothers are referred to the Virology Laboratory for HBsAG/Anti-HBe testing. Mothers who are e antigen positive and those who are surface antigen positive and e antigen negative are at high risk for passing their infection to their baby. A dose of hepatitis B immunoglobulin is placed in the delivery suite refrigerator to be given to the babies of these mothers.

3 At birth, 200 mg of HEPATITIS B IMMUNOGLOBULIN (HBIG) IS GIVEN INTRAMUSCULARLY AS SOON AS POSSIBLE AFTER BIRTH.

4 Between 24 h and 3 days after birth the first dose of hepatitis B vaccine is given. The dose given is 0.5 ml ($^1/_2$ bottle). The baby is seen at 1 month and 6 months of age, when the same dose is given.

5 The baby is seen again at 12 months of age for paediatric assessment and a blood sample is taken to check for hepatitis B markers.

6 HBsAG-positive mothers who have 'e' antibody are at lower risk of infecting their babies. There is dispute as to whether their babies should receive vaccine and immunoglobulin, but they may very occasionally develop acute fulminating hepatitis; immunoglobulin should therefore be given. These children are still at risk for later becoming chronic carriers, by horizontal infection, and should be started on a course of vaccine.

Herpes simplex virus infection

HSV in baby units

Herpes simplex virus infection may cause a problem in neonatal units in different ways:

Herpes labialis in medical and nursing staff

Doctors and nurses with herpetic lesions should not handle babies. Any member of staff who develops a 'cold sore' should treat this with 35% idoxuridine (5-iodo-2'-deoxyuridine) in DMSO. The liquid is applied to the lesion five times a day for not more than 3 days. After 24 h treatment, work may be resumed.

A mother with active herpes labialis

Her baby should be isolated from other babies. The mother should be treated as above, and be discouraged from kissing her baby during the time of treatment.

Maternal genital herpes

A primary herpetic infection of the genital tract is a potent source of infection of the baby. Active recurrent genital herpes is less worrying as the baby receives protective maternal antibody transplacentally. The incidence of neonatal herpes infection in Oxford is very low. Pregnant mothers with a history of genital herpes should be examined periodically and virus cultures of any lesions made. Caesarean section seems rational when there is confirmed active maternal genital herpes, although it has not always prevented the baby from being infected.

35% Idoxuridine in DMSO

The preparation of idoxuridine (IOU) available from general practitioners is 5% (Herpid) which the makers claim is unstable; 35% idoxuridine in DMSO supplied by the hospital pharmacy is stable and may be kept for treating recurrent attacks.

If local or generalized herpes simplex infection is suspected in the newborn, the appropriate cultures and blood samples should be sent immediately to the virus laboratory, and the virologists and paediatric infectious disease team should be consulted.

Even local HSV (vesicular or bullous skin lesions) carries a high risk of dissemination to cause devastating disease, and the neonatal consultant should be urgently informed if this is suspected.

References

Adams, B. G. and Marrie, T. J. (1982) Hand carriage of aerobic gram-negative rods may not be transient. *J. Hyg.*, **89**, 33–46

Adams, J. M., Speer, M. E. and Rudolph, A. J. (1980) Bacterial colonization of radial artery catheters. *Pediatrics*, **65**, 94–97

Adelstein, A. M. and Donovan, J. W. (1972) Malignant disease in children whose mothers had chickenpox, mumps, or rubella in pregnancy. *Br. Med. J.*, **4**, 629–631

Ahlfors, K., Ivarsson, S. A., Johnsson, T. and Svanberg, L. (1979) A prospective study on congenital and acquired cytomegalovirus infections in infants. *Scand. J. Infect. Dis.*, **11**, 177–178

Ahlfors, K., Ivarsson, S. A., Johnson, T. *et al.* (1981) Risk of cytomegalovirus infection in nurses and congenital infection in their offspring. *Acta Paediatr. Scand.*, **70**, 819–823

Ahlfors, K., Ivarsson, S. A., Harris, S. *et al.* (1984) Congenital cytomegalovirus infection and disease in Sweden and the relative importance of primary and secondary maternal infections. *Scand. J. Infect. Dis.*, **16**, 129–137

Ahonkhai, V. I., Cyhan, G. M., Wilson, S. E. and Brown, K. R. (1989) Imipenem-cilastatin in pediatric patients: an overview of safety and efficacy studies conducted in the United States. *Pediatr. Infect. Dis. J.*, **8**, 740–744

Albers, W. H., Tyler, C. W. and Boxerbaum, B. (1966) Asymptomatic bacteremia in the newborn infant. *J. Pediatr.*, **69**, 193–197

Alford, C. A., Stagno, S. and Reynolds, D. W. (1974) Congenital toxoplasmosis: clinical, laboratory and therapeutic considerations, with special reference to subclinical disease. *Bull. N.Y. Acad. Med.*, **50**, 160–181

Alkalay, A. L., Pomerance, J. J. and Rimoin, D. (1987) Fetal varicella syndrome. *J. Pediatr.*, **111**, 320–323

American Academy of Pediatrics (1987) Committee on Infectious Diseases. Ribavirin therapy of respiratory syncytial virus disease. *Pediatrics*, **79**, 475–478

Anderson, S. G. and Gilbert, G. L. (1990) Neonatal gram-negative meningitis; a ten year review; with reference to outcome and relapse of infection. *J. Paed. Child Health*, **26**, 212–216

Anthony, B. F. and Okada, D. M. (1977) The emergence of group B streptococci in infections of the newborn. *Annu. Rev. Med.*, **28**, 335–369

Aperia, A. and Zetterstrom, R. (1982) Renal control of fluid homeostasis in the newborn infant. *Clin. Perinatol.*, **9**, 523–533

Ardati, K. O., Thirumoorthi, M. C. and Dajani, A. S. (1979) Intravenous trimethoprim–sulfamethoxazole in the treatment of serious infections in children. *J. Pediatr.*, **95**, 801–806

Armstrong, J. H., Zacarias, F. and Rein, M. F. (1976) Ophthalmia neonatorum: a chart review. *Pediatrics*, **57**, 84–92

Ascuitto, R. J., Gerber, M. A., Cates, K. L. and Tilton, R. C. (1985) Buffy coat smears of blood drawn through central venous catheters as an aid to rapid diagnosis of systemic fungal infections. *J. Pediatr.*, **106**, 445–447

Ash, J. M. and Gilday, D. L. (1980) The futility of bone scanning in neonatal osteomyelitis: concise communication. *J. Nucl. Med.*, **21**, 417–420

Assael, B. M., Cavanna, G., Jusko, W. J. *et al.* (1980) Multiexponential elimination of gentamicin. A kinetic study during development. *Dev. Pharmacol. Ther.*, **1**, 171–181

Athavale, V. B. and Pai, P. N. (1965) Tetanus neonatorum – clinical manifestations. *J. Pediatr.*, **67**, 649–657

Aula, P. (1964) Chromosomes and viral infections. *Lancet*, **i**, 720–721

Axline, S. G., Yaffee, S. J. and Simon, H. J. (1967) Clinical pharmacology of antimicrobials in premature infants. II. Ampicillin, methicillin, oxacillin, neomycin and colistin. *Pediatrics*, **39**, 97–107

Bai, P. V. A. and John, T. J. (1979) Congenital skin ulcers following varicella in late pregnancy. *J. Pediatr.*, **94**, 65–67

Baker, C. J. and Edwards, M. S. (1990) Group B streptococcal infections. In *Infectious Diseases of the Fetus and Newborn Infant*, 3rd edn (eds J. S. Remington and J. O. Klein), W. B. Saunders, Philadelphia, pp. 742–811

Baker, C. J., Rench, M. A., Edwards, M. S. *et al.* (1988) Immunisation of pregnant women with a polysaccharide vaccine of group B streptococcus. *N. Engl. J. Med.*, **319**, 1180–1185

Baker, C. J., Rench, M. and Kasper, D. L. (1990) Response to type III polysaccharide in women whose infants have had invasive group B streptococcal infection. *N. Engl. J. Med.*, **322**, 1857–1860

Baley, J. E., Kliegman, R. M. and Fanaroff, A. A. (1984a) Disseminated fungal infections in very low birth-weight infants: clinical manifestations and epidemiology. *Pediatrics*, **73**, 144–152

Baley, J. E., Kliegman, R. M. and Fanaroff, A. A. (1984b) Disseminated fungal infections in very low-birth-weight infants: therapeutic toxicity. *Pediatrics*, **73**, 153–157

Baley, J. E., Stork, E. K., Warkentin, P. I. and Shurin, S. B. (1987) Buffy coat transfusions in neutropenic neonates with presumed sepsis: a prospective, randomized trial. *Pediatrics*, **80**, 712–720

Baley, J. E., Meyers, C., Kliegman, R. M. *et al.* (1990) Pharmacokinetics, outcome of treatment, and toxic effects of amphotericin B and 5-fluorocytosine in neonates. *J. Pediatr.*, **116**, 791–797

Bannon, M. J., Stutchfield, P. R., Weindling, A. M. and Damjanovic, V. (1989) Ciprofloxacin in neonatal *Enterobacter cloacae* septicaemia. *Arch. Dis. Child.*, **64**, 1388–1391

Barnard, J. A., Cotton, R. B. and Lutin, W. (1985) Necrotizing enterocolitis. Variables associated with the severity of disease. *Am. J. Dis. Child.*, **139**, 375–377

Barter, R. (1953) The histopathology of congenital pneumonia. A clinical and experimental study. *J. Pathol. Bacteriol.*, **66**, 407–415

Barter, R. A. and Hudson, J. A. (1974) Bacteriological findings in perinatal pneumonia. *Pathology*, **6**, 223–230

Bass, J. W. and Zacher, L. L. (1989) Do newborn infants have passive immunity to pertussis? *Pediatr. Infect. Dis. J.*, **8**, 352–353

Bates, T. (1955) Poliomyelitis in pregnancy, fetus and newborn. *Am. J. Dis. Child.*, **90**, 189–195

Beasley, R. P., Hwang, L.-Y., Lin, C.-C. *et al.* (1981) Hepatitis B immune globulin (HBIG) efficacy in the interruption of perinatal transmission of hepatitis B carrier state. *Lancet*, **ii**, 388–393

Beasley, R. P., Hwang, L. Y., Stevens, C. E. *et al.* (1983a) Efficacy of hepatitis B immune globulin for prevention of perinatal transmission of the hepatitis B virus-carrier state: final report of a randomized, double-blind, placebo-controlled trial. *Hepatology*, **3**, 135–141

Beasley, R. P., Hwang, L. Y., Lee, G. C. Y. *et al.* (1983b) Prevention of perinatally transmitted hepatitis B virus infections with hepatitis B immune globulin and hepatitis B vaccine. *Lancet*, **ii**, 1099–1102

Becroft, D. M. O., Farmer, K., Seddon, R. J. *et al.* (1971) Epidemic listeriosis in the newborn. *Br. Med. J.*, **iii**, 747–751

Beem, M. O. and Saxon, E. M. (1977) Respiratory tract colonization and a distinct pneumonia syndrome in infants infected with *Chlamydia trachomatis*. *N. Engl. J. Med.*, **296**, 306–310

Bell, M. J., Ternberg, J. L. and Feigin, R. D. (1978) Neonatal necrotising enterocolitis: therapeutic decisions based upon clinical staging. *Ann. Surg.*, **187**, 1–7

Belton, E. M. and Jones, R. V. (1965) Haemolytic anaemia due to nalidixic acid. *Lancet*, **ii**, 691

Benirschke, K. (1960) Routes and types of infection in the fetus and newborn. *Am. J. Dis. Child.*, **99**, 714–721

Benirschke, K. and Driscoll, S. G. (1967) *The Pathology of the Human Placenta*, Springer, Berlin

Bennhagen, R., Svenningsen, N. W. and Bekassy, A. N. (1987) Changing pattern of neonatal meningitis in Sweden. *Scand. J. Infect. Dis.*, **19**, 587–593

Bergman, I., Painter, M. J., Wald, E. R. *et al.* (1987) Outcome in children with enteroviral meningitis during the first year of life. *J. Pediatr.*, **110**, 705–709

Bergstrom, T., Larson, H., Lincoln, K. and Winberg, J. (1972) Neonatal urinary tract infections. *J. Pediatr.*, **80**, 859–866

Best, J. E., Banatvala, J. E., Morgan-Capner, P. and Miller, E. (1989) Fetal infection after maternal reinfection with rubella: criterion for defining reinfection. *Br. Med. J.*, **299**, 773–775

Besunder, J. B., Reed, M. D. and Blumer, J. L. (1988) Principles of drug biodisposition in the neonate. *Clin. Pharmacokinet.*, **14**, 189–216

Binkin, N. J., Koplan, J. P. and Cates, W. (1984) Preventing neonatal herpes: the value of weekly viral cultures in pregnant women with recurrent genital herpes. *JAMA*, **251**, 2816–2821

Birnbaum, G., Lynch, J. I., Margileth, A. M. *et al.* (1969) Cytomegalovirus infections in newborn infants. *J. Pediatr.*, **75**, 789–795

Biron, C. A., Byron, K. S. and Sullivan, J. L. (1989) Severe herpesvirus infections in an adolescent without natural killer cells. *N. Engl. J. Med.*, **320**, 1731–1735

Boe, R. W., Williams, C. P. S., Bennet, J. V. and Oliver, T. K. (1967) Serum levels of methicillin and ampicillin in newborn and premature infants in relation to postnatal age. *Pediatrics*, **39**, 194–201

Bollgren, I. and Winberg, J. (1976) The periurethral aerobic bacterial flora in healthy boys and girls. *Acta Paediatr. Scand.*, **65**, 74–80

Bortolussi, R., Thompson, T. R. and Ferrieri, P. (1977) Early-onset pneumococcal sepsis in newborn infants. *Pediatrics*, **60**, 352–355

Boyer, K. M. and Gotoff, S. P. (1986) Prevention of early-onset neonatal group B streptococcal disease with selective intrapartum chemoprophylaxis. *N. Engl. J. Med.*, **314**, 1665–1669

Boyer K. M., Gadzala C. A., Burd, L. I. *et al.* (1983) Selective intrapartum chemoprophylaxis of group B streptococcal early-onset disease. I. Epidemiologic rationale. *J. Infect. Dis.*, **148**, 795–801

Boyle, R. J., Chandler, B. D., Stonestreet, B. S. and Oh, W. (1978) Early identification of sepsis in infants with respiratory distress. *Pediatrics*, **62**, 744–750

Brasfield, D. M., Stagno, S., Whitley, R. J. *et al.* (1987) Infant pneumonitis associated with cytomegalovirus, *Chlamydia, Pneumocystis* and *Ureaplasma*: follow-up. *Pediatrics*, **79**, 76–83

Bressler, E. L., Conway, J. J. and Weiss, S. C. (1984) Neonatal osteomyelitis examined by bone scintigraphy. *Radiology*, **152**, 685–688

Brice, J. E. H. (1976) Congenital varicella resulting from infection during second trimester of pregnancy. *Arch. Dis. Child.*, **51**, 474–476

British Paediatric Association (1984) *Categories of Babies Receiving Neonatal Care*, British Paediatric Association, London

British Paediatric Association (1989) *HIV Infection in Infancy and Childhood. Report of the BPA Working Party*, British Paediatric Association, London

Broome, C. V., Ciesielski, C. A., Linnan, M. J. and Hightower, A. W. (1986) Listeriosis in the United States. *J. Fd. Prot.*, **49**, 848

Brown, E. G. and Sweet, A. Y. (1978) Preventing necrotizing enterocolitis in neonates. *JAMA*, **240**, 2452–2454

Brown, Z. A., Vontver, L. A., Benedetti, J. *et al.* (1987) Effects on infants of a first episode of genital herpes during pregnancy. *N. Engl. J. Med.*, **317**, 1246–1251

Brumfitt, W., Dixson, S. and Hamilton-Miller, J. M. T. (1985) Resistance to antiseptics in methicillin and gentamicin resistant *Staphylococcus aureus*. *Lancet*, **i**, 422–423

Brunell, P. A., Bass, J. W., Daum, R. S. *et al.* (1985) Prevention of neonatal hepatitis B virus infections. *Pediatrics*, **75**, 362–364

Buchanan, N. (1985) Aminoglycoside monitoring in neonates – a reappraisal. *Aust. N.Z. J. Med.*, **15**, 457–459

Burns, L. E., Hodgman, J. E. and Cass, A. B. (1959) Fatal circulatory collapse in premature infants receiving chloramphenicol. *N. Engl. J. Med.*, **261**, 1318–1321

Butler, K. M., Rench, M. A. and Baker, C. J. (1990) Amphotericin B as a single agent in the treatment of systemic candidiasis in neonates. *Pediatr. Infect. Dis. J.*, **9**, 51–56

Cairo, M. S., Rucker, R., Bennetts, G. A. *et al.* (1984) Improved survival of newborns receiving leukocyte transfusions for sepsis. *Pediatrics*, **74**, 887–892

Cassell, G. H., Waites, K. B., Crouse, D. T. *et al.* (1988) Association of *Ureaplasma urealyticum* infection of the lower respiratory tract with chronic lung disease and death in very low-birth-weight infants. *Lancet*, **ii**, 240–245

Cattermole, H. E. J. and Rivers, R. P. A. (1987) Neonatal candida septicaemia: diagnosis on buffy coat smear. *Arch. Dis. Child.*, **62**, 302–304

Centers for Disease Control (1987) Rubella and congenital rubella – United States, 1984–6. *MMWR*, **36**, 457

Centers for Disease Control (1988a) Guidelines for the prevention and control of congenital syphilis. *MMWR*, **37** (Suppl. S-1), 1–13

Centers for Disease Control (1988b) Sept. 12, *AIDS Weekly Surveillance Report*

Challacombe, D. (1974) Bacterial microflora in infants receiving nasojejunal tube feeding. *J. Pediatr.*, **85**, 113

Chirico, G., Rondini G., Plebani, A. *et al.* (1987) Intravenous gammaglobulin therapy for prophylaxis of infection in high-risk neonates. *J. Pediatr.*, **110**, 437–442

Christensen, K. K. and Christensen, P. (1986) Intravenous gammaglobulin in the treatment of neonatal sepsis with special reference to Group B streptococci and pharmacokinetics. *Pediatr. Infect. Dis. J.*, **5**, S189–192

Christensen, R.D., Rothstein, G., Anstall, H. B. and Bybee, B. (1982) Granulocyte transfusions in newborns with bacterial infection, neutropenia and depletion of mature marrow neutrophils. *Pediatrics*, **70**, 1–6

Clarke, M., Davies, D. P., Odds, F. and Mitchell, C. (1980) Neonatal systemic candidiasis treatment with miconazole. *Br. Med. J.*, **281**, 354

Cohen, P. and Scadron, S. J. (1943) The placental transmission of protective antibodies against whooping cough by inoculation of the pregnant mother. *JAMA*, **121**, 656–662

Cohlan, S. Q., Bevelander, G. and Tiamsic, T. (1963) Growth inhibition of prematures receiving tetracycline. *Am. J. Dis. Child.*, **105**, 453–461

Committee on fetus and newborn (1980) Perinatal herpes simplex virus infection. *Pediatrics*, **66**, 147–148

Conway, N. and Birt, D. N. (1965) Streptomycin in pregnancy: effect on the foetal ear. *Br. Med. J.*, **2**, 260–263

Coudron, P. E., Mayhall, C. G., Facklam, R. R. *et al.* (1984) *Streptococcus faecium* outbreak in a neonatal intensive care unit. *J. Clin. Microbiol.*, **20**, 1044–1048

Craig, W. S. (1962) *Care of the Newly Born Infant*, Williams and Wilkins, Baltimore

Daffos, F., Forestier, F., Grangeot-Keros, L. *et al.* (1984) Prenatal diagnosis of congenital rubella. *Lancet*, **ii**, 1–3

Daffos, F., Forestier, F., Capella-Pavlovsky, M. *et al.* (1988) Prenatal management of 746 pregnancies at risk for congenital toxoplasmosis. *N. Engl. J. Med.*, **318**, 271–275

Davey, P. (1985) Aminoglycosides and neonatal deafness. *Lancet*, **ii**, 612

Davies, E. A., Emmerson, A. M., Hogg, G. M. *et al.* (1987) An outbreak of infection with a methicillin-resistant *Staphylococcus aureus* in a special care baby unit. *J. Hosp. Infect.*, **10**, 120–128

Davies, P. A. and Aherne, W. (1962) Congenital pneumonia. *Arch. Dis. Child.*, **37**, 598–602

Davis, L. E., James, C. G., Fiber, F. and MacLaren, L. C. (1979) Cytomegalovirus isolation from a human ear. *Ann. Otol. Rhinol. Laryngol.*, **88**, 424–426

de Man, P., Claeson, I., Johanson, I. M. *et al.* (1989) Bacterial attachment as a predictor of renal abnormalities in boys with urinary tract infection. *J. Pediatr.*, **115**, 915–922

de Nicola, L. K. and Hanshaw, J. B. (1979) Congenital and neonatal varicella. *J. Pediatr.*, **94**, 175–176

de Virgilis, S., Frau, F., Sanna, G. *et al.* (1985) Perinatal hepatitis B virus detection by hepatitis B virus-DNA analysis. *Arch. Dis. Child.*, **60**, 56–58

Decker, M. D. and Edwards, K. M. (1988) Central venous catheter infections. *Pediatr. Clin. North Am.*, **35**, 579–612

Dennis, J. E., Rhodes, K. H., Cooney, D. R. *et al.* (1980) Nosocomial *Rhizopus* infection (zygomycosis) in children. *J. Pediatr.*, **96**, 824–828

Desmonts, G., Daffos, F., Forestier, F. *et al.* (1985) Prenatal diagnosis of congenital toxoplasmosis. *Lancet*, **i**, 500–504

DHSS (1989) *(PL/CMO (89)4 and PL/CNO (89)3). HIV Infection, Breast Feeding and Human Milk Banking in the United Kingdom*, DHSS, London

Dietzman, D. E., Fischer, G. W. and Schoenknecht, F. D. (1974) Neonatal *Escherichia coli* septicemia – bacterial counts in blood. *J. Pediatr.*, **85**, 128–130

Dobson, S. R. M. and Baker, C. J. (1990) Enterococcal sepsis in neonates: features by age at onset and occurrence of focal infection. *Pediatrics*, **85**, 165–171

Dormer, B. A., Harrison, I., Swart, J. A. *et al.* (1959) Prophylactic isoniazid protection of infants in a tuberculosis hospital. *Lancet*, **ii**, 902–903

Dunham, E. C. (1933) Septicemia in newborn. *Am. J. Dis. Child.*, **45**, 229–253

Dupuy, J. M., Frommel, D. and Alagille, D. (1975) Severe viral hepatitis in infancy. *Lancet*, i, 191–194

Dvorak, A. M. and Gavaller, B. (1964) Congenital systemic candidiasis: report of a case. *N. Engl. J. Med.*, **274**, 540–543

Dworsky, M., Welch, K., Cassady, G. *et al.* (1983) Occupational risk for primary cytomegalovirus infection among paediatric health-care workers. *N. Engl. J. Med.*, **309**, 950–953

Dwyer, D. E., O'Flaherty, S., Packham, D. and Cunningham, A. L. (1986) Herpes simplex encephalitis in infants. *Med. J. Aust.*, **144**, 714–715

Dyer, I. (1940) Measles complicating pregnancy. Report of 24 cases with three instances of congenital measles. *South. Med. J.*, **33**, 601–606

Editorial (1985a) A nasty shock from antibiotics? *Lancet*, ii, 594

Editorial (1985b) What's to be done about resistant staphylococci? *Lancet*, ii, 189–190

Editorial (1986) Avoiding the danger of enteroviruses in newborn babies. *Lancet*, i, 194–196

Editorial (1989) Cerebrospinal fluid shunt infections. *Lancet*, i, 1304–1305

Edouard, L. and Alberman, E. (1980) National trends in the certified causes of perinatal mortality, 1966 to 1978. *Br. J. Obstet. Gynaecol.*, **87**, 833–838

Edwards, M. S., Baker, C. J., Wagner, M. L. *et al.* (1978) An etiologic shift in infantile osteomyelitis: the emergence of the group B streptococcus. *J. Pediatr.*, **93**, 578–583

Edwards, M. S., Rench, M. A., Haffar, A. A. M. *et al.* (1985) Long-term sequelae of group B streptococcal meningitis in infants. *J. Pediatr.*, **106**, 717–722

Eglin, R. P. and Wilkinson, A. R. (1987) HIV infection and pasteurisation of breast milk. *Lancet*, i, 1093

Eibl, M. M., Welf, H. M., Furnkranz, H. and Rosenkranz, A. (1988) Prevention of necrotizing enterocolitis in low-birth-weight infants by IgA–IgG feeding. *N. Engl. J. Med.*, **319**, 1–7

Eichenwald, H. F., Kotsevalov, O. and Fasso, L. A. (1960) The 'cloud baby': an example of bacterial–viral interaction. *Am. J. Dis. Child.*, **100**, 161–173

Eilard, T. and Strannegard, O. (1974) Rubella reinfection in pregnancy followed by transmission to the fetus. *J. Infect. Dis.*, **129**, 594–596

Enders, G. (1984) Varicella–zoster virus infection in pregnancy. *Progr. Med. Virol.*, **29**, 166–196

Erlich, R. M., Turner, J. A. P. and Clarke, M. (1958) Neonatal varicella. *J. Pediatr.*, **53**, 139–147

Ermocilla, R., Cassady, G. and Ceballos, R. (1974) Otitis media in the pathogenesis of neonatal meningitis with group B beta-hemolytic streptococcus. *Pediatrics*, **54**, 643–644

European Collaborative Study (1988) Mother-to-child transmission of HIV infection. *Lancet*, ii, 1039–1042

Evans, M. E., Schaffner, W., Federspiel, C. F. *et al.* (1988) Sensitivity, specificity and predictive value of body surface cultures in a neonatal intensive care unit. *JAMA*, **259**, 248–252

Eviatar, L. and Eviatar, E. (1982) Development of head control and vestibular responses in infants treated with aminoglycosides. *Dev. Med. Child. Neurol.*, **24**, 372–379

Faden, H. S. (1976) Early diagnosis of neonatal bacteremia by buffy-coat examination. *J. Pediatr.*, **88**, 1032–1034

Faix, R. G., Polley, T. Z. and Grasela, T. H. (1988) A randomized, controlled trial of parenteral clindamycin in neonatal necrotizing enterocolitis. *J. Pediatr.*, **112**, 271–277

Falloon, J., Eddy, J., Wiener, L. and Pizzo, P. A. (1989) Human immunodeficiency virus infection in children. *J. Pediatr.*, **114**, 1–30

Fallot, M. E., Boyd, J. L. and Oski, F. A. (1980) Breast-feeding reduces incidence of hospital admissions for infection in infants. *Pediatrics*, **65**, 1121–1124

Faix, R. G. (1984) Systemic candida infections in infants in intensive care nurseries: high incidence of central nervous system involvement. *J. Pediatr.*, **105**, 616–622

Farmer, K., MacArthur, B. A. and Clay, M. M. (1975) A follow-up study of 15 cases of neonatal meningoencephalitis due to coxsackie B5. *J. Pediatr.*, **87**, 568–571

Feldman, W. E. (1976) *Bacteroides fragilis* ventriculitis and meningitis. *Am. J. Dis. Child.*, **13**, 880–883

Field, D. J., Isaacs, D. and Stroobant, J. (1989) *Tutorials in Paediatric Differential Diagnosis*, Churchill Livingstone, Edinburgh

Fine, P. E. M., Adelstein, A. M., Snowman, J. *et al.* (1985) Long term effects of exposure to viral infection *in utero*. *Br. Med. J.*, **290**, 509–511

Finitzo-Heiber, T., McCracken, G. H. and Brown, K. C. (1985) Prospective controlled evaluation of auditory function in neonates given netilmicin or amikacin. *J. Pediatr.*, **106**, 129–136

Fleet, W. F., Benz, E. W., Karzon, D. T. *et al.* (1974) Fetal consequences of maternal rubella immunisation. *JAMA*, **227**, 621–627

Flemming, D. W., Cochi, S. L., McDonald, K. L. *et al.* (1985) Pasteurised milk as a vehicle of infection in an outbreak of listeriosis. *N. Engl. J. Med.*, **312**, 406–407

Forfar, J. O. and Arneil, G. C. (1991) *Textbook of Paediatrics*, 4th edn, Churchill Livingstone, Edinburgh

Forsgren, M., Carlstrom, G. and Strangert, K. (1979) Congenital rubella after maternal reinfection. *Scand. J. Infect. Dis.*, **11**, 81–83

Fox, L. and Sprunt, K. (1978) Neonatal osteomyelitis. *Pediatrics*, **62**, 535–542

Fransen, L., Nsawze, H., Klauss, V. *et al.* (1986) Ophthalmia neonatorum in Nairobi, Kenya: the roles of *Neisseria gonorrhoeae* and *Chlamydia trachomatis*. *J. Infect. Dis.*, **153**, 862–869

Fransen, L., van den Berghe, P., Mertens, A. *et al.* (1987) Incidence and bacterial aetiology of neonatal conjunctivitis. *Eur. J. Pediatr.*, **146**, 152–155

Freedman, R. M., Ingram, D. L., Gross, I. *et al.* (1981) A half century of neonatal sepsis at Yale. *Am. J. Dis. Child.*, **135**, 140–144

Friedman, H. M., Lewis, M. R., Nemerofsky, D. M. and Plotkin, S. A. (1984) Acquisition of cytomegalovirus infection among female employees at a pediatric hospital. *Pediatr. Infect. Dis. J.*, **3**, 233–235

Fujikura, T. and Froehlich, L. A. (1967) Intrauterine pneumonia in relation to birth, weight and race. *Am. J. Obstet. Gynecol.*, **97**, 81–84

Fuquay, D., Koup, J. and Smith, A. L. (1981) Management of neonatal gentamicin over-dosage. *J. Pediatr.*, **99**, 473–476

Fulginiti, V. A. and Ray, C. G. (1988) Body surface cultures in the newborn infant. An exercise in futility, wastefulness and inappropriate practice. *Am. J. Dis. Child.*, **142**, 19–20

Fussel, E. N., Kaack, B., Cherry, R. and Roberts, J. A. (1988) Adherence of bacteria to human foreskins. *J. Urol.*, **140**, 997–1001

Galazka, A., Gasse, F. and Henderson, R. H. (1987) Neonatal tetanus in the world and the global expanded programme on immunisation. In *Proceedings of the VII International Conference on Tetanus, Leningrad*, WHO, Geneva

Gall, L. S. (1968) The role of intestinal flora in gas formation. *Ann. N.Y. Acad. Sci.*, **150**, 27–30

Gilbert, G. L., Hayes, K., Hudson, I. L. *et al.* (1989) Prevention of transfusion-acquired cytomegalovirus infection in infants by blood filtration to remove leucocytes. *Lancet*, **i**, 1228–1231

Ginsburg, C. M. and McCracken, G. H. (1982) Urinary tract infections in young infants. *Pediatrics*, **69**, 409–412

Gitlin, D., Kumate, J., Urrusti, J. and Morales, C. (1964) The selectivity of the human placenta in the transfer of plasma proteins from mother to fetus. *J. Clin. Invest.*, **43**, 1938–1951

Glennon, J., Ryan, P. J., Keane, C. T. and Rees, J. P. R. (1988) Circumcision and periurethral carriage of *Proteus mirabilis* in boys. *Arch. Dis. Child.*, **63**, 556–557

Gluck, L., Wood, H. F. and Fousek, M. D. (1966) Septicemia of the newborn. *Pediatr. Clin. North Am.*, **13**, 1131–1148

Goldacre, M. J. (1976) Acute bacterial meningitis in childhood: incidence and mortality in a defined population. *Lancet*, **i**, 28–31

Goldmann, D. A., Leclair, J. and Macone, A. (1978) Bacterial colonization of neonates admitted to an intensive care unit. *J. Pediatr.*, **69**, 193–197

Goldmann, D. A., Durbin, W. A. and Freeman, J. (1981) Nosocomial infections in a neonatal intensive care unit. *J. Infect. Dis.*, **144**, 449–459

Goossens, H., Henocque, G., Kremp, L. *et al.* (1986) Nosocomial outbreak of *Campylobacter jejuni* meningitis in newborn infants. *Lancet*, **ii**, 146–149

Granstrom, G., Sterner, G., Nord, C. E. and Granstrom, M. (1987) Use of erythromycin to prevent pertussis in newborns of mothers with pertussis. *J. Infect. Dis.*, **155**, 1210–1214

Grant, S., Edmond, E. and Syme, J. (1981) A prospective study of primary cytomegalovirus infection during pregnancy. *J. Infect*, **3**, 24–31

Graves, G. R. and Rhodes, P. G. (1984) Tachycardia as a sign of early onset neonatal sepsis. *Pediatr. Infect. Dis. J.*, **3**, 404–406

Gray, E. S., Lloyd, D. J., Miller, S. S. *et al.* (1981) Evidence for an immune complex vasculitis in neonatal necrotising enterocolitis. *J. Clin. Pathol.*, **34**, 759–763

Greenwood, D. (1989) *Antimicrobial Chemotherapy*, 2nd edn, Oxford University Press, Oxford

Greffe, B. S., Dooley, S. L., Deddish, R. B. and Krasny, H. C. (1986) Transplacental passage of acyclovir. *J. Pediatr.*, **108**, 1020–1021

Griffiths, P. D. and Baboonian, C. (1984) A prospective study of primary cytomegalovirus infection during pregnancy: final report. *Br. J. Obstet. Gynaecol.*, **91**, 307–315

Griffiths, P. D., Campbell-Benzie, A. and Heath, R. B. (1980) A prospective study of cytomegalovirus infection in pregnancy. *Br. J. Obstet. Gynaecol.*, **87**, 308–314

Grossman, M. and Ticknor, W. (1965) Serum levels of ampicillin, cephalothin, cloxacillin and nafcillin in the newborn infant. *Antimicrob. Agents Chemother.*, **5**, 214–219

Guignard, J. P. and John, E. G. (1986) Renal function in the tiny, premature infant. *Clin. Perinatol.*, **13**, 377–401

Gustafson, T. L., Shehab, Z. and Brunell, P. A. (1984) Outbreak of varicella in a newborn intensive care nursery. *Am. J. Dis. Child.*, **138**, 548–550

Gutman, L. T., Idriss, Z. H., Gehlbach, S. and Blackmon, L. (1976) Neonatal staphylococcal enterocolitis: association with indwelling feeding catheters and *S. aureus* colonization. *J. Pediatr.*, **88**, 836–839

Gyllensward, A. and Malmstrom, S. (1962) The cerebrospinal fluid in immature infants. *Acta Paediatr. Scand.*, **51** (Suppl. 35), 54–62

Haldane, E. V., van Rooyan, C. E., Embil, J. A. *et al.* (1968) A search for transmissible birth defects of virologic origin in members of the nursing profession. *Am. J. Obstet. Gynecol.*, **105**, 1032–1040

Haley, R. W. and Bregman, D. A. (1982) The role of understaffing and overcrowding in recurrent outbreaks of staphylococcal infection in a neonatal intensive care unit. *J. Infect. Dis.*, **145**, 875–885

Hall, C. B. and Douglas, R. G. (1981) Modes of transmission of respiratory syncytial virus. *J. Pediatr.*, **99**, 100–102

Hall, C. B., Kopelman, A. E., Douglas, R. G. *et al.* (1979) Neonatal respiratory syncytial virus infection. *N. Engl. J. Med.*, **300**, 393–396

Hall, P., Kaye, C. M., McIntosh, N. and Steele, J. (1983) Intravenous metronidazole in the newborn. *Arch. Dis. Child.*, **58**, 529–531

Hall, R. T., Hall, S. L., Barnes, W. G. *et al.* (1987) Characteristics of coagulase-negative staphylococci from infants with bacteremia. *Pediatr. Infect. Dis. J.*, **6**, 377–383

Hall, S. and Glickman, M. (1988) The British Paediatric Surveillance Unit. *Arch. Dis. Child.*, **63**, 344–346

Hall, S. M., Crofts, N., Gilbert, R. J. *et al.* (1988) Epidemiology of listeriosis in England and Wales. *Lancet*, **ii**, 502–503

Halperin, S. A., Hendley, J. O., Nosal, C. and Roizman, B. (1980) DNA finger-printing in investigation of apparent nosocomial acquisition of neonatal herpes simplex. *J. Pediatr.*, **97**, 91–93

Hammerberg, O., Watts, J., Chernesky M. *et al.* (1983) An outbreak of herpes simplex virus type 1 in an intensive care nursery. *Pediatr. Infect. Dis.*, **2**, 290–294

Haneberg, B., Bertnes, E. and Haukenes, G. (1980) Antibodies to cytomegalovirus among personnel at a children's hospital. *Acta Paediatr. Scand.*, **69**, 407–409

Hanngren, K., Grandien, M. and Granstrom, G. (1985) Effect of zoster immunoglobulin for varicella prophylaxis in the newborn. *Scand. J. Infect. Dis.*, **17**, 343–347

Hanshaw, J. B., Scheiner, A. P., Moxley, A. W. *et al.* (1976) School failure and deafness after 'silent' congenital cytomegalovirus infection. *N. Engl. J. Med.*, **295**, 468–470

Haque, K. N., Zaidi, M. H., Haque, S. K. *et al.* (1986) Intravenous immunoglobulin for prevention of sepsis in preterm and low birth weight infants. *Pediatr. Infect. Dis. J.*, **5**, 622–625

Haque, K. N., Zaidi, M. H. and Bahakim, H. (1988) IgM-enriched intravenous immunoglobulin therapy in neonatal sepsis. *Am. J. Dis. Child.*, **142**, 1293–1296

Harley, J. D. and Robin, H. (1962) 'Late' neonatal jaundice in infants with glucose-6-phosphate dehydrogenase deficient erythrocytes. *Aust. Ann. Med.*, **11**, 148–155

Harris, H., Wirtshaffer, D. and Cassady, G. (1976) Endotracheal intubation and its relationship to bacterial colonization and systemic infection of newborn infants. *Pediatrics*, **58**, 816–823

Harrison, H. R., English, M. G., Lee, C. K. and Alexander, E. R. (1978) *Chlamydia trachomatis* infant pneumonitis: comparison with matched controls and other infant pneumonitis. *N. Engl. J. Med.*, **298**, 702–708

Harrison, H. R., Taussig, L. M. and Fulginiti, V. A. (1982) *Chlamydia trachomatis* and chronic respiratory disease in childhood. *Pediatr. Infect. Dis. J.*, **1**, 29–33

Haukenes, G. and Haram, K. O. (1972) Clinical rubella after reinfection. *N. Engl. J. Med.*, **287**, 1204

Heckmatt, J. Z. (1976) Coliform meningitis in the newborn. *Arch. Dis. Child.*, **51**, 569–573

Hinman, A. R., Foster, S. O. and Wassilak, S. G. F. (1987) Neonatal tetanus: potential for elimination in the world. *Pediatr. Infect. Dis. J.*, **6**, 813–816

Hohlfeld, P., Daffos, F., Thulliez, P. *et al.* (1989) Fetal toxoplasmosis: outcome of pregnancy and infant follow-up after in utero treatment. *J. Pediatr.*, **115**, 765–769

Holland, P., Isaacs, D. and Moxon, E. R. (1986) Fatal neonatal varicella infection. *Lancet*, **ii**, 1156

Hummell, D. S., Swift, A. J., Tomasz, A. *et al.* (1985) Activation of the alternative pathway of complement pathway by pneumococcal lipoteichoic acid. *Infect. Immun.*, **47**, 384–387

Ingram, D. L., Pengergrass, E. L., Bromberger, P. I. *et al.* (1980) Group B streptococcal disease: its diagnosis with use of antigen detection, Gram's stain, and the presence of apnea, hypotension. *Am. J. Dis. Child.*, **134**, 754–758

Iosub, S., Bamji, M., Stone, R. K. *et al.* (1987) More on human immunodeficiency virus embryopathy. *Pediatrics*, **80**, 512–516

Isaacs, D. (1989) Impact of AIDS on neonatal care. *Arch. Dis. Child.*, **64**, 892

Isaacs, D. and Wilkinson, A. R. (1987) Antibiotic use in the neonatal unit. *Arch. Dis. Child.*, **62**, 204–208

Isaacs, D., Bower, B. D. and Moxon, E. R. (1986a) Neonatal osteomyelitis presenting as nerve palsy. *Br. Med. J.*, **292**, 1071

Isaacs, D., Slack, M. P. E., Wilkinson, A. R. and Westwood, A. W. (1986b) Successful treatment of pseudomonas ventriculitis with ciprofloxacin. *J. Antimicrob. Chemother.*, **17**, 535–538

Isaacs, D., Wilkinson, A. R. and Moxon, E. R. (1987a) Surveillance of colonisation and late-onset septicaemia in neonates. *J. Hosp. Infect.*, **10**, 114–119

Isaacs, D., Wilkinson, A. R. and Moxon, E. R. (1987b) Duration of antibiotic courses for neonates. *Arch. Dis. Child.*, **62**, 727–728

Isaacs, D., Bangham, C. R. M. and McMichael, A. J. (1987c) Cell-mediated cytotoxic response to respiratory syncytial virus in infants with bronchiolitis. *Lancet*, **ii**, 769–771

Isaacs, D., North, J., Lindsell, D. and Wilkinson, A. R. (1987d) Serum acute phase reactants in necrotizing enterocolitis. *Acta Paediatr. Scand.*, **76**, 923–927

Isaacs, D., Catterson, J., Hope, P. L. *et al.* (1988a) Factors influencing colonisation with gentamicin resistant Gram negative organisms in the neonatal unit. *Arch. Dis. Child.*, **63**, 533–535

Isaacs, D., Moxon, E. R., Harvey, D. *et al.* (1988b) Ribavirin in respiratory syncytial virus infection. *Arch. Dis. Child.*, **63**, 986–990

Isaacs, D., Dobson, S. R. M., Wilkinson, A. R. *et al.* (1989) Conservative management of an echovirus 11 outbreak in a neonatal unit. *Lancet*, **i**, 543–545

Italian Multicentre Study (1988) Epidemiology, clinical features and prognostic factors of paediatric HIV infection. *Lancet*, **ii**, 1043–1045

Jager-Roman, E., Doyle, P. E., Baird-Lambert, J. *et al.* (1982) Pharmacokinetics and tissue distribution of metronidazole in the newborn infant. *J. Pediatr.*, **100**, 651–654

Jeannel, D., Costagliola, D., Niel, G. *et al.* (1990) What is known about the prevention of congenital toxoplasmosis. *Lancet*, **336**, 359–361

Jeffery, H., Mitchinson, R., Wigglesworth, J. S. and Davies, P. A. (1977) Early neonatal bacteraemia. *Arch. Dis. Child.*, **52**, 683–686

Johnson, D. and McKenna, H. (1975) Bacteria in ophthalmia neonatorum. *Pathology*, **7**, 199–201

Johnson, D., Thompson, T., Green, T. and Ferrieri, P. (1984) Systemic candidiasis in very low-birth-weight infants (less than 1500 grams). *Pediatrics*, **73**, 138–143

Jones, H. C. (1973) Intrauterine ototoxicity: a case report and review of literature. *J. Natl. Med. Assoc.*, **65**, 201–204

Jones, J. F., Ray, G. G. and Fulginiti, V. A. (1980) Perinatal mumps infection. *J. Pediatr.*, **96**, 912–914

Kafetzis, D. A., Brater, D. C., Kapiki, A. N. *et al.* (1982) Treatment of severe neonatal infections with cefotaxime: efficacy and pharmacokinetics. *J. Pediatr.*, **100**, 438–439

Kahlon, J. and Whitley, R. J. (1988) Antibody response of the newborn after herpes simplex virus infection. *J. Infect. Dis.*, **158**, 925–933

Kaijser, B., Hanson, L. A., Jodal, U. *et al.* (1977) Frequency of E. *coli* K antigens in urinary-tract infections in children. *Lancet*, **i**, 663–666

Kaplan, M. H., Klein, S. W., McPhee, J. and Harper, R. G. (1983) Group B Coxsackievirus infections in infants younger than three months of age: a serious childhood illness. *Rev. Infect. Dis.*, **5**, 1019–1032

Katzenstein, A.-L., Davis, C. and Braude, A. (1976) Pulmonary changes in neonatal sepsis due to Group B beta-haemolytic streptococcus: relation to hyaline membrane disease. *J. Infect. Dis.*, **133**, 430–435

Kendig, E. I. (1969) The place of BCG vaccine in the management of infants born to tuberculous mothers. *N. Engl. J. Med.*, **281**, 520–523

Kerr, K. G., Dealler, S. F. and Lacey, R. W. (1988) Listeria in cook–chill food. *Lancet*, **ii**, 37–38

Kleiman, M. B., Reynolds, J. K., Schreiner, R. L. *et al.* (1984) Rapid diagnosis of neonatal bacteremia with acridine orange-stained buffy coat smears. *J. Pediatr.*, **105**, 419–421

Klein, J. O. (1990a) Bacterial infections of the urinary tract. In *Infectious Diseases of the Fetus and Newborn Infant*, 3rd edn (eds J. S. Remington and J. O. Klein), W. B. Saunders, Philadelphia, pp. 690–699

Klein, J. O. (1990b) Bacterial infections of the respiratory tract. In *Infectious Diseases of the Fetus and Newborn Infant*, 3rd edn (eds J. S. Remington and J. O. Klein), W. B. Saunders, Philadelphia, pp. 657–673

Klein, J. O. and Marcy, S. M. (1990) Bacterial sepsis and meningitis. In *Infectious Diseases of the Fetus and Newborn Infant*, 3rd edn (eds J. S. Remington and J. O. Klein), W. B. Saunders, Philadelphia, pp. 601–656

Kliegman, R. M. and Fanaroff, A. A. (1981) Neonatal necrotising enterocolitis: a nine-year experience. I. Epidemiology and uncommon observations. *Am. J. Dis. Child.*, **135**, 603–607

Kliegman, R. M. and Fanaroff, A. A. (1984) Necrotising enterocolitis. *N. Engl. J. Med.*, **310**, 1093–1103

Kline, A. H., Blattner, R. J. and Lunin, M. (1964) Transplacental effect of tetracyclines on teeth. *JAMA*, **188**, 178–180

Kohl, S. (1989) The neonatal human's immune response to herpes simplex infection: a critical view. *Pediatr. Infect. Dis. J.*, **8**, 67–74

Kohn, J. L. (1933) Measles in newborn infants (maternal infection). *J. Pediatr.*, **3**, 176–179

Korzeniowski, O. and Sande, M. A. (1982) Combination antimicrobial therapy for *Staphylococcus aureus* endocarditis inpatients addicted to parenteral drugs and in non-addicts. A prospective study. *Ann. Intern. Med.*, **97**, 496–503

Kozinn, P. J., Taschdjian, C. L., Wiener, H. *et al.* (1958) Neonatal candidiasis. *Pediatr. Clin. North Am.*, **5**, 803–815

Kumar, M. L., Nakervis, G. A., Cooper, A. R. and Gold, E. (1984a) Postnatally acquired cytomegalovirus infections in infants of CMV-excreting mothers. *J. Pediatr.*, **104**, 669–673

Kumar, M. L., Nankervis, G. A., Jacobs, I. B. *et al.* (1984b) Congenital and post-natally acquired cytomegalovirus infections: long-term follow-up. *J. Pediatr.*, **104**, 674–679

Kumari, S., Bhargava, S. K., Baijal, V. N. and Ghosh, S. (1978) Neonatal osteomyelitis: a clinical and follow-up study. *Indian Pediatr.*, **15**, 393–397

Lacey, R. W. (1984) Evolution of microorganisms and antibiotic resistance. *Lancet*, **ii**, 1022–1025

La Gamma, E. F., Drusin, L. M., Mackles, A. W. *et al.* (1983) Neonatal infections: an important determinant of late NICU mortality in infants less than 1000g at birth. *Am. J. Dis. Child.*, **137**, 838–841

La Gamma, E. F., Ostertag, S. G. and Birenbaum, H. (1985) Failure of delayed oral feedings to prevent necrotizing enterocolitis. *Am. J. Dis. Child.*, **139**, 385–389

Lake, A. M. and Walker, A. A. (1977) Neonatal necrotizing enterocolitis: a disease of altered host defense. *Clin. Gastroenterol.*, **6**, 463–480

Larson, E. (1988) A causal link between handwashing and risk of infection? Examination of the evidence. *Infect. Control Hosp. Epidemiol.*, **9**, 28–36

Laure, F., Courgnaud, V., Rouzioux, C. *et al.* (1988) Detection of HIV-1 DNA in infants and children by means of the polymerase chain reaction. *Lancet*, **ii**, 538–541

Laurenti, F., Ferro, R., Isacchi, G. *et al.* (1981) Polymorphonuclear leukocyte transfusion for the treatment of sepsis in the newborn infant. *J. Pediatr.*, **98**, 118–123

Lawrence, G., Bates, J. and Gaul, A. (1982) Pathogenesis of neonatal necrotising enterocolitis. *Lancet*, **i**, 137–139

Lepage, P., Van de Perre, P., Carael, M. *et al.* (1987) Postnatal transmission of HIV from mother to child. *Lancet*, **ii**, 400

Leslie, G. I., Scurr, R. D. and Barr, P. A. (1981) Early-onset bacterial pneumonia: a comparison with severe hyaline membrane disease. *Aust. Paediatr. J.*, **17**, 202–206

Light, I. J. (1979) Postnatal acquisition of herpes simplex virus by the newborn infant: a review of the literature. *Pediatrics*, **63**, 480–482

Likitnukul, S., McCracken, G. H., Threlkeld, N. *et al.* (1987) Pharmacokinetics and plasma bactericidal activity of aztreonam in low birth weight infants. *Antimicrob. Agents Chemother.*, **31**, 81–83

Lim, M. O., Gresham, E. L., Franken, E. A. and Leake, R. D. (1977) Osteomyelitis as a complication of umbilical artery catheterization. *Am. J. Dis. Child.*, **131**, 142–144

Lincoln, K. and Winberg, J. (1964a) Studies of urinary tract infections in infancy and childhood. II. Quantitative estimation of bacteriuria in unselected neonates with special reference to the occurrence of asymptomatic infections. *Acta Paediatr. Scand.*, **53**, 307–316

Lincoln, K. and Winberg, J. (1964b) Studies of urinary tract infection in infancy and childhood. III. Quantitative estimation of cellular excretion in unselected neonates. *Acta Paediatr. Scand.*, **53**, 447–453

Linnemann, C. C., Buchman, T. G., Light, I. J. and Ballard, J. L. (1978) Transmission of herpes-simplex virus type 1 in a nursery for the newborn. Identification of viral isolates by DNA 'fingerprinting'. *Lancet*, **i**, 964–966

Lissauer, T. (1989) The impact of AIDS on neonatal care. *Arch. Dis. Child.*, **64**, 4–7

Littlewood, J. M., Kite, P. and Kite, B. A. (1969) Incidence of neonatal urinary tract infection. *Arch. Dis. Child.*, **44**, 617–620

Lohrer, R. and Belohradsky, B. H. (1987) Bacterial endophthalmitis in neonates. *Eur. J. Pediatr.*, **146**, 354–359

Loke, H. L., Verber, I., Szymonowicz, W. and Yu, V. H. (1988) Systemic candidiasis and pneumonia in preterm infants. *Aust. Paediatr. J.*, **24**, 138–142

Lomberg, H., Hanson, L. A., Jacobsson, B. *et al.* (1983) Correlation of P blood group, vesicoureteral reflux, and bacterial attachment in patients with recurrent pyelonephritis. *N. Engl. J. Med.*, **308**, 1189–1192

Luginbuhl, L. M., Rotbart, H. A., Facklam, R. R. *et al.* (1987) Neonatal enterococcal sepsis: case-control study and description of an outbreak. *Pediatr. Infect. Dis. J.*, **6**, 1022–1030

McCabe, R. and Remington, J. S. (1988) Toxoplasmosis: the time has come. *N. Engl. J. Med.*, **318**, 313–315

McCracken, G. H. (1972) The rate of bacteriologic response to antimicrobial therapy in neonatal meningitis. *Am. J. Dis. Child.*, **123**, 547–553

McCracken, G. H. and Feldman, W. E. (1976) Editorial comment. *J. Pediatr.*, **89**, 203–204

McCracken, G. H. and Mize, S. G. (1976) A controlled study of intrathecal antibiotic therapy in gram-negative enteric meningitis of infancy. *J. Pediatr.*, **89**, 66–72

McCracken, G. H. and Nelson, J. D. (1983) *Antimicrobial Therapy for Newborns*, 2nd edn, Grune and Stratton, New York

McCracken, G. H. and Freij, B. J. (1990) Clinical pharmacology of antimicrobial agents. In *Infectious Diseases of the Fetus and Newborn Infant*, 3rd edn (eds J. S. Remington and J. O Klein), W. B. Saunders, Philadelphia, pp. 1020–1078

McCracken G. H., Ginsberg, C., Chrane D. F. *et al.* (1973) Clinical pharmacology of penicillin in newborn infants. *Pediatrics*, **82**, 692–698

McCracken, G. H., Ginsberg, C. M., Clahsen, J. C. and Thomas, M. L. (1978) Pharmacologic evaluation of orally administered antibiotics in the newborn infant. *Antimicrob. Agents Chemother.*, **5**, 214–219

McCracken, G. H., Mize, S. G. and Threlkeld, N. (1980) Intraventricular gentamicin therapy in gram-negative bacillary meningitis of infancy. *Lancet*, **i**, 787–791

McCracken, G. H., Threlkeld, N, Mize, S. *et al.* (1984) Moxalactam therapy for neonatal meningitis due to gram-negative enteric bacilli. A prospective controlled evaluation. *JAMA*, **252**, 1427–1432

McDougall, P. N., Fleming, P. J., Speller, D. C. E. *et al.* (1982) Neonatal systemic neonatal candidiasis: a failure to respond to intravenous miconazole in two infants. *Arch. Dis. Child.*, **57**, 884–886

Macfarlane, D. E. (1987) Neonatal group B streptococcal septicaemia in a developing country. *Acta Paediatr. Scand.*, **76**, 470–473

McGill, R. E. T. (1979) Neonatal eye infections. *Communicable Diseases (Scotland) Weekly Report*, **22**, 12

McLaughlin, J. (1987) *Listeria monocytogenes*, recent advances in the taxonomy and epidemiology of listeriosis in humans. *J. Appl. Bacteriol.*, **63**, 1–11

Maherzi, M., Guignard, J.-P. and Torrado, A. (1978) Urinary tract infection in high-risk newborn infants. *Pediatrics*, **62**, 521–523

Manroe, B. L., Weinberg, A. G., Rosenfeld, C. R. *et al.* (1979) The neonatal blood count in health and disease. I. Reference values for neutrophilic cells. *J. Pediatr.*, **95**, 89–98

Marild, S., Jodal, U., Orskov, I. *et al.* (1989) Special virulence of the *Escherichia coli* O1:K1:H7 clone in acute pyelonephritis. *J. Pediatr.*, **115**, 40–45

Marion, R. W., Wiznia, A. A., Hutcheon, R. G. and Rubinstein, A. (1986) Human T-cell lymphotropic virus type III (HTLV-III) embryopathy: a new dysmorphic syndrome associated with intrauterine HTLV-III infection. *Am. J. Dis. Child.*, **140**, 638–640

Marion, R. W., Wiznia, A. A., Hutcheon, R. G. and Rubinstein, A. (1987) Fetal AIDS syndrome score: correlation between severity of dysmorphism and age at diagnosis of immunodeficiency. *Am. J. Dis. Child.*, **141**, 429–431

Mason, W. H., Andrews, R., Ross, L. A. and Wright, H. T. (1989) Omphalitis in the newborn infant. *Pediatr. Infect. Dis. J.*, **8**, 521–525

Maupas, P., Chiron, J.-P., Barim, F. *et al.* (1981) Efficacy of hepatitis B vaccine in prevention of HBsAG carrier state in children. Controlled trial in an endemic area. *Lancet*, **i**, 289–292

Maybe, D. C. W. and Whittle, H. C. (1982) Genital and neonatal chlamydial infection in a trachoma endemic area, Gambia. *Lancet*, **ii**, 300–301

Meheus, A., Delgadillo, R., Widy-Wirsky, R. and Piot, P. (1982) Chlamydial ophthalmia neonatorum in Central Africa. *Lancet*, **ii**, 882

Meissner, H. C., Murray, S. A., Kiernan, M. A. *et al.* (1984) A simultaneous outbreak of respiratory syncytial virus and parainfluenza virus type 3 in a newborn nursery. *J. Pediatr.*, **104**, 680–684

Messaritakis, J., Anagnostakis, D., Laskari, H. and Katerelos, C. (1990) Rectal–skin temperature difference in septicaemic newborn infants. *Arch. Dis. Child.*, **65**, 380–382

Mifsud, A., Seal, D., Wall, R. and Valman, B. (1988) Reduced neonatal mortality from infection after introduction of respiratory monitoring. *Br. Med. J.*, **296**, 17–18

Millar, M. R., Keyworth, N., Lincoln, C. *et al.* (1987) 'Methicillin-resistant' *Staphylococcus aureus* in a regional neonatology unit. *J. Hosp. Infect.*, **10**, 187–197

Miller, E., Cradock-Watson, J. E. and Pollock, T. M. (1982) Consequences of confirmed maternal rubella at successive stages of pregnancy. *Lancet*, **ii**, 781–784

Miller, E., Cradock-Watson, J. E. and Ridehalgh, M. K. S. (1989) Outcome of newborn babies given anti-varicella–zoster immunoglobulin after perinatal maternal infection with varicella–zoster virus. *Lancet*, **ii**, 371–373

Miller, M. E. (1978) *Host Defenses in the Human Neonate*, Grune and Stratton, New York

Milne, L. M., Isaacs, D. and Crook, P. J. (1988) Neonatal infections with *Haemophilus* species. *Arch. Dis. Child.*, **63**, 83–85

Mintz, L., Ballard, R. A., Sniderman, S. H. *et al.* (1979) Nosocomial respiratory syncytial virus infections in an intensive care nursery: rapid diagnosis by direct immunofluorescence. *Pediatrics*, **64**, 149–153

Modi, N., Damjanovic, V. and Cooke, R. W. (1987) Outbreak of cephalosporin resistant *Enterobacter cloacae* infection in a neonatal intensive care unit. *Arch. Dis. Child.*, **62**, 148–151

Modlin, J. F. (1986) Perinatal echovirus infection: insights from a literature review of 61 cases of serious infection and 16 outbreaks in nurseries. *Rev. Infect. Dis.*, **8**, 918–926

Modlin, J. F., Hermann, K., Brandling-Bennett, A. D. *et al.* (1976) Risk of congenital abnormality after inadvertent rubella vaccination of pregnant women. *N. Engl. J. Med.*, **294**, 972–974

Mok, J. Q., Giaquinto, C., de Rossi, A. *et al.* (1987) Infants born to mothers seropositive for human immunodeficiency virus. *Lancet*, **i**, 1164–1167

Mok, J. Y. G., Hague, R. A., Yap, P. L. *et al.* (1989) Vertical transmission of HIV: a prospective study. *Arch. Dis. Child.*, **64**, 1140–1145

Moller, M., Thomsen, A. C., Borch, K. *et al.* (1984) Rupture of fetal membranes and premature delivery associated with group-B streptococci in urine of pregnant women. *Lancet*, **ii**, 69–70

Morrison, A. J. and Wenzel, R. P. (1984) Epidemiology of infections due to *Pseudomonas aeruginosa*. *Rev. Infect. Dis.*, **6** (Suppl.), 627–642

Morrison, J. E. (1970) *Foetal and Neonatal Pathology*, 3rd edn, Butterworth, Washington DC

Moxon, E. R. and Ostrow, P. T. (1977) *Haemophilus influenzae* meningitis in infant rats: role of bacteremia in pathogenesis of age-dependent inflammatory responses in cerebrospinal fluid. *J. Infect. Dis.*, **135**, 303–307

Moxon, E. R., Smith, A. L., Averill, D. R. and Smith, D. H. (1974) *Haemophilus influenzae* meningitis in infant rats after intranasal inoculation. *J. Infect. Dis.*, **129**, 154–162

Mulhall, A., de Louvois, J. and Hurley, R. (1983a) Efficacy of chloramphenicol in the treatment of neonatal and infantile meningitis: a study of 70 cases. *Lancet*, **i**, 284–287

Mulhall, A., de Louvois, J. and Hurley, R. (1983b) Chloramphenicol toxicity in neonates: its incidence and prevention. *Br. Med. J.*, **287**, 1424–1427

Murphy, N., Buchanan, C. R., Damjanovic, V. *et al.* (1986) Infection and colonisation of neonates by *Hansenula anomala*. *Lancet*, **i**, 291–293

Myers, J. D. (1974) Congenital varicella in term infants: risks reconsidered. *J. Infect. Dis.*, **129**, 215–217

Naeye, R. L. (1977) Causes of perinatal morbidity in the US Collaborative Perinatal Project. *JAMA*, **238**, 228–229

Naeye, R. L. and Peters, E. C. (1978) Amniotic fluid infections with intact membranes leading to perinatal death: a prospective study. *Paediatrics*, **61**, 171–177

Naeye, R. L., Dellinger, W. S., and Blanc, W. A. (1971) Fetal and maternal features of antenatal bacterial infections. *J. Pediatr.*, **79**, 733–739

Naeye, R. L., Tafari, N., Judge, D. *et al.* (1977) Amniotic fluid infections in an African city. *J. Pediatr.*, **90**, 965–970

Nagington, J., Gandy, G., Walker, J. and Gray, J. J. (1983) Use of normal immunoglobulin in an echovirus 11 outbreak in a special-care baby unit. *Lancet*, **ii**, 443–446

Nahmias, A. J., Josey, W. E., Naib, Z. M. *et al.* (1971) Perinatal risk factors associated with maternal genital herpes simplex virus infection. *Am. J. Obstet. Gynecol.*, **110**, 825–833

Nahmias, A. J., Whitley, R. J., Visitine, A. N. *et al.* (1982) Herpes simplex virus encephalitis: laboratory evaluations and their diagnostic significance. *J. Infect. Dis.*, **145**, 829–836

Nahmias, A. J., Keyserling, H. L. and Kerrick, G. M. (1983) Herpes simplex. In *Infectious Diseases of the Fetus and Newborn Infant*, 2nd edn (eds J. S. Remington and J. O. Klein), W. B. Saunders, Philadelphia, pp. 636–678

Naidoo, B. T. (1968) The cerebrospinal fluid in the newborn infant. *South Afr. Med. J.*, **42**, 933–935

Naqvi, S. H., Maxwell, M. A. and Dunkle, L. M. (1985) Cefotaxime therapy of neonatal Gram-negative bacillary meningitis. *Pediatr. Infect. Dis.*, **4**, 499–502

Nelson, J. D. (1983) Control of infection acquired in the nursery. In *Infectious Diseases of the Fetus and Newborn Infant*, 2nd edn (eds J. S. Remington and J. O. Klein), W. B. Saunders, Philadelphia, pp. 1035–1052

Nilsby, I. and Norden, A. (1949) Studies of occurrence of *Candida albicans*. *Acta Med. Scand.*, **133**, 340–345

Northrop, R. L., Gardner, W. M. and Geittmann, W. F. (1972) Rubella reinfection during early pregnancy: a case report. *Obstet. Gynecol.*, **39**, 524–526

Nota, F. J. D., Rench, M. A., Metzger, T. G. *et al.* (1987) Unusual occurrence of an epidemic of Ib/c group B streptococcal sepsis in a neonatal intensive care unit. *J. Infect. Dis.*, **155**, 1135–1144

Numazaki, Y., Yano, N., Morizuka, T. *et al.* (1970) Primary infection with cytomegalovirus: virus isolation from healthy infants and pregnant women. *Am. J. Epidemiol.*, **91**, 410–417

Odds, F. C. (1981) The pathogenesis of candidosis. *Hospital Update*, **7**, 935–945

Ogden, J. A. and Lister, G. (1975) The pathology of neonatal osteomyelitis. *Pediatrics*, **55**, 474–478

Oh, W. (1981) Renal functions and clinical disorders in the neonate. *Clin. Perinatol.*, **8**, 215–223

Otiti, J. M. L. (1975) Ophthalmia neonatorum in Mbale Hospital, Uganda. *East Afr. Med. J.*, **52**, 644–647

Oxtoby, M. J. (1988) HIV and other viruses in human milk: placing the issue in broader perspective. *Pediatr. Infect. Dis. J.*, **7**, 825–835

Paredes, A., Wong, P. and Yow, M. D. (1976) Failure of penicillin to eradicate the carrier state of group B streptococcus in infants. *J. Pediatr.*, **89**, 191–193

Paryani, S. G. and Arvin, A. M. (1986) Intrauterine infection with varicella–zoster virus after maternal varicella. *N. Engl. J. Med.*, **314**, 1542–1546

Pass, M. A., Khare, S. and Dillon, H. C. Jr (1980) Twin pregnancies: Incidence of group B streptococcal colonization and disease. *J. Pediatr.*, **97**, 635–637

Patrick, C. C., Kaplan, S. L., Baker, C. J. *et al.* (1989) Persistent bacteraemia due to coagulase-negative staphylococci in low birth weight neonates. *Pediatrics*, **84**, 977–985

Payne, N. R., Burke, B. A., Day, D. L. *et al.* (1988) Correlation of clinical and pathologic findings in early onset neonatal Group B streptococcal infection with disease severity and prediction of outcome. *Pediatr. Infect. Dis. J.*, **7**, 836–847

Peckham, C. S., Coleman, J. C., Hurley, R. *et al.* (1983) Cytomegalovirus infection in pregnancy: preliminary findings from a prospective study. *Lancet*, **i**, 1352–1355

Pedersen, G. T. (1964) Yeasts isolated from the throat, rectum and vagina in 60 women examined during pregnancy and half to one year after labour. *Acta Obstet. Gynaecol. Scand.*, **42** (suppl. 6), 47–51

Philip, A. G. S. and Hewitt, J. R. (1980) Early diagnosis of neonatal sepsis. *Pediatrics*, **65**, 1036–1041

Pichichero, M. D. and Todd, J. K. (1979) Detection of neonatal bacteremia. *J. Pediatr.*, **94**, 958–960

Pierce, J. M., Ward, M. E. and Seal, D. V. (1982) Ophthalmia neonatorum in the 1980's: incidence, aetiology and treatment. *Br. J. Ophthalmol.*, **66**, 728–731

Polakoff, S. (1985) Hepatitis B virus DNA and e antigen in serum from blood donors positive for HBsAg. *Br. Med. J.*, **290**, 1211–1212

Pole, J. R. and McAllister, T. A. (1975) Gastric aspirate analysis in the newborn. *Acta Paediatr. Scand.*, **64**, 109–112

Pourcyrous, M., Korones, S. B., Bada, H. S. *et al.* (1988) Indwelling umbilical arterial catheter: a preferred sampling site for blood culture. *Pediatrics*, **81**, 821–825

Preblud, S. R., Stetler, H. C., Frank, J. A. *et al.* (1981) Fetal risk associated with rubella vaccine. *JAMA*, **246**, 1413–1417

Preblud, S. R., Orenstein, W. A. and Bart, K. J. (1984) Varicella: clinical manifestations, epidemiology and health impact in children. *Pediatr. Infect. Dis. J.*, **3**, 505–509

Preblud, S. R., Bregman, D. J. and Vernon, L. L. (1985) Deaths from varicella in infants. *Pediatr. Infect. Dis. J.*, **4**, 503–507

Preblud, S. R., Cochi, S. L. and Orenstein, W. A. (1986) Varicella–zoster infection in pregnancy. *N. Engl. J. Med.*, **315**, 1416–1417

Preece, P. M., Pearl, K. N. and Peckham, C. S. (1984) Congenital cytomegalovirus infection. *Arch. Dis. Child.*, **59**, 1120–1126

Preece, P. M., Tookey, P., Ades, A. and Peckham, C. S. (1986) Congenital cytomegalovirus infection: predisposing maternal factors. *J. Epidemiol. Community Health*, **40**, 205–209

Prentice, M. J., Hutchinson, C. R. and Taylor-Robinson, D. (1977) A microbiological study of neonatal conjunctivae and conjunctivitis. *Br. J. Ophthalmol.*, **61**, 601–607

Prince, G. A., Hemming, V. G. and Chanock, R. M. (1986) The use of purified immunoglobulin in the therapy of respiratory syncytial virus infection. *Pediatr. Infect. Dis. J.*, **5**, 201–203

Prober, C. G. and Yeager, A. S. (1979) Use of the serum bactericidal titer to assess the adequacy of oral antibiotic therapy in the treatment of acute haematogenous osteomyelitis. *J. Pediatr.*, **95**, 131–135

Prober, C. G., Sullender, W. M., Yasukawa, L. L. *et al.* (1987) Low risk of herpes simplex virus infections in neonates exposed to the virus at the time of vaginal delivery to mothers with recurrent genital herpes simplex virus infection. *N. Engl. J. Med.*, **316**, 240–244

Prober, C. G., Hensleigh, P. A., Boucher, F. D. *et al.* (1988) Use of routine viral cultures at delivery to identify neonates exposed to herpes simplex virus. *N. Engl. J. Med.*, **318**, 887–891

Prober, C. G., Stevenson, D. K. and Benitz, W. E. (1990) The use of antibiotics in neonates weighing less than 1200 grams. *Pediatr. Infect. Dis. J.*, **9**, 111–121

Pyati, S. P., Pildes, R. S., Jacobs, N. M. *et al.* (1983) Penicillin in infants weighing two kilograms or less with early-onset group B streptococcal disease. *N. Engl. J. Med.*, **308**, 1383–1389

Qasi, Q. H., Sheikh, T. M., Fikrig, S. and Menikoff, H. (1988) Lack of evidence for craniofacial dysmorphism in perinatal human immunodeficiency virus infection. *J. Pediatr.*, **112**, 7–11

Rajchgot, P., Prober, C. G., Soldin, S. J. *et al.* (1983) Toward optimization of therapy in the neonate. *Clin. Pharmacol. Ther.*, **33**, 551–555

Rapoza, P. A., Quinn, T. C., Kiessling, L. A. and Taylor, H. R. (1986) Epidemiology of neonatal conjunctivitis. *Ophthalmology*, **93**, 456–461

Raz, R., Sharir, R., Shmilowitz, L. *et al.* (1987) The elimination of gentamicin-resistant gram-negative bacteria in a newborn intensive care unit. *Infection*, **15**, 32–34

RCOG Sub-Committee (1987) *Report on Problems Associated with AIDS in Relation to Obstetrics and Gynaecology*, Royal College of Obstetricians and Gynaecologists, London

Rees, E., Tait, I. A., Hobson, D. *et al.* (1977) Neonatal conjunctivitis caused by *Neisseria gonorrhoeae* and *Chlamydia trachomatis*. *Br. J. Vener. Dis.*, **53**, 173–179

Regan, J. A., Chao, S. and James, L. S. (1981) Premature rupture of membranes, preterm delivery and group B streptococcal colonization of mothers. *Am. J. Obstet. Gynecol.*, **141**, 184–186

Reman, O., Freymuth, F., Laloum, D. and Boute, J. P. (1986) Neonatal respiratory distress due to mumps. *Arch. Dis. Child.*, **61**, 80–81

Remington, J. S. and Desmonts, G. (1990) Toxoplasmosis. In *Infectious Diseases of the Fetus and Newborn Infant*, 3rd edn (eds J. S. Remington and J. O. Klein), W. B. Saunders, Philadelphia, pp. 89–195

Reynolds, D. W., Stagno, S., Stubbs, K. G. *et al.* (1974) Inapparent congenital cytomegalovirus infection with elevated cord blood IgM levels: causal relation with auditory and mental deficiency. *N. Engl. J. Med.*, **290**, 291–296

Richardson, D. L. (1920) Measles contracted *in utero*. *Rhode Island Med. J.*, **3**, 13–16

Robbins, J. B., McCracken, G. H., Gotschlich, E. C. *et al.* (1974) *Escherichia coli* Kl capsular polysaccharide associated with neonatal meningitis. *N. Engl. J. Med.*, **290**, 1216–1220

Robertson, A., Fink, S. and Karp, W. (1988) Effect of cephalosporins on bilirubin–albumin binding. *J. Pediatr.*, **112**, 291–294

Robinson, G. C. and Cambon, K. G. (1964) Hearing loss in infants of tuberculous mothers treated with streptomycin in pregnancy. *N. Engl. J. Med.*, **271**, 949–951

Rodwell, R. L., Leslie, A. L. and Tudehope, D. I. (1988) Early diagnosis of neonatal sepsis using a hematologic scoring system. *J. Pediatr.*, **112**, 761–767

Rodwell, R. L., Leslie, A. L. and Tudehope, D. I. (1989) Evaluation of direct and buffy coat films of peripheral blood for the early detection of bacteraemia. *Aust. Paediatr. J.*, **25**, 83–85

Rolleston, G. L., Shannon, F. T. and Utley, W. L. F. (1970) Relationship of infantile vesicoureteric reflux to renal damage. *Br. Med. J.*, **1**, 460–463

Rozycki. H. J., Stahl, G. E. and Baumgart, S. (1987) Impaired sensitivity of a single early leukocyte count in screening for neonatal sepsis. *Pediatr. Infect. Dis. J.*, **6**, 440–442

Rubin, L., Leggiadro, R., Elie, M. T. and Lipsitz, P. (1986) Disseminated varicella in a neonate: implications for immunoprophylaxis of neonates exposed to varicella. *Pediatr. Infect. Dis. J.*, **5**, 100–102

Rubinstein, A. (1986) Pediatric AIDS. *Curr. Probl. Pediatr.*, **16**, 361–409

Rudd, P. T. and Carrington, D. (1984) A prospective study of chlamydial, mycoplasmal and viral infections in a neonatal intensive care unit. *Arch. Dis. Child.*, **59**, 120–125

Rudd, P. T., Waites, K. B., Duffy, L. B. *et al.* (1986) *Ureaplasma urealyticum* and its possible role in pneumonia during the neonatal period and infancy. *Pediatr. Infect. Dis. J.*, **5**, S288–S291

Rutter, D., Griffiths, P. and Trompeter, R. S. (1985) Cytomegalovirus inclusion disease after recurrent maternal infection. *Lancet*, **ii**, 1182

Ryder, R. W., Shelton, J. D. and Guinan, M. E. (1980) Committee on necrotising enterocolitis. Necrotising enterocolitis: a prospective multicenter study. *Am. J. Epidemiol.*, **112**, 113–123

Sabel, K. G. and Brandberg, A. (1975) Treatment of meningitis and septicemia in infancy with a sulfamethoxazole–trimethoprim combination. *Acta Pediatr. Scand.*, **64**, 25–32

Sabel, K. G. and Hanson, L. A. (1974) The clinical usefulness of C-reactive protein (CRP) determinations in bacterial meningitis and septicaemia in infancy. *Acta Paediatr. Scand.*, **63**, 381–388

Sabin, A. B. (1942) Toxoplasmosis: recently recognized disease of human beings. V. Clinical manifestations of toxoplasmosis in man. *Adv. Pediatr.*, **1**, 1–56

Saccharow, L. and Pryles, C. V. (1969) Further experience with the use of percutaneous suprapubic aspiration of the urinary bladder. Bacteriologic studies in 654 infants and children. *Pediatrics*, **43**, 1018–1024

Sadiq, H. F., Devaskar, S., Keenan, W. J. and Weber, T. R. (1987) Broviac catheterisation in low birth weight infants: incidence and treatment of associated complications. *Crit. Care Med.*, **15**, 47–50

Saigal, S., Lunyk, O., Larke, R. P. B. and Chernesky, M. A. (1982) The outcome in children with congenital cytomegalovirus infection. *Am. J. Dis. Child.*, **136**, 896–901

Salimpour, R. (1977) Cause of death in tetanus neonatorum. Study of 233 cases with 54 necropsies. *Arch. Dis. Child.*, **52**, 587–594

Sande, M. A., Scheld, W. M., McCracken, G. H. *et al.* (1987) Report of a workshop: pathophysiology of bacterial meningitis – implications for new management strategies. *Pediatr. Infect. Dis. J.*, 6 Suppl, 1143–1171

Sandstrom, I. (1987) Etiology and diagnosis of neonatal conjunctivitis. *Acta Paediatr. Scand.*, **76**, 221–227

Sandstrom, I., Bell, T. A., Chandler, J. W. *et al.* (1984) Microbial causes of neonatal conjunctivitis. *J. Pediatr.*, **105**, 706–711

Sarff, L. D., Platt, L. H. and McCracken, G. H. (1976) Cerebrospinal fluid evaluation in neonates: comparison of high-risk infants with and without meningitis. *J. Pediatr.*, **88**, 473–477

Schaad, U. B., McCracken, G. H. and Nelson, J. D. (1980) Clinical pharmacology and efficacy of vancomycin in pediatrics. *J. Pediatr.*, **96**, 119–126

Schaad, U. B., McCracken, G. H., Threlkeld, N. *et al.* (1981) Clinical evaluation of a new broad-spectrum oxa-beta-lactam, moxalactam, in neonates and infants. *J. Pediatr.*, **98**, 129–36

Schachter, J. and Grossman, M. (1981) Chlamydial infections. *Ann. Rev. Med.*, **32**, 45–61

Scheifele, D. W., Bjornson, G. L., Dyer, R. A. and Dimmick, J. E. (1987) Delta-like toxin produced by coagulase-negative staphylococci is associated with neonatal necrotizing enterocolitis. *Infect. Immun.*, **55**, 2268–2273

Schlech, W. F., Lavigne, P. M., Bortolussi, R. A. *et al.* (1983) Epidemic listeriosis – evidence for transmission by food. *N. Engl. J. Med.*, **308**, 203–206

Schoenbaum, S. C., Gardner, P. and Shillito, J. (1975) Infections of cerebrospinal fluid shunts: epidemiology, clinical manifestations and therapy. *J. Infect. Dis.*, **131**, 543–552

Schopfer, K., Lauber, E. and Krech, U. (1978) Congenital cytomegalovirus infection in newborn infants of mothers infected before pregnancy. *Arch. Dis. Child.*, **53**, 536–539

Schopfner, C. F. (1970) Modern concepts of lower urinary tract obstruction in pediatric patients. *Pediatrics*, **45**, 194–196

Schreiber, J. R., Maynard, E. and Lew, M. A. (1984) Candida antigen detection in two premature neonates with disseminated candidiasis. *Pediatrics*, **74**, 838–841

Schwartz, B., Ciesielski, C. A., Broome, C. V. *et al.* (1988) Association of sporadic listeriosis with consumption of uncooked hot dogs and undercooked chicken. *Lancet*, **ii**, 779–782

Schweitzer, I. L., Wing, A., McPeak, C. and Spears, R. L. (1972) Hepatitis and hepatitis-associated antigen in 56 mother–infant pairs. *JAMA*, **220**, 1092–1095

Schweitzer, I. L., Dunn, A. E., Peters, R. L. and Spears, R. L. (1973) Viral hepatitis B in neonates and infants. *Am. J. Med.*, **55**, 762–771

Scotto, J., Hadchouel, M. and Hery, C. (1983) Detection of hepatitis B virus DNA in serum by a simple spot hybridization technique. Comparison with results for other viral markers. *Hepatology*, **3**, 279–284

Seelig, M. S. (1966) The role of antibiotics in the pathogenesis of *Candida* infections. *Am. J. Med.*, **40**, 887–917

Sells, C. J., Carpenter, R. L. and Ray, C. G. (1975) Sequelae of central nervous system enterovirus infections. *N. Engl. J. Med.*, **293**, 1–4

Sever, J. A. and White, L. R. (1968) Intrauterine viral infections. *Ann. Rev. Med.*, **19**, 471–486

Sherman, M. P., Goetzman, B. W., Ahlfors, C. E. and Wennberg, R. P. (1980) Tracheal aspiration and its clinical correlates in the diagnosis of congenital pneumonia. *Pediatrics*, **65**, 258–263

Sherman, M. P., Chance, K. H. and Goetzman, B. W. (1984) Gram's stains of tracheal secretions predict neonatal bacteremia. *Am. J. Dis. Child.*, **138**, 848–850

Shiraki, K., Yoshi, N., Sakurai, M. *et al.* (1980) Acute hepatitis B in infants born to carrier mothers with the antibody to hepatitis B e antigen. *J. Pediatr.*, **97**, 768–770

Shirkey, H. C. (1970) Therapeutic orphans: who speaks for children? *South. Med. J.*, **63**, 1361–1363

Sidiropoulos, D., Boehme, U., von Muralt, G. *et al.* (1981) Immunoglobulinsubstitution bei der Behandling der neonatalen sepsis. *Schweiz. Med. Wochenschr.*, **111**, 1649–1655

Siegel, J. D. and McCracken, G. H. (1981) Sepsis neonatorum. *N. Engl. J. Med.*, **304**, 642–647

Siegel, J. D., McCracken, G. H., Threlkeld N. *et al.* (1980) Single-dose penicillin prophylaxis against neonatal group B streptococcal infections. A controlled trial in 18, 738 newborn infants. *N. Engl. J. Med.*, **303**, 769–775

Siegel, M. (1973) Congenital malformations following chickenpox, measles, mumps and hepatitis. *JAMA*, **226**, 1521–1524

Siegel, M., Fuerst, H. T. and Peress, N. S. (1966) Comparative fetal mortality in maternal virus diseases. A prospective study on rubella, measles, mumps, chickenpox and hepatitis. *N. Engl. J. Med.*, **274**, 768–771

Silverman, W. A., Andersen, D. M., Blanc, W. A. *et al.* (1956) A difference in mortality rate and incidence of kernicterus among premature infants allotted to two prophylactic antibacterial regimens. *Pediatrics*, **18**, 614–624

Sims, M. E., Yoo, Y., You, H. *et al.* (1988) Prophylactic oral nystatin and fungal infections in very-low-birth weight infants. *Am. J. Perinatol.*, **5**, 33–36

Sinatra, F. R., Shah, P., Weissman, J. Y. *et al.* (1982) Perinatal transmitted acute icteric hepatitis B in infants born to hepatitis B surface antigen-positive and anti-hepatitis Be-positive carrier mothers. *Pediatrics*, **70**, 557–559

Slagle, T. A., Bifano, E. M., Wolf, J. W. and Gross, S. J. (1989) Routine endotracheal cultures for the prediction of sepsis in ventilated babies. *Arch. Dis. Child.*, **64**, 34–38

Small, P. M., Tauber, M. G., Hackbarth, C. J. *et al.* (1986) Influence of body temperature on bacterial growth rates in experimental pneumococcal meningitis in rabbits. *Infect. Immun.*, **52**, 484–487

Smythe, P. M., Bowie, M. D. and Voss, T. J. V. (1974) Treatment of tetanus neonatorum with muscle relaxants and intermittent positive-pressure ventilation. *Br. Med. J.*, **1**, 223–226

Sowa, S., Sowa, J. and Collier, L. H. (1968) Investigation of neonatal conjunctivitis in the Gambia. *Lancet*, **ii**, 243–247

Spritzer, R., Kamp, H. J. V. D, Dzolvic, G. and Sauer, P. J. J. (1990) Five years of cefotaxime use in a neonatal intensive care unit. *Pediatr. Infect. Dis. J.*, **9**, 92–96

Sprunt, K., Redman, W. and Leidy, G. (1973) Antibacterial effectiveness of routine hand-washing. *Pediatrics*, **52**, 264–267

Sprunt, K., Leidy, G. and Redman, W. (1978) Abnormal colonization of neonates in an intensive care unit: means of identifying neonates at risk of infection. *Pediatr. Res.*, **12**, 998–1002

Squire, E., Favara, B. and Todd, J. (1979) Diagnosis of neonatal bacterial infection: hematologic and pathologic findings in fatal and non-fatal cases. *Pediatrics*, **64**, 60–64

Srouji, M. N. and Buck, B. E. (1978) Neonatal appendicitis: ischemic infarction in incarcerated inguinal hernia. *J. Pediatr. Surg.*, **13**, 177–179

Stabile, A., Miceli, A., Sopo, S. *et al.* (1988) Intravenous immunoglobulin for prophylaxis of neonatal sepsis in premature infants. *Arch. Dis. Child.*, **63**, 441–443

Stagno, S., Reynolds, D. W., Huang, E. S. *et al.* (1977) Congenital cytomegalovirus infection. Occurrence in an immune population. *N. Engl. J. Med.*, **296**, 1254–1258

Stagno, S., Reynolds, D. W., Pass, R. F. and Alford, C. A. (1980) Breast milk and the risk of cytomegalovirus infection. *N. Engl. J. Med.*, **302**, 1073–1076

Stagno, S., Brasfield, D. M., Brown, M. B. *et al.* (1981) Infant pneumonitis associated with cytomegalovirus, *Chlamydia*, *Pneumocystis* and *Ureaplasma*: a prospective study. *Pediatrics*, **68**, 322–329

Stagno, S., Pass, R. F., Dworsky, M. E. *et al.* (1982) Congenital cytomegalovirus infection. The relative importance of primary and recurrent maternal infection. *N. Engl. J. Med.*, **306**, 945–949

Stagno, S., Pass, R. F., Cloud, G. *et al.* (1986) Primary cytomegalovirus infection in pregnancy. *JAMA*, **256**, 1904–1908

Steele, R. W. (1984) Ceftriaxone therapy of meningitis and serious infections. *Am. J. Med.*, **77**, 50–53

Steer, P. L., Marks, M. I., Klite, P. D. and Eickhoff, T. C. (1972) 5-Fluorocytosine: an oral antifungal compound. A report on clinical and laboratory experience. *Ann. Intern. Med.*, **76**, 15–22

Stevens, C. E., Beasley, R. P., Tsui, J. *et al.* (1975) Vertical transmission of hepatitis B antigen in Taiwan. *N. Engl. J. Med.*, **292**, 771–774

Stevens, C. E., Neurath, R. A., Beasley, P. and Szmuness, W. (1979) HBeAg and anti HBe detection by radioimmunoassay – correlation with vertical transmission of HBV in Taiwan. *J. Med. Virol.*, **3**, 237–241

Stewardson-Krieger, P. B. and Gotoff, S. P. (1978) Risk factors in early-onset neonatal group B streptococcal infections. *Infection*, **6**, 50–53

Stoll, B. J., Kanto, W. P., Glassri, R. I. *et al.* (1980) Epidemiology of neonatal necrotising enterocolitis: a case control study. *J. Pediatr.*, **96**, 447–451

Stone, J. W. and Das, B. C. (1985) Investigation of an outbreak of infection with *Acinetobacter calcoaceticus* in a special care baby unit. *J. Hosp. Infection*, **6**, 42–48

Storm, W. (1980) Transient bacteremia following endotracheal suctioning in ventilated newborns. *Pediatrics*, **65**, 487–490

Strannegard, O., Holm, S. E., Hermodsson, S. *et al.* (1970) Case of apparent reinfection with rubella. *Lancet*, **i**, 240–241

Strausbaugh, L. J., Murray, T. W. and Sande, M. A. (1980) Comparative penetration of six antibiotics into the cerebrospinal fluid of rabbits with experimental staphylococcal meningitis. *J. Antimicrob. Chemother.*, **6**, 363–371

Stray-Pederson, B. (1983) Economic evaluation of maternal screening to prevent congenital syphilis. *Sex. Transm. Dis.*, **10**, 167–172

Sullender, W. M., Miller, J. L., Yasukawa, L. L. *et al.* (1987) Humoral and cell-mediated immunity in neonates with herpes simplex virus infection. *J. Infect. Dis.*, **155**, 28–37

Syriopoulou, V. P. and Smith, A. L. (1987) Osteomyelitis and septic arthritis. In *Textbook of Pediatric Infectious Diseases*. 2nd edn (eds R. D. Feigin and J. D. Cherry), W. B. Saunders, Philadelphia, pp. 759–779

Szmuness, W., Prince, A. M., Hirsch, R. L. and Brotman, B. (1973) Familial clustering of hepatitis B infection within families. *N. Engl. J. Med.*, **289**, 1162–1166

Tauber, M. G., Khayam-Bashi, H. and Sande, M. A. (1985) Effects of ampicillin and corticosteroids on brain water content, cerebrospinal fluid pressure, and cerebrospinal fluid lactate levels in experimental pneumococcal meningitis. *J. Infect. Dis.*, **151**, 528–534

Teberg, A. J., Yonekura, M. L., Salminen, C. and Pavlova, Z. (1987) Clinical manifestations of epidemic neonatal listeriosis. *Pediatr. Infect. Dis. J.*, **6**, 817–820

Thiry, L., Sprecher-Goldberger, S., Jonckheer, T. *et al.* (1985) Isolation of AIDS virus from cell-free breast milk of three healthy virus carriers. *Lancet*, **ii**, 891–892

Thomas, D. F. M., Fernie, D. S., Bayston, R. and Spitz, L. (1984a) Clostridial toxins in neonatal necrotising enterocolitis. *Arch. Dis. Child.*, **59**, 270–272

Thomas, P. A., Jaffe, H. W., Spira, T. J. *et al.* (1984b) Unexplained immunodeficiency in children. *JAMA*, **252**, 639–644

Thomsen, A. C., Morup, L. and Hansen, K. B. (1987) Antibiotic elimination of group-B streptococci in urine in prevention of preterm labour. *Lancet*, **i**, 591–593

Tipple, M., Beem, M. O. and Saxon, E. (1979) Clinical characteristics of the afebrile pneumonia associated with *Chlamydia trachomatis* infection in infants less than 6 months of age. *Pediatrics*, **63**, 192–197

Tong, M. J., Sinatra, F. R., Thomas, D. W. *et al.* (1984) Need for immunoprophylaxis in infants born to HBsAg-positive carrier mothers who are HBe Ag negative. *J. Pediatr.*, **105**, 945–947

Totterman, L. E. and Saxen, L. (1969) Incorporation of tetracycline into human foetal bones after maternal drug administration. *Acta Obstet. Gynaecol. Scand.*, **48**, 542–549

Traverso, H. P., Bennett, J. V., Kahn, A. J. *et al.* (1989) Ghee applications to the umbilical cord: a risk factor for neonatal tetanus. *Lancet*, **i**, 486–488

Trueta, J. (1959) The three types of acute haematogenous osteomyelitis: a clinical and vascular study. *J. Bone Jt Surg.*, **41**, 671–680

Tullus, K. and Burman, L. G. (1989) Ecological impact of ampicillin and cefuroxime in neonatal units. *Lancet*, **i**, 1405–1407

Umana, M. A., Odio, C. M., Castro, E. *et al.* (1990) Evaluation of aztreonam and ampicillin vs. amikacin and ampicillin for treatment of neonatal bacterial infections. *Pediatr. Infect. Dis. J.*, **9**, 175–180

Vaheri, A., Vesikari, T., Oker-Blom, N. *et al.* (1972) Isolation of attenuated rubella-vaccine virus from human products of conception. *N. Engl. J. Med.*, **286**, 1071–1074

Vain, N. D., Mazlumian, J. R., Swarner, O. W. *et al.* (1980) Role of exchange transfusion in the treatment of severe septicemia. *Pediatrics*, **66**, 693–697

Vaisanen-Rhen, V., Elo, J., Vaisanen, E. *et al.* (1984) P-fimbriated clones among uropathogenic *Escherichia coli* strains. *Infect. Immun.*, **43**, 149–155

Valenti, W. M., Clarke, T. A., Hall, C. B. *et al.* (1982) Concurrent outbreaks of rhinovirus and respiratory syncytial virus in an intensive care nursery. *J. Pediatr.*, **100**, 722–726

Valvano, M. A., Hartstein, A. I., Morthland, V. H. *et al.* (1988) Plasmid DNA analysis of *Staphylococcus epidermidis* isolated from blood and colonization cultures in very low birth weight infants. *Pediatr. Infect. Dis. J.*, **7**, 116–120

Visser, V. E. and Hall, R. T. (1979) Urine culture in the evaluation of suspected neonatal sepsis. *J. Pediatr.*, **94**, 635–638

Visser, V. E. and Hall, R. T. (1980) Lumbar puncture in the evaluation of suspected neonatal sepsis. *J. Pediatr.*, **96**, 1063–1067

Waites, K. B., Crouse, D. T., Philips, J. B. *et al.* (1989) Ureaplasmal pneumonia and sepsis associated with persistent pulmonary hypertension of the newborn. *Pediatrics*, **83**, 79–85

Wallace, R. J., Baker, C. J., Quinones, F. J. *et al.* (1983) Nontypable *Haemophilus influenzae* (Biotype 4) as a neonatal, maternal and genital pathogen. *Rev. Infect. Dis.*, **5**, 123–136

Webber, S., Lindsell, D., Wilkinson, A. R. *et al.* (1990) Neonatal pneumonia. *Arch. Dis. Child.*, **65**, 207–211

Webster, M. H. and Smith, C. S. (1977) Congenital abnormalities and maternal herpes zoster. *Br. Med. J.*, **2**, 1193

Weese-Mayer, D. E., Fondriest, D. W., Brouillette, R. T. and Shulman, S. T. (1987) Risk factors associated with candidemia in the neonatal intensive care unit: a case-control study. *Pediatr. Infect. Dis. J.*, **6**, 190–196

Welliver, R. C., Wong, D. T., Sun, M. *et al.* (1981) The development of respiratory syncytial virus-specific IgE and the release of histamine in nasopharyngeal secretions after infection. *N. Engl. J. Med.*, **305**, 841–846

White, R. D., Townsend, T. R., Stephens, M. A. and Moxon, E. R. (1981) Are surveillance of resistant enteric bacilli and antimicrobial usage among neonates in a newborn intensive care unit useful? *Pediatrics*, **68**, 1–4

Whitelaw, A. (1990) Treatment of sepsis with IgG in very low birth weight infants. *Arch. Dis. Child.*, **65**, 347–348

Whitley, R. J. (1990) Herpes simplex virus infections. In *Infectious Diseases of the Fetus and Newborn Infant*, 3rd edn (eds J. S. Remington and J. O. Klein), W. B. Saunders, Philadelphia, pp. 282–305

Whitley, R. J., Nahmias, A. J., Visintine, A. M. *et al.* (1980) The natural history of herpes simplex virus infection of mother and newborn. *Pediatrics*, **66**, 489–494

Whitley, R. J., Corey, L., Arvin, A. *et al.* (1988) Changing presentation of herpes simplex virus infection in neonates. *J. Infect. Dis.*, **158**, 109–116

Whitley, R. J., Arvin, A., Prober, C. *et al.* (1991) A controlled trial comprising vidarabine with acyclovir in neonatal herpes simplex virus infection. *N. Engl. J. Med.*, **324**, 444–449

Wild, N. J., Sheppard, S. and Smithells, R. W. (1986) The consequences of antenatal rubella testing. *Health Trends*, **18**, 9–10

Wilfert, C. M., Thompson, R. J., Jr, Sunder, T. R. O. *et al.* (1981) Longitudinal assessment of children with enterovirus meningitis during the first three months of life. *Pediatrics*, **67**, 811–815

Wilson, C. B. (1986) Immunologic basis for increased susceptibility of the neonate to infection. *J. Pediatr.*, **108**, 1–12

Wilson, R., Kanto, W. P., McCarthy, B. J. *et al.* (1981) Epidemiological characteristics of necrotising enterocolitis: a population based study. *Am. J. Epidemiol.*, **114**, 880–887

Wiswell, T. E. and Roscelli, J. D. (1986) Corroborative evidence for the decreased incidence of urinary tract infections in circumcised male infants. *Pediatrics*, **78**, 96–99

Wiswell, T. E., Smith, F. R. and Bass, J. W. (1985) Decreased incidence of urinary tract infections in circumcised male infants. *Pediatrics*, **75**, 901–903

Wiswell, T. E., Enzenauer, R. W., Holton, M. E. *et al.* (1987) Declining frequency of circumcision: implications for changes in the absolute incidence and male to female sex ratio of urinary tract infections in early infancy. *Pediatrics*, **79**, 338–342

Wiswell, T. E., Miller, G. M., Gelston, H. M. *et al.* (1988) Effect of circumcision status on periurethral bacterial flora during the first year of life. *J. Pediatrics*, **113**, 442–446

Wong, V. C. W., Ip, H. M. H., Reesink, H. W. *et al.* (1984) Prevention of the HBsAG carrier state in newborn infants of mothers who are chronic carriers of HBsAG and HBeAG by administration of hepatitis B vaccine and heptatitis B immunoglobulin. *Lancet*, **i**, 921–926

Woody, R. C. and Ross, E. M. (1989) Neonatal tetanus (St Kilda, 19th century). *Lancet*, **i**, 1339

Yeager, A. S. (1974) Transfusion-acquired cytomegalovirus infections in newborn infants. *Am. J. Dis. Child.*, **128**, 478–483

Yeager, A. S. (1975) Longitudinal, serological study of cytomegalovirus infections in nurses and in personnel without patient contact. *J. Clin. Microbiol.*, **2**, 448–452

Yeager, A. and Arvin, A. (1984) Reasons for the absence of a history of recurrent genital infections in mothers of neonates infected with herpes simplex virus. *Pediatrics*, **73**, 188–193

Yeager, A. S., Hafleigh, M. T., Arvin, A. M. *et al.* (1981) Prevention of transfusion-acquired cytomegalovirus infection in newborn infants. *J. Pediatr.*, **98**, 281–287

Yeung, C. Y. and Tam, A. S. Y. (1972) Gastric aspirate findings in neonatal pneumonia. *Arch. Dis. Child.*, **47**, 735–740

Young, A. B., Reid, D. and Grist, N. R. (1983) Is cytomegalovirus a serious hazard to female staff? *Lancet*, **i**, 975–976

Yow, M. D., Tengg, N. E., Bangs, J. *et al.* (1962) The ototoxic effects of kanamycin sulfate in infants and in children. *J. Pediatr.*, **60**, 230–242

Yu, V. H., Joseph, R., Bajuk, B. *et al.* (1984) Perinatal risk factors for necrotising enterocolitis. *Arch. Dis. Child.*, **59**, 430–434

Ziegler, J. B., Cooper, D. A., Johnson, R. O. and Gold, J. (1985) Postnatal transmission of AIDS-associated retrovirus from mother to infant. *Lancet*, **i**, 896–898.

Index

THE WOMAN
I WANTED TO BE

THE WOMAN
I WANTED TO BE

Diane von Furstenberg

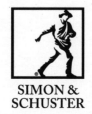

**SIMON &
SCHUSTER**

London · New York · Sydney · Toronto · New Delhi

A CBS COMPANY

First published in Great Britain by Simon & Schuster UK Ltd, 2014
A CBS COMPANY

Copyright © 2014 by Diane von Furstenberg

1 3 5 7 9 10 8 6 4 2

Simon & Schuster UK Ltd
1st Floor
222 Gray's Inn Road
London WC1X 8HB

www.simonandschuster.co.uk

Simon & Schuster Australia, Sydney
Simon & Schuster India, New Delhi

A CIP catalogue record for this book
is available from the British Library

ISBN: 978-1-47114-027-3
ISBN: 978-1-47114-028-0 (Trade Paperback)
ISBN: 978-1-47114-030-3 (ebook)

Interior design by Ruth Lee-Mui
Jacket art (chain link print) © DVF Studio, LLC
Front cover photograph by Peter Lindbergh
Back flap photograph by Hans Dorsinville

Printed and bound by CPI Group (UK) Ltd, Croydon, CR0 4YY

To Alexandre, Tatiana, Talita, Antonia, Tassilo, and Leon.
I will always protect you.
And to Barry, for protecting all of us.

If you wish to be loved, love!

—*Seneca*

Contents

Acknowledgments

I want to thank all of the people who helped to bring this project to life.

Linda Bird Francke for her patience and dedication as she collected my memories and structured this book, and for her friendship for the last four decades.

Genevieve Ernst for reading and correcting it with me over and over and putting up with me and my endless changes.

I could not have done it without you both.

Alice Mayhew for her macro support and knowledge, and Andrew Wylie for being the best agent. Franca Dantes for her incredible archival skills, Peter Lindbergh for the cover photo, and Tara Romeo for her assistance with the cover design. Lisa Watson for transcribing my rambling, Jonathan Cox for keeping all of the chapters straight, and Liz McDaniel for helping with the book jacket.

THE WOMAN
I WANTED TO BE

Introduction

When I was a child, studying for my exams, I would pretend I was teaching imaginary students. It was my way to learn.

Living is learning, and as I look back at the many layers of experience I collected, I feel ready to share some of the lessons I learned along the way.

Living also means aging. The good thing about aging is that you have a past, a history. If you like your past and stand by it, then you know you have lived fully and learned from your life.

Those were the lessons that allowed me to be the woman I am.

As a girl, I did not know what I wanted to do but I knew the kind of woman I wanted to be. I wanted to be my own person, independent and free. I knew that freedom could only be achieved if I took full responsibility for myself and my actions, if I were true to truth, if I became my very best friend.

Life is not always a smooth ride. Landscapes change, people come in and out, obstacles appear and disrupt the planned itinerary, but one thing you know for sure is that you will always have yourself.

I have arranged this book into chapters on what has inspired me the most and continues to give me strength: family, love, beauty, and the business of fashion. But I must single out the person who was the most important in shaping my life, in making me the woman I wanted to be . . . my mother. That is where this memoir begins.

THE
WOMAN
I AM

1

ROOTS

There is a large frame on the bookshelf in my bedroom in New York. In it is a page torn from a German magazine of 1952. It is a photo of an elegant woman and her small daughter in the train station of Basel, Switzerland, waiting for the Orient Express. The little girl is nestled in her mother's tented coat and is eating a brioche. That was the first time, at the age of five, that I had my photo in a magazine. It is a sweet picture. My mother's older sister, Juliette, gave it to me when I was first married, but it is only recently that I realized its true importance.

On the surface, it is a photograph of a glamorous, apparently wealthy woman en route to a ski holiday with her curly-haired little girl. The woman is not looking into the camera, but there is a hint of a smile as she knows she is being photographed. Her appearance is elegant. Nothing would indicate that only a few years before, she was in another German-speaking railroad station coming back from the Nazi concentration camps where she had been a prisoner for thirteen months, a bunch of bones, close to death from starvation and exhaustion.

How did she feel when the photographer asked her name to be put in the magazine? Proud, I imagine, to be noticed for her style and elegance. Only seven years had passed. She was not a number anymore. She had a name; warm, beautiful, clean clothes; and most of all she had a daughter, a healthy little girl. "God has saved my life so that I can give you life," she used to write me every New Year on my birthday. "By giving you life, you gave me my life back. You are my torch, my flag of freedom."

My voice catches each time I speak publicly about my mother, and I do in every speech I make, aware that I wouldn't be giving that speech if Lily Nahmias had not been my mother. Sometimes it feels odd that I always bring up her story, but somehow I am compelled to. It explains the child I was, the woman I became.

"I want to tell you the story of a young girl who, at twenty-two years old, weighed fifty-nine pounds, barely the weight of her bones," I say to a seminar at Harvard about girls' health. "The reason she weighed fifty-nine pounds is that she had just spent thirteen months in the Nazi death camps of Auschwitz and Ravensbrück. It was a true miracle that that young girl didn't die, though she came very close. When she was liberated and returned to her family in Belgium, her mother fed her like a little bird, every fifteen minutes a tiny bit of food, and then a little bit more, making her feel as if she was being slowly blown up like a balloon. Within a few months her weight was close to normal."

There are always murmurs in the audience when I get to that point in my mother's story, perhaps because it is so shocking and unexpected or maybe because I am living history to a young audience that has heard only vaguely about Auschwitz. It must be hard to imagine the high-energy, healthy woman speaking to them having a mother who weighed fifty-nine pounds. Whatever it is, I want and need to honor my mother, her courage and her strength. It is what made me the woman she wanted me to be.

"God has saved my life so that I can give you life." Her words resonate with me every day of my life. I feel it is my duty to make up for all the suffering she endured, to always celebrate freedom and live fully. My birth was her triumph. She was not supposed to survive; I was not supposed to be born. We proved them wrong. We both won the day I was born.

I repeat a few of the lessons my mother drummed into me that have served me well. "Fear is not an option." "Don't dwell on the dark side of things, but look for the light and build around it. If one door closes, look for another one to open." "Never, ever, blame others for what befalls you, no matter how horrible it might be. Trust you, and only you, to be responsible for your own life." She lived those lessons. In spite of what she endured, she never wanted others to feel that she was a victim.

I didn't used to talk nearly as much about my mother. I took her for granted, as children do their mothers. It was not until she died in 2000 that I fully realized what an incredibly huge influence she had been on me and how much I owe her. Like any child, I hadn't paid much attention. "OK, OK, you told me that already," I'd brush her off, or even pretend not to hear. I bridled, too, at the unsolicited advice she persisted in giving my friends. In fact, it annoyed me. Now, of course, I feel I have had the experience and earned the wisdom to hand out my own unsolicited advice, and I press every lesson my mother taught me on my children, grandchildren, and anyone I talk to. I have become her.

I didn't know, as a very little girl in Brussels, why my mother had two lines of blue tattooed numbers on her left arm. I remember thinking they were some sort of decoration and wished I had them, too, so my arms wouldn't look so plain. I didn't understand why the housekeeper often told me not to bother her when she was lying down in her bedroom. I instinctively knew my mother needed her rest and I would tiptoe around the house so I wouldn't disturb her.

Sometimes I'd ignore the housekeeper's instructions and, gathering my beloved little picture books, I would sneak into her darkened room in the hope she would smile and read them to me. More often than not she did. She loved books and taught me to cherish them. She read my little picture books to me so many times I memorized them. One of my favorite things to do was to fake reading them, carefully turning the pages at the right time and showing off, pretending that I could read.

My mother was very strict. I never doubted that she loved me, but if I said something she didn't approve of or failed to live up to her expectations, she would give me a severe look or pinch me. I would be sent to the corner, my face to the wall. Sometimes I would go to the corner by myself, knowing I had done wrong. She spent a lot of time with me, sometimes playing, but mostly teaching me anything she could think of. She read me fairy tales and would tease me when I got scared. I remember how she amused herself by telling me that I was an abandoned child she had found in the garbage. I would cry until she took me in her arms, consoling me. She wanted me to be strong and not be afraid. She was very demanding. Before I had learned how to read, she had me memorize and recite the seventeenth-century fables of La Fontaine. As soon as I was old enough to write, she insisted I write stories and letters with perfect spelling and grammar. I remember how proud I was when she praised me.

To train me never to succumb to shyness, she made me give a speech at every family gathering, teaching me to be comfortable speaking in public no matter the audience. Like many children I was scared of the dark, but unlike most mothers, she shut me in a dark closet and waited outside so I would learn for myself that there was nothing to be afraid of. That was just one of the times she'd say "Fear is not an option."

My mother did not believe in coddling children too much or overprotecting them. She wanted me to be independent and responsible for myself. My earliest memories are of traveling with my parents and being left alone in the hotel room while they went out to dinner. I did not mind nor did I feel lonely. I was so proud that they trusted me to stay alone. I liked entertaining myself and feeling grown up. To this day, I have the same feeling and sense of freedom when I check into a hotel room alone.

When my parents allowed me to join them in a restaurant, my mother often encouraged me to get up and check out the room, and sometimes, even to go outside and report to her what I'd seen, who I had met. That instilled curiosity in me—watch what other people do, make friends with people I do not know. When I was nine, she sent me on the train from Brussels to Paris all by myself to visit her sister, my favorite aunt, Mathilde. I felt so proud to be responsible for myself. I think, deep down, I was a bit nervous, but I would never admit it and pride overcame the fear.

I still like to travel alone, and at times prefer it. Even on business trips, I don't like traveling with an entourage because it limits my freedom and reduces the fun of the unpredictable. I love the adventure, that feeling of excitement and satisfaction I had when I was a little girl. To be alone on the road, in an airport, with my bag, my passport, my credit cards, my phone, and a camera makes me feel so free and happy. I thank my mother for always encouraging me to "go."

Independence. Freedom. Self-reliance. Those were the values she was drumming into me, and she did it with such naturalness that I never questioned or resisted her. There was no other way but to be responsible for myself. As much as I loved and respected her, I was certainly a little frightened of her, and never wanted to displease her. I understand now that she was processing all of her past frustrations and unhappy experiences and putting them into a package of strength and positivity. That is the gift she prepared for me. It felt occasionally like a heavy burden, but I never questioned it, even if I sometimes wished I belonged to some other family.

Happily she let up on me somewhat when I was six and my baby brother, Philippe, was born. I adored him. To my surprise, having never played with dolls, I felt maternal, and to this day I think of him as my first child. As the older sister, I played with him and sometimes tortured him a bit, but as my mother had done to me, I taught him everything I knew and was very protective. When we played doctor, I asked him to urinate into a little bottle, only to then laugh at him that he had actually done it. We also used to play travel agency with my parents' airline brochures, scheduling and booking imaginary trips all over the world.

Philippe says he realized that I loved him the day I transcribed all the words from a Beatles record while I was at boarding school in England, and sent them to him. There were no computers then, no Internet, no iTunes, just a doting sister with pen and paper, listening to the lyrics and transcribing them. We're still extremely close, and he is still my baby brother, whom I always try to impress and tease. Philippe is a successful businessman in Brussels, has two amazing daughters, Sarah and Kelly, and his wife, Greta, launched and runs DVF Belgium. Philippe and I talk on the phone every weekend and whenever I miss my parents, I call him.

I don't think my mother was half as hard on him as she'd been with me. He was a boy, after all, and we are much softer and less demanding toward boys in our family. It was I she related to, the daughter she was determined would survive whatever life threw at her. As I grew older, I understood. Independence and freedom were key to her because she had lost both. Self-reliance had kept her alive.

My mother was twenty and engaged to my father in 1944 when the Nazi SS arrested her on May 17 for working in the Belgian Resistance. She was living in a "safe house" and her job was to go around Brussels on her bicycle to deliver documents and fake papers to those who needed them. Immediately after her arrest, she was thrown onto a crowded truck, which took her and many other suspected saboteurs to a prison in Malines, Flanders, a city twenty-five kilometers from Brussels. To avoid being tortured into giving information about others in the resistance, she said she knew nothing and that she was hiding in the safe house because she was Jewish. The woman who was interrogating her advised her not to say she was Jewish. She ignored it and was deported on the twenty-fifth transport, which left Malines on May 19, 1944. She was sent to Auschwitz and given prisoner number 5199.

My mother often told me how she'd written her parents a note on a scrap of paper and dropped it from the truck onto the street. She hoped but had no idea whether anyone ever picked it up and delivered it. It wasn't until after her death that I found out that the message had been delivered. I'd loaned the house she'd owned on Harbour Island in the Bahamas to my first cousin Salvator. Salvator left me a thick envelope full of family photographs, in the midst of which was a sealed envelope marked "Lily, 1944." Inside was a piece of torn paper with faint handwriting. I stared at it until I finally made out the words:

Dear Mommy and Daddy,

I am writing to tell you that your little Lily is leaving. Where, she does not know, but God is everywhere isn't he? So she will never be alone or unhappy.

I want you both to be courageous, and not forget that you have to be in good health for my wedding. I am counting more than ever in having a beautiful ceremony.

I want you to know that I am leaving with a smile, I promise. I love you very very much and will soon kiss you more than ever.

Your little daughter,
Lily

I couldn't breathe. Could I be holding the actual note my mother had told me she had written to her parents on that truck, using a burnt match for a pencil? On the other side of the note was a plea for anybody finding the piece of paper to please deliver it to her parents' address. Somebody had found it and delivered it to her parents and my aunt Juliette, Salvator's mother, had kept it in a sealed envelope all these years!

I was in shock; I'd only half-believed her story of the note. All these stories about her arrest and deportation seemed surreal, more like a movie script, and yet they were true. She had always told me that she was more worried about her parents than herself. I held the proof in my shaky hands.

I walked out of the house in a daze and across the beach into the clear blue water. "This explains who I am," I said out loud to myself. "I am the daughter of a woman who went to the concentration camps with a smile."

The sayings she had drummed into me as a child and which had sometimes annoyed me took on whole new meanings. She had often illustrated one of her favorites—"you never really know what is good for you; what may seem the absolute worst thing to happen to you can, in fact, be the best"—by her story of the inhuman train ride to Auschwitz and her arrival.

No food. No water. No air. No toilet. Four days jammed in a cattle car. An "older woman" in her forties who spoke a little German comforted my mother and gave her a sense of protection. My mother made sure never to leave her side, especially when they arrived at Auschwitz and were unloaded onto a ramp. Women with children were immediately separated from the rest and sent toward long, low buildings while the others were forced into a long line. At the head of the line, a soldier directed the prisoners into two groups. Looking on, from the top of the ramp, was an officer in white.

When it came her turn, the older woman was directed to the group being formed on the left and my mother quickly followed her. The soldier did not stop her, but the white-coated officer, who had not interfered until then, did. Striding down the ramp, he walked directly to my mother, yanked her away from her friend, and threw her into the group on the right. My mother always said that she'd never felt such sheer hatred for anyone as she felt for that man.

That man was Dr. Josef Mengele, she found out later, the notorious Angel of Death, who killed or mutilated many, many prisoners in medical experiments, especially children and twins. Why did he go through the trouble of saving her? Did she remind him of someone he cared about? However evil or not his intentions were, he saved her life. The group the older woman was assigned to went directly to the gas chamber. The group my mother was thrust into did not.

I always use that story when I want to console anyone, just as my mother told it so often to me: You never know how something that seems the worst thing turns out to be the best.

After that, she was determined to survive, no matter the horror. Even when the unmistakable smell of the smoke coming from the camp crematorium seemed unbearable and her fellow prisoners would say "We're all going to die," my mother would insist: "No, we're not. We're going to live." Fear was not an option.

Nearly one million Jews were murdered at Auschwitz, many in the gas chamber. Others were executed, or killed in Dr. Mengele's experiments, or died from starvation and exhaustion from slave labor. My mother was fortunate, if anyone could have been considered fortunate in those unimaginably cruel surroundings. She was put to work on the twelve-hour night shift in the nearby weapons factory making bullets; so long as she worked she was useful and was kept alive. She was tiny, barely five feet tall, and naturally slender. She had never eaten much and could exist, albeit barely, on the miniscule rations of bread and watery soup she and other prisoners were given. Heavier prisoners, radically deprived of anything close to the amount of food they were used to, she told me, were the first to succumb to starvation.

If ever I think I'm too lazy to do a necessary chore, if I hesitate to go out because of the cold or complain about having to wait in line, I remember my mother. I envision her being marched out of Auschwitz with sixty thousand others in the winter of 1945, just nine days before the Soviet troops reached the camp. The SS hastily executed thousands of inmates and marched the others fifty kilometers through the snow to a train depot where they were stuffed into freight cars and sent to Ravensbrück in the north, and from there force-marched again to their new camps, in my mother's case to Neustadt-Glewe in Germany. Some fifteen thousand prisoners died on that Death March, of exposure, exhaustion, illness, or being shot by the SS for falling or lagging behind.

In what can only be described as a miracle, my tiny mother survived it all. She was one of the 1,244 who survived the camps out of the 25,631 Belgian Jews who were deported. Her will and spirit to live were her defiance of the evil she had endured, a declaration of her future. When Neustadt-Glewe was liberated a few months later by the Russians, followed closely by the Americans, my mother's weight was barely the weight of her bones.

She was hospitalized at an American base and wasn't expected to live. She defied the odds again. When she was stable enough to return home to Belgium she had to fill out a form, as did all survivors returning to their countries. I found that form. It had her name and date of birth on it and a question: "in what condition" she was returning from her thirteen months in captivity. Her astonishing answer was, in impeccable handwriting: "en très bonne santé" ("in very good health").

My father, Leon Halfin, was very different from my mother. Where she was strict and somewhat distant, he was relaxed and affectionate. In his eyes I could do no wrong and he loved me unconditionally. As a child I loved him much more than my demanding mother, though maybe I respected her a little more. When I needed to get up to go to the bathroom in the middle of the night, I would call for my father and that made him laugh. "Why do you call me and not your mother?" he'd ask. And I would reply: "Because I don't want to disturb her."

My father never scolded me. He simply adored me and I adored him. I was as affectionate toward him as he was to me. I loved to sit on his lap, covering him with kisses and drinking all of his after-dinner lemon tea. To my father I was the most beautiful thing in the world and I felt entitled to his love and devotion.

My father and I looked alike and we had the same kind of relentless energy. He loved American cars, and when I was nine or ten he would often take me for a drive in his beautiful, sky-blue and navy American Chevrolet Impala convertible, a bicolor combination that was very popular in the late fifties. In that era, before seat belts were common, I would kneel on the front seat instead of sitting, because I thought that that would make people think I was a grown-up. I always, always wanted to be older than my age. I never wanted to be a little girl. I wanted to be a woman, a sophisticated woman, a glamorous woman. I wanted to be important.

My father, unknowingly, hastened that wish. When he came to say good night to me and kiss me in my bed, he was often cautioned by my mother. "Be careful, don't wake up her senses," she'd say. My father used to think my mother's warning was hysterically funny. How could he, a man, wake up the senses of a little girl? Looking back now, however, no matter how funny he thought it was, he did wake up my senses. My father made me feel like a woman, so my mother was clever actually to say that.

The feelings were not sexual. It was the awareness that he was a man and that my relationship with him was therefore different from one I'd have with a woman. How lucky I was that this first man in my life loved me uncritically, unguardedly, without judging. I did not have to work for his love, I did not have to please him; his approval required no effort. That made an important impact on my life, and though I didn't know it then, I now know it has made my relationships with men much easier. What I owe my father, and what I am so thankful for, is how comfortable I always feel with men. He gave me confidence.

That first love and affection marks the way I presume men feel toward me. I simply take their fondness for granted, neither expecting nor looking for it. The biggest gift my father gave me was not to be needy. I had so much love from him that I didn't really need any more. In fact, I sometimes had to push it away because his display of affection in front of people embarrassed me.

My father was a successful businessman, a distributor of General Electric electronic tubes and semiconductors. He did well, so we lived very comfortably.

My parents were a striking couple. My father was very good-looking with high cheekbones and a mischievous smile. My mother had an elegant build and beautiful legs. She dressed very well and had a lot of allure. She was very much the boss of the house and I always saw her as the brains of the family. As much as I adored my father it was to her I went for advice.

She was not a traditional housewife, and only on Sundays, the housekeeper's day off, did I occasionally see her in the kitchen. She would make a delicious grilled chicken with crispy potatoes and my father would bring pastries for dessert. My favorite petit gâteau was called a Merveilleux and was made of meringue, chocolate, and whipped cream. We were, after all, in Belgium, the land of chocolate. In fact, most of what my mother did at home was to instruct everyone else, but she did it very well. Our apartment was beautifully decorated, full of antiques she had collected. I have a clear memory of her looking for and finally finding the Empire chandelier she so desired. It now illuminates my Mayfair shop in London.

Since my mother died, my father having died six years before, I have searched for clues in my parents' lives as to what formed them and why I am who I am. That quest has taken me to Eastern Europe and the city of Kishinev, then the capital of Bessarabia, now the capital of Moldova, where my father was born in 1912, and to Salonika, Greece, where my mother was born in 1922.

Both my parents' families were in the textile business. My father's father, a wealthy Russian merchant whose relatives included many intellectuals and artists—one relative, Lewis Milestone, directed the 1930 Academy Award–winning war film *All Quiet on the Western Front*—owned several fabric stores in Kishinev. My mother's father, Moshe Nahmias, a Sephardic Jew (a Jew of Spanish origin), moved his family from Salonika to Brussels when my mother was seven and ran La Maison Dorée, the large department store owned by his brother-in-law, Simon Haim. My maternal grandmother's sister, my great-aunt Line, was married to the wealthy Simon Haim and had urged her sister to join her in Brussels with her family. So, although I had never made the connection before, I do indeed have a legacy of the fashion and retail business from both sides of my family.

There is nothing I could find in my mother's childhood that would give her the unimaginable strength to survive the death camps. As far as I could tell, she had a pleasant, uneventful young life in Brussels, rather spoiled as the youngest of three girls in the family. The only challenge for her and her two older sisters, who had gone to an Italian school in Greece, was to become more fluent in French when they moved to Brussels so they could do well at school. My maternal grandparents, who spoke Ladino, the language of the Sephardic Jews, at home, changed the birthdates of the girls when the family arrived in Brussels, passing them off as two years younger so they would have more time to adapt, learn French, and be successful at school. My mother went to the Lycée Dachsbeck, the same school I went to years later, and we even had the same kindergarten teacher and the same headmistress, Mademoiselle Gilette. I found out recently that Mlle. Gilette had ignored the racial laws of the Nazi occupation and allowed my mother to graduate from high school. It is probably why she chose me to blow out the candles on the cake at the school's seventy-fifth anniversary in 1952; I was the daughter of an alumna who went to the death camps and survived.

My father arrived in Brussels two years after my mother and her family moved to Belgium. He was seventeen in 1929 and was planning to follow in his brother's footsteps and train to be a textile engineer, when something went very wrong in Kishinev. My grandfather's business went bankrupt, which actually killed him, and my grandmother was no longer able to send money to my future father. He stopped studying, although I am not sure he ever officially entered school in Belgium, and went to work, taking any job he could find. He had no plan to go back home and enjoyed his freedom as a young, good-looking man even though his life as a refugee was not always easy.

It was the war that brought my parents together. When Germany invaded and occupied Belgium in 1940, many people fled south in what was called L'Exode. Thousands of cars jammed the roads escaping from the occupation. My father and his best friend, Fima, drove south to France and settled, temporarily, in a small hotel in Toulouse. They were young and very handsome and even though it was wartime and the situation was serious, they laughed a lot and had many women along the way. My mother also arrived in Toulouse with her aunt Line and uncle Simon. They made the trip rather regally in a Cadillac with a driver.

Fima had money but my father did not. He hated being dependent on his friend, so every morning he went around on a bicycle looking for the jobs that had been posted, but in every place he arrived, the job had been taken. "Try the train station," a sympathetic would-have-been employer suggested. There he met a man named Jean who began the sequence of events that would draw my mother and father together.

"I know someone who needs to go back to Belgium and has to sell a very large amount of dollars because Belgium won't allow anyone to bring in foreign currency," Jean told him. "Do you know anyone who wants to buy dollars? He paid thirty-four French francs for them and is willing to sell at thirty-three." My father certainly didn't know anyone who wanted to buy dollars, so he paid little attention. A few days later, completely by accident, he met another man called Maurice who had a friend looking to buy dollars and was willing to pay a rate of seventy-six French francs for them.

My father couldn't believe his ears. Was he understanding right? Jean had a seller at thirty-three and Maurice had a buyer at seventy-six. So much profit could be made with the difference. The problem was that my father had no idea how to find Jean. He didn't know his last name or where he lived, so he raced around Toulouse on his bicycle for three days and three nights, looking for him. On the fourth day, my father went to the cinema and, realizing he had left his newspaper when he came out of the theater, went back for it—and bumped into Jean!

It took days to smooth out the many complications and finalize the transaction, because the sum was very large and my father had to prove he could deliver the money. He had to borrow some from his friend Fima to do a small sample transaction first, to prove he was trustworthy and, after a few days, completed the whole exchange. Overnight he went from having no money at all to actually being rich. In his diary my father recalls feeling so ashamed of his worn-out suit during the transaction that the day it was completed he bought three suits, six shirts, and two pairs of shoes. His good fortune didn't end there. As fate would have it, the man who was buying the dollars turned out to be my mother's uncle Simon. And that is how my parents met.

Theirs was not an immediate romance. Leon Halfin was twenty-nine, ten years older than my mother, and very interested in being a ladies' man. But Lily was a Jewish girl, and as far as he was concerned, you didn't touch Jewish girls—you married them.

The news from Belgium was that things weren't so bad under the German occupation, and in October 1941, my parents returned separately to Belgium. My mother couldn't go to university because of the racial laws, so she went to fashion school, studied millinery, and learned how to make hats. My father, who now had a lot of money, did not go back to Tungsram, the electronics company he had worked for, but became an independent businessman in the radio field in Brussels. They saw each other at gatherings of older relatives and family friends, but my father always treated my mother like a little girl, teasing her and pinching her cheeks. There was no romance although they clearly liked each other. Leon didn't know my mother had a secret crush on him.

It wasn't until the summer of 1942, when the SS started rounding up Jews in Belgium and deporting them that the danger began in earnest. Lucie, my father's very good friend and ex-colleague at Tungsram, advised him to get out of Belgium and flee to Switzerland.

He bought fake papers from the Belgian underground and began to plan his escape under the assumed and typical Belgian name of Leon Desmedt. He did not go alone. Lucie arranged for Gaston Buyne, a nineteen-year-old Christian boy to accompany him through France to the Swiss border. In a surprising turn of events, they were joined by Renée, a nineteen-year-old girl my father had just met. She was a Belgian Catholic girl who had fallen in love with my father and wanted to run away with him. Her mother had recently died and she didn't like the woman her father had taken up with. That was the unlikely trio who set out together on August 6, 1942.

The train ride to Nancy, where they would transfer to another train to Belfort, was very dangerous. Gaston, a Belgian with legal papers, carried a lot of Leon's money—banknotes in his shoulder pads, gold coins in his shoes and socks, and more Swiss notes in his toiletry bag. Because Gaston looked Jewish, much more so than Leon, he turned out to be the perfect foil. There were many, many checkpoints at which the German SS would randomly order male passengers to pull down their trousers to check whether they were circumcised. Gaston was ordered to drop his pants. "Sorry," the SS man apologized to him, and didn't bother with my father who was sitting next to him.

They arrived in Nancy at night and checked into a hotel. The train to Belfort left at 5:15 a.m. and they had another run-in on board with a young SS soldier who wanted both Gaston and Leon to drop their pants. This time it was Renée who saved Leon by smiling coquettishly at the young soldier until he moved on to other passengers.

Belfort was even more dangerous. There were many, many Jewish refugees checking into the same hotel, but my father's fake ID saved him. The German SS raided the hotel that night and arrested all the Jews, but not Leon Desmedt. (My father's diary records that he made love to Renée twice that night.) Later they heard that all the people arrested that night were killed.

Leon and Renée parted ways with Gaston the next morning as they approached the Swiss border. They took a bus to Hérimoncourt, at which point Leon hired a local guide to lead them through the mountains and pastures into Switzerland just six kilometers away. That last leg of the escape cost fifteen hundred French francs with no guarantee of success. A few more refugees joined in as they met the guide at five a.m., among them a woman with a baby. She gave the baby a sleeping pill so he wouldn't cry, and they set out on foot through the alpine mountains to the border. "Run, run, run in that direction," the guide pointed and sent them off on their own. I remember my father telling me that it was the cows and their noisy bells that made their escape possible. By following the bells, Leon and Renée arrived at the Swiss border town of Damvant on August 8, 1942.

"Why do you carry so much money?" the border police asked my father. He told them that he was an industrialist from Belgium, but the police did not believe his story. "Your papers are fake," they said. They confiscated his money but did allow him to enter Switzerland. "You can claim it back when you leave," the police told him.

My father was very lucky. Although he remained under surveillance by the Swiss authorities, and was unable to travel freely or have access to his money without going through long bureaucratic requests, he spent a few fairly pleasant years there. He separated from Renée, who eloped with a policeman soon after their arrival, and began to miss Lily, the vivacious "little" girl he'd left behind in Belgium. The occupation of Brussels had become very severe and he was worried about her. Lily and her parents had to abandon their apartment and live separately. She was hiding in a resistance house where she worked. My aunt Juliette sent her son, my cousin Salvator, to live with his Christian Belgian nanny.

Curious Lily went to her family's apartment one day and discovered that the SS had ransacked it and stolen all their belongings. She also discovered something that would change her life. There was a letter in the mailbox, an unexpected letter from Switzerland, from Leon, the man she had met in Toulouse and never forgotten. After reading and rereading it many times, she responded. It started a daily correspondence between them, carefully crafted because all the letters had to go through censors as the wide blue stripe across the stationery indicated. I am lucky to possess those letters, which, over time, became more and more intimate and passionate. They wrote about their love and about the moment they would meet again after the war, that they would marry, build a life together, have a family, and be happy forever. It was all about hope and love.

Then, suddenly, Lily's letters stopped. (It was then, I recall my father telling me, that the mirror in his bedroom, on which he had taped a photo of my mother, fell and broke.)

He wrote to her again and again, begging in vain for an answer. On July 15, two months after my mother's arrest, he received a letter from Juliette, my mother's older sister, written in code to get through the censors.

"Dear Leon," she wrote. "I have very bad news. Lily has been hospitalized."

When my mother returned from Germany in June 1945, my father was still in Switzerland. By the time he came back to Brussels four months later, she had gained back much of the weight she had lost, but she wasn't the same naïve, mischievous, fun-loving, passionate girl he had been corresponding with and planned to marry. That girl was gone forever. This new young woman had endured true horrors and would carry the wounds forever.

In his diary, my father wrote with great honesty about their reunion. He admitted that he barely recognized the girl he had been separated from for more than two years. She was different, a stranger to him. Lily sensed his unease and told him he was under no obligation to marry her. The love was still there, he reassured her as he hid his doubts away. They were married on November 29, 1945.

The doctor warned them, "No matter what, you have to wait a few years before having a baby. Lily isn't strong enough for childbirth and the baby may not be healthy." Six months later, I was accidentally conceived. Remembering the doctor's warning, both my mother and father were concerned. They thought they could get rid of the pregnancy by taking long rides on his motorcycle over the cobblestoned streets, but it didn't work. Finally one morning my father brought home some pills to induce a miscarriage. My mother threw those pills out the window.

I was born healthy and strong in Brussels on New Year's Eve, December 31, 1946, a miracle. Because of the price my mother paid for that miracle, I never felt I had the right to question her, complain, or make her life more difficult. I was always a very, very good little grown-up girl, and for some reason felt it was my role to protect her. In his diaries, my father confesses that at first he was disappointed that I was not a boy, but within a few days he had totally accepted me and fallen in love with my mother again.

I have long suspected that if I hadn't been born, my mother might have killed herself. If nothing else, my existence gave her a focus and a reason to keep going. For all the strength and determination of her personality, she was extremely fragile. She hid it very well, and when people were around she was always light and fun. But when she was alone, she was often overtaken by uncontrollable sadness. When I came home from school in the afternoons, I would sometimes find her sitting in her darkened bedroom, weeping. Other times, when she picked me up from school, she'd take me to have a patisserie, or antiques shopping, laughing with me and giving no hint of her painful memories.

The people who went to the camps didn't want to talk about it and the people who weren't in the camps didn't want to hear about it, so I sensed she often felt like a stranger or an alien. When she did talk about it to me, she would only emphasize the good—the friendships, the laughter, the will to go back home and the dream of a plate of spaghetti. If I asked her how she endured, she would joke and say, "Imagine it is raining and you run in between the drops!" She always told me to trust the goodness of people. She wanted to protect me, but I realized that it is also how she protected herself . . . denying the bad . . . always denying the bad and demanding that the good forces win and, no matter what, never appearing a victim.

She did the best she could to put the war behind her. She had the two sets of tattooed numbers removed. And in a wonderful gesture of defiance, and to override her memory of the bitter cold she'd endured, she bought a very expensive, warm sable coat with the restitution money she got from the German government.

I spent a lot of time alone as a child, reading and imagining a grand life for myself. My childhood went smoothly, though life in Brussels was often gray and boring. I loved my big school, I loved my books, and I was a very good student. I loved my brother and my girlfriends,

Mireille Dutry and Myriam Wittamer, whose parents owned the best patisserie in Brussels. On the weekends, our family spent Sundays in the country at my great-great-aunt and -uncle's villa. They had a beautiful house on the edge of a large forest, the Forêt de Soignes. I loved walking in the woods, picking chestnuts in the winters and berries in the summers. My father would play cards with the men and my mother gossiped with the women. We ate a lot of good food. On the long, gray days, I lost myself reading Stendhal, Maupassant, Zola, and, on a lighter note, my favorite, *The Adventures of Tintin,* comic books about a daring young boy reporter created by the Belgian cartoonist Hergé. I lived vicariously through Tintin's travels and exploits. Would I ever discover all these exotic places in the world? It seemed like nothing would ever happen to me.

When I had a few days off from school and my parents could not travel, I would often visit my aunt Mathilde in Paris. She had an elegant boutique off the Faubourg Saint-Honoré catering to a loyal, international clientele. She sold printed cashmere sweaters and jersey dresses and suits. I would spend entire days in the shop. My job was to fold the clothes and put them back in order. It was my first encounter with fashion, retail, and the secret virtues of jersey fabrics.

In Paris, I also visited my cousins, Eliane and Nadia Neiman, the two daughters of my father's rich cousin Abraham, who had invented the theft alarm for cars. The girls spoke perfect Russian, gave piano recitals, and were very sophisticated. I felt terribly awkward and provincial when I visited them for tea or lunch at their villa in Neuilly. During the summers, my brother and I would go to summer camp near Montreux in the Swiss Alps or in the North Sea resort of Le Coq-sur-Mer in Belgium. We would also go on trips with my parents and my aunts and uncles to the South of France or the Swiss mountains.

My parents were a good-looking couple, and they loved each other very much, but my father wasn't as sensitive around my mother as he should have been. He didn't want to acknowledge her wounds, so he ignored them. He was a hardworking, generous man, but he could be indifferent and sometimes verbally harsh. I don't think he had any real love affairs after he married my mother. He traveled frequently on business, and I am sure he did not always spend his nights alone, but that was not the problem between my parents. It was his insensitivity toward her that made her feel vulnerable. So the scene was set for what came next. And what came next was a man named Hans Muller.

The letter, addressed to my mother, was on the table in our front hall that day when I came back from school. For reasons that I still cannot fathom, I opened the blue envelope with the very clear handwriting. It was from someone named Hans Muller, who, I realized as I read, was a friend of hers. I did not know who this Hans was and I do not recall what the letter said, but I remember that my heart started to beat fast. I felt something major had happened, something that would change all of our lives, and that something was Hans. Knowing I had done something wrong, I carefully put the letter back in the blue envelope and left it on the table, but the damage was done. My mother came home, saw the envelope, and I confessed I'd opened it. I had never seen her so upset and angry. Though I was twelve at the time, she reacted in a very violent way, slapping me across the face with all her strength. I was desperate, I was in pain, I was ashamed. Whatever had come upon me to open that letter?

My face was only a little bruised the next day when I went to class, but my insides were crushed. I had disappointed my mother. I had betrayed her trust. We never discussed it again and I am not sure what she told my father that night when he came home. Was he home anyway or was he traveling? I don't remember. I felt terrible, and to this day I have never again opened a letter or looked at a document or an email that was not addressed to me.

The following year, over my father's objections but to my own excitement, my mother sent me to Pensionnat Cuche, a private boarding school by the Lake Sauvabelin in Lausanne, Switzerland. It did not escape me that Lausanne is very close to Geneva, where Mr. Muller lived.

During the two wonderful years I spent at that school, living my own life, making many friends, and for the first time relishing my independence from my parents, I pieced together the story of my mother and Hans Muller. My father traveled a lot for his business, often taking my mother with him. When the travel entailed planes, they flew separately as insurance for my brother and me in case anything happened.

Hans Muller was my mother's seatmate on one of those trips, a long flight from Brussels to New York. He was a very handsome young Swiss German businessman who worked in the fruit business. Separated from his wife, he lived with his small son, Martin, who was the same age as my brother, Philippe. Monsieur Muller was polite and considerate, a stark contrast to my father, whose manners could be coarse and who sometimes belittled my mother in public. Hans was quite a bit younger than my mother and very taken with her. He would tell me, over the years, that he had never met a woman so attractive, interesting, and intelligent. They developed a friendship, which eventually led to a secret love affair and later to a long relationship.

I was not happy when my father insisted I be brought back to Brussels after my two years at boarding school in Switzerland. There I was, stuck at home again, and not a pleasant home at all. My mother and my father argued all the time and there was a lot of tension. I was relieved when they decided to officially separate. I think they both expected me to be upset that the family was splitting up. I wasn't, but I felt sad for my little brother. He was only nine and my parents would continue to fight over him for years after their separation and divorce.

As for me, I was fifteen in 1962. I felt grown up and secure, eager for whatever change lay ahead. Never once did I make my mother feel guilty about leaving my father, but instead I encouraged her and supported her completely. What she wanted, I'm convinced, was her freedom and independence after sixteen years of marriage, and I felt she deserved it. Was Hans an excuse or the reason? I never knew for sure. "Go on," I said. In turn, she would never make me feel guilty about anything either. When, years later, I told her I was leaving my husband, Egon, her response was "All right" and that was the end of it.

My father was devastated when my mother left him. His whole life revolved around his work and his family. I was not very sympathetic. Though I looked exactly like him and I loved him so very much, it was my mother I identified with. She wanted to move on, to experience life, to travel, learn, grow, expand her horizons, meet people, live her life. I understood it.

And so my parents parted and my childhood ended. One door closed, many others opened. I went on to another boarding school, this one in England, for two years and later to the University of Madrid in Spain. My mother lived with Hans for the next twenty years before separating from him, too. And I, with my mother as my role model, started to become the woman I wanted to be.

If anyone had the right to be bitter, my mother did, but never, ever did I hear her express any bitterness. She looked for the good in everything and everyone.

I'm often asked what was the worst thing that ever happened to me, what were my biggest challenges. I find it difficult to answer because I have this habit I inherited from my mother that somehow transforms what's bad into something good, so in the end, I don't remember what was bad. When I have an obstacle in front of me, especially of someone else's making, I say "OK. I don't like it, but I can't change it, so let's find a way around it." Then I find a different path to a solution, which so satisfies me that I forget what the problem was in the first place. Of all the lessons my mother drummed into me, that was perhaps the most important. How could you possibly better yourself if you didn't face your challenges up front or if you laid your problems off on someone or something else and didn't learn from them? I offer that lesson often in my talks to young women. "Don't blame your parents, don't blame your boyfriend, don't blame the weather. Accept the reality, embrace the challenge, and deal with it. Be in charge of your own life. Turn negatives into positives and be proud to be a woman."

It doesn't happen overnight, of course, and I never stopped learning from my mother. Over and over, she reinforced the lessons she'd taught me as a child.

When I was in my thirties, I suddenly developed a fear of flying, but when I told her I was afraid, she looked at me, smiling, and said, "Tell me, what does it mean to be afraid?" When once I was conflicted about starting a new business, she said, "Don't be ridiculous. You know how to do it." When I was diagnosed with cancer at forty-seven, predictably she told me not to worry, that I had nothing to fear. I wanted to believe her, but I had my doubts. Because she never showed any sign even in private that she was afraid, I wasn't either. When my treatment was all done, she collapsed, and I realized that she had, in fact, been afraid for me, but by never showing it to me, she had made me strong and trusting that I would be fine.

After Egon and I married in 1969, she spent several months each year living with us in New York and formed close, loving relationships with my children, Alexandre and Tatiana. Her relationship with them was very different from the relationship she had had with me. She had never been very affectionate to me and there had always been a distance between us. As a result, I was reserved around her and never told her my intimate thoughts, except in letters. It was much easier for me to open up in letters, and I think easier for her, too. In her letters to me at boarding school in Switzerland and then in England, she would often call me her "pride," but actually she never told me that to my face until much, much later when she was about to die.

She was much more open with my daughter as a grandmother and my daughter was more open with her than with me. They had an amazing complicity and spent hours together on her bed, telling each other stories. Tatiana became an excellent storyteller and filmmaker.

My mother was superb at handling money. She had taken half my father's assets with her when she left him and invested them so well that she was, in her later years, able to feel secure and buy herself a beautiful house on the beach in Harbour Island, Bahamas. Had she been born at a different time and under different circumstances, she would have made a sought-after investment banker.

My son, Alexandre, benefited greatly from her financial skills. She taught him what stocks and bonds were, what kinds of companies were good investments, and about yields and dividends. Every afternoon when he came home from school, the two of them studied the stock market pages in the afternoon edition of the *New York Post* so he could see which stocks were going up and which down. When he was six or seven, my new boyfriend, Barry Diller, wanted to give him one share of stock for his birthday and told him he could choose which one. "Choose the most expensive," my mother advised him. Alexandre chose IBM.

There is no doubt the financial education she gave him turned him into the financier he is today. He manages the family money, sits on prestigious boards, and has proven to be a superb adviser to all of us.

My mother was my rock. For all that I thought I'd conquered my fear of flying, I remember a very scary, bumpy flight to Harbour Island with her and Alexandre when she had just gotten out of the hospital. When the plane dropped suddenly and made loud creaking noises, I closed my eyes and thought, "OK, I am afraid. Where do I go for strength? Do I take the hand of my big, strong son or of my weak, dying mother?" And there was no question that I would go to my mother for strength. I put my hand over hers.

At about the same time as that plane trip, I remember being anxious when my daughter, Tatiana, was about to give birth. It's one thing when your son has a child, but for some reason, when your daughter has a child, you feel it in your own flesh. It is physical agony. I was frightened for my little girl, thinking of all the things that could go wrong. I called my mother, in tears, while driving to the hospital. She was very frail, but she summoned the strength to make me strong, though happily it turned out I didn't need it. Antonia was born without any complication and Tatiana was fine. In yet another testament to her strength, my mother clung to life so that she could see Tatiana's baby. Though her body was almost nonexistent, her mind and her will were strong. So many times in her life she was ill and on the verge of dying, but her incredible strength and determination kept her alive.

We had already welcomed her first great-grandchild, Talita, the daughter of Alexandre and his then wife, Alexandra Miller, and just as intense in my memory is the astonishing day when Alexandre brought the one-year-old Talita in her carriage to visit me and my mother in the Carlyle hotel in New York. It was Mother's Day and Alexandre gallantly brought each of us a bouquet of flowers. All our eyes were on the adorable little girl who pulled herself upright, clinging to a chair, then suddenly launched off on her own and took her first steps! We all clapped and praised her, but then something unbelievable took place. I was watching my old mother, wrinkled and sick in her chair, looking at this little girl on the floor and that little girl looking back at her, when suddenly I saw a flash of something white, almost like lightning coming out of my mother and going into Talita. I believe that that day my mother's energy and spirit transferred to my granddaughter. I saw it happen, that white flash going from my mother into Talita. I saw it.

My mother did not die peacefully. I think she was reliving the horrors of the camps and fighting giving in to death, as she had in Auschwitz. It was not the first time she'd relived those horrors. As much as she had tried to bury the past and concentrate on looking forward to life, she had had a breakdown twenty years before during a visit to Germany with Hans and some clients of his. My heart had nearly stopped when Hans called me in New York to tell me he'd woken up that morning in the hotel to find my mother missing. He'd finally found her hiding in the lobby of the hotel, underneath the concierge's desk, disoriented, speaking loudly and making little sense. "Why? What happened?" I'd asked him, in a panic myself. He thought it must have been the dinner they'd had the night before with his clients at a restaurant. It was very hot and the people at the tables around her were speaking loudly in German. I suspected that she and Hans had also had a fight, but whatever the reason, she'd completely come apart.

Hans thought she might snap out of it if I talked to her and I tried to talk calmly to her over the phone, but all she could do was babble nonsensically. Hans drove her back to Switzerland and put her in the psychiatric ward of the hospital and we all flew to her side—my brother and I and even my father—but she remained very confused, laughing one minute, crying the next, raving and incoherent. She wouldn't eat and she wouldn't drink nor would she surrender the fur coat she insisted on wearing in her hospital bed. We thought we'd lost her. But she was a survivor through and through, and three weeks later she was well enough to leave the hospital to convalesce in a clinic. She was a miracle once again, coming back to life from far away.

In her final illness in 2000, even though lovingly cared for by Lorna, her nurse, she no longer had the strength to fight off death or the demons that had always haunted her.

My brother, Philippe, and I buried her in Brussels, beside our father. She knew there was a spot for her there, and was happy about it. They had been each other's big loves in life, even though they separated, and it was appropriate that they end up together. We had our father's headstone engraved: "Thank you for your love," and our mother's: "Thank you for your strength."

The Mullers did not come to the service. Hans had married after they separated and in our agitation after my mother's death, we did not manage to reach his son, Martin, in time for the funeral . . . I feel very bad about that because Martin had remained very close to her; I love him and Lily was a mother to him.

"Today, we're taking Lily, my mother, for her eternal rest," I wrote to her friends and my friends who couldn't be there. "Our hearts are heavy but they should also be light because she has been liberated from all pain and has left on her eternal adventure surrounded by so much love.

"Fifty-five years almost to the day, Lily was liberated from the death camps. Twenty-two years old and less than 28 kilos. In that little package of bones, there was a flame, a flame that was life. Doctors forbade her to have children, she had two. She taught them everything, how to see, question, learn, understand and more important, never to be afraid.

"She touched all the ones that she met, listened to their problems, brought solutions and inspired them to find *joie de vivre* again. She looked so frail and fragile but she was strong and courageous, always curious to discover new horizons. She lived fully and will continue to do so through her children, her grandchildren, her great-grandchildren and her friends who loved her so."

I signed the letter from all of us—"Diane, Philippe, Alexandre, Tatiana, Sarah, Kelly, Talita, and Antonia." (My grandsons Tassilo and Leon were not born yet.)

I found a sweet note among many others my mother had written to herself, had it printed with an embossed lily of the valley because it was her favorite flower, and included it with what I had written.

"God gave me life and luck with my life," she'd written. "During my life, I've kept my luck all along. I have felt it like a shadow. It follows me everywhere and so I take it wherever I go, saying, 'Thank you, my luck. Thank you, my life. Thank you. Thank you.'"

2

LOVE

"Love is life is love is life . . ." I first wrote these words inside a heart when asked to design a T-shirt for a charity years ago, in the early nineties. I don't remember which charity it was for, but I do remember taking a photo of the T-shirt on Roffredo Gaetani, an aristocratic, muscular, good-looking Italian ex-boyfriend of mine, cropping his head and turning the photo into a postcard. I still have some of those postcards, and that same drawing marches across my computer screen, has appeared on DVF iPhone cases, canvas shopping bags, graffiti wrap dresses, even babyGap bodysuits. The words from my heart have become my personal mantra and the signature motto for the company.

Love is life is love. There is no way to envision life without love, and at this point in my life, I don't think there is anything more important—love of family, love of nature, love of travel, love of learning, love of life in every way—all of it. Love is being thankful, love is paying attention, love is being open and compassionate. Love is using all the privileges you possess to help those who are in need. Love is giving voice to those who don't have one. Love is a way of feeling alive and respecting life.

I have been in love many times, but I know now that being in love does not always mean you know how to love. Being in love can be a need, a fantasy, or an obsession, whereas loving truly is a much calmer and happier state. I agree with George Sand, the nineteenth-century French novelist: "There is only one happiness in life, to love and be loved," she wrote. I've enjoyed that happiness many times, but what I discovered with age is that true love is unconditional, and that is bliss.

Love is about relationships, yet the most important relationship is the one you have with yourself. Who else is with you at all times? Who else feels the pain when you are hurt? The shame when you are humiliated? Who can smile at your small satisfactions and laugh at your victories but you? Who understands your moments of fear and loneliness better? Who can console you better than you? You are the one who possesses the keys to your being. You carry the passport to your own happiness.

You cannot have a good relationship with anyone, unless you first have it with yourself. Once you have that, any other relationship is a plus, and not a must. "Take time this summer to really get to know yourself," I told a graduating class of high school girls as they were about to start their own journey of life. "Become your best friend; it is well worth it. It takes a lot of work and it can be painful because it requires honesty and discipline. It means you have to accept who you are, see all your faults and weaknesses. Having done that, you can correct, improve, and little by little discover the things you do like about yourself and start to design your life. There is no love un- less there is truth and there is nothing truer than discovering and accepting who you really are. By being critical, you will find things you dislike as well as things you like, and the whole package is who you are. The whole package is what you must embrace and the whole package is what you have control of. It is you! Everything you think, do, like, becomes the person you are and the whole thing weaves into a life, your life."

I finished my talk with an ancient quotation:

> *Beware of your thoughts for they become words,*
> *beware of your words for they become actions,*
> *beware of your actions for they become habits,*
> *beware of your habits for they become character,*
> *beware of your character for it becomes your destiny.*

I was lucky to start a relationship with myself very early in life. I am not sure why; maybe because I had no sibling until the age of six and I was alone a lot, or maybe because I was taught from an early age to be responsible for myself and for my actions.

I remember discovering that little "me" person in the reflection of my mother's vanity mirror and being intrigued by it. Not that I loved my image, but as I made funny and ugly faces at my own reflection, I enjoyed the control I had over it; I could make it do anything I wanted. I was absorbed by that little "me" person and wanted to discover more about her. Later, when I learned to write, I wrote stories about this character and the fantasies I imagined for her. The fictional stories became rarer as I turned to writing my diaries, recounting my experiences, my frustrations, my sense of cosmic emptiness, or my desire to conquer. My diary became my friend, my refuge.

My teenage diaries got lost and though I wish I still had them,

I rarely look back at the ones I do have. Their importance was in the moment, of having a friend to confide in. At this point in my life, I seldom write in my diaries. I have replaced the writing with a visual diary. I carry a camera with me everywhere and take pictures of what I want to store in my memory—people, nature, objects, architecture. Often I use those photos for inspiration.

I also learned how critical it is for me to have time alone to recharge and strengthen that inner connection. It is easy to lose oneself when you are with people all the time. I need silence and solitude to create a buffer against the daily barrage of information and challenges. Sometimes, in a big crowd, even at parties that I host, I find myself disappearing for a few minutes to be alone. I used to feel sad and out of place in those moments, lonely and disconnected. I don't anymore. I use these moments to reconnect with myself and build my strength.

Equally soothing and crucial is my love and need for nature. Nothing is more nourishing than seeing the day appear from the night, the strength of the waves, the majesty of the trees. Walking in the woods, being lost in nature reminds me of how small we are in the universe and somehow that reassures me. I remember one day walking in the country with my then very small son, Alexandre. I was lost in thought and when he inquired what those thoughts were, I responded, "I wonder what will happen to us." Very wisely little Alexandre answered, "I know what will happen, Mommy. Spring will come and the leaves will cover the trees again, then it will be summer, then autumn and the leaves will change color and fall. Winter and snow will follow." I smiled and took his hand. "Of course that is what will happen," I answered. I never forgot that moment.

Love is life is love and like most mothers, my strongest love has always been for my children. I'll never forget the intense rush I felt the first time I saw Alexandre. Not only was he my firstborn, I felt as if I already knew him. I had had many long conversations with him before he was born and I have always felt he was my partner as much as my son.

Alexandre was also the answer to my dream as a young girl—to have a little American son when I grew up. As a European girl, I always thought American boys were cooler, more casual and more boyish. Boys in Europe seemed serious and sometimes even repressed and I loved that American boys, who watched football and played sports endlessly, were not. Anyway, I got exactly what I wanted: a real little American boy, though he carries Egon's title of "prince." However, as I've watched the grown Alexandre raise his own American boys, I've realized that I failed him at least in one thing—I did not pay enough attention to his athletic life and seldom went to his games when he was growing up. I was never the Soccer Mom he secretly wished for.

In many respects I didn't know what I was doing when he was a baby, because, like any young mother, I had no experience. I was a little intimidated and relied heavily on our Italian nanny until I happened upon her handling Alexandre roughly in the bath—and fired her. From then on, no longer intimidated, I followed my common sense.

Beautiful, mischievous Princess Tatiana Desiree von und zu Furstenberg followed her brother thirteen months later. She was something else. I said from the beginning that she was the drop of oil you put into egg yolks and mustard to make mayonnaise happen. She was the magic that turned we three into a real family. When Tatiana was born, it wasn't Egon and me having a child, it was Egon, Alexandre, and me becoming a full family. And though the marriage didn't last, we remained a family forever.

I have great empathy with working mothers and the tug of war they feel, as I did, between staying with my children and going off to work. It never occurred to me to give up my growing business because I insisted on paying all my bills and took no money from Egon when we separated, but it was always wrenching to walk out the door. Once outside, however, I felt free, energized, and focused on making a good life for all of us. And it quickly came true all because of that little wrap dress.

With the first money I earned, I bought Cloudwalk, an astonishingly beautiful property in Connecticut for my twenty-seventh birthday so we could spend relaxed time together in a setting where we could also feel free. And we did. I spent much time there with the children and their school friends, cooking for them and often transporting one of them to the emergency room to see if a cut needed stitches or an arm was more than just bruised. During the week I'd be a tycooness in New York again, striding out the door in my high heels and fishnet stockings. I winked in the mirror, smiled at my shadow, and off I went, to make a living and become the woman I wanted to be.

From the beginning, I treated Alexandre and Tatiana more as people than as children. I never talked down to them and always encouraged them to express their opinions and take responsibility for themselves. Making me independent is what my mother did for me, and I was, for sure, going to do that for my children. Just as I had started keeping a journal in my childhood, I urged them to start recording their lives and thoughts. They began even before they were old enough to read and write, drawing the events of their days in pictures. We ended the day by exchanging news about what they'd done at school and what I'd done at work during "discussion time" on their beds. I involved them in every facet of my life, including my business.

"I have my job and school is your job," I told them. "We all go to work, we all have our own lives, we all have our responsibilities. You deliver on yours and I'll deliver on mine." It turned out to be a very good approach. Tatiana excelled at school, Alex did very well, and I managed all right at work.

I took them with me on trips as often as I could and, in spite of themselves, they became very good travelers. They would often complain or be upset about traveling conditions that seemed dangerous or boring to them at the moment, but those moments from their unusual adventures ended up being wonderful memories and great stories to tell. I remember a trip to the very isolated, prehistoric island of Nias across from Sumatra in the Indonesian archipelago. The tiny little local boat we took was fragile, to say the least. The return crossing in the middle of the night was rough, hot, and buggy. We kept silent as I prayed that we would make it safely to the mainland. Exotic it was, but maybe too exotic, risky, and dangerous, but we made it. That trip ended up in both their college applications in answer to the question: "What was one of the most riveting and adventurous things you've done in your life?"

In such extreme circumstances, and in other, calmer ones, I treasured traveling with my children. Traveling with children is unique because it is about discovering together. You are equal in front of new things and experiences. I always found it a great period of closeness, and I recommend it to parents. You lose the power role a bit and become companions. You don't have to say look at this and look at that because you're discovering at the same time—the landscapes you see, the people you encounter, the lines for tickets, the stop for lunch, the unexpected.

Could I have become the woman I wanted to be without having children? I certainly would not have been the same person. In fact, it's very hard, impossible really, for me to imagine what my life would have been without them. We actually grew up together. I was twenty-four when I had them both, barely a grown-up myself. I wasn't old enough to have yearned for children, yet suddenly there they were and my responsibility. I loved them with an intensity I'd never felt before. They were a part of me forever.

I was helped enormously by their two amazing grandmothers, both of whom were very present in my children's lives. My mother came to live with us in New York for months during the school year and struck her own loving relationship with them. Egon's mother, Clara Agnelli Nuvoletti, was just as attentive. The children spent almost every vacation with her, either on the island of Capri, at her house outside Venice, or in the mountain chalet in Cortina. My mother had become a very good friend of Clara's, and often she went along so my children had two fantastic grandmothers with them.

How wonderful it was, especially for Tatiana. Alexandre started going off on various adventures like glacier skiing and sailing, but Tatiana preferred staying with her grandmothers. She learned French from my mother and Italian and cooking from Clara. Her second husband, Giovanni Nuvoletti, was the president of the culinary academy of Italy and Clara wrote several cookbooks. Tatiana became an excellent cook and often cooks for us now. She also had long philosophical discussions with both of her grandmothers about love and the meaning of life. Clara would make her laugh with the gossip of her very privileged life and my mother would remind her of the challenges of adversity.

Unlike me, the grandmothers had nothing but time, which was wonderful for the children and wonderful for me. They had such a strong and very important influence: They were teachers, role models, active participants, and, above all, loving family members. Both had memories to share, both had great senses of humor, and both were great storytellers.

In a house with three women—my mother, Tatiana, and me—Alexandre was always considered the man of the house. He was the one we trained to be counted on. Now that he is a grown man, he has become all the things I had wished him to be. He watches over our assets and has become very valuable to the growth of DVF. Tatiana also became an important protector of the family: a specialist in diagnosing illnesses and best at giving advice. Now they both watch over Barry and me. We all sit on the board of DVF and we share the Diller–von Furstenberg Family Foundation. My children are the bookends that support me. We talk on the phone every day, sometimes more than once. "I love you," "I love you, too," we end each conversation.

If I have one regret in my life, it is that I didn't pay more attention to Tatiana when, in fact, she was the one who needed it more. In contrast to Alexandre, who was quite a wild boy and reduced me to pleading tears when he became a very fast teenage driver, Tatiana was such a good girl and caused so few problems that I took her for granted. This was a mistake. I didn't realize until much later that because she so rarely did anything to draw attention to herself, she felt I cared less about her than I did her brother. That brought an ache to my heart because I love them both with equal intensity, but I could see how she felt that way. Alexandre did get more of my attention because Tatiana didn't seem to need it. I was completely wrong.

From the time she could walk, Tatiana's legs seemed quite stiff. She could certainly get around all right, but she was never able to run. Her condition grew more noticeable when she began school and had difficulty with sports. I took her to several orthopedists, who checked her bones and looked to see if she had scoliosis, but they said there was nothing the matter with her, that her muscles were just stiffer than others and she would probably grow out of it. She didn't. Instead she hid her suffering from all of us for years until one day in her early twenties when she tried to run across Park Avenue and collapsed on the pavement. What a wrenching sight she was with two black eyes and a hugely swollen lip because she couldn't raise her arms in time to block her fall. Tatiana had just completed her master's degree in psychology at the time and remembered a reference to neuromuscular disorders. A neurologist at Columbia Presbyterian finally gave her a diagnosis: myotonia, a genetic muscular disorder that delays the muscles from relaxing after any exercise, especially in cold weather.

"Why didn't your mother know this before?" the doctor asked in wonderment, a question that stabbed my heart. We'd been going to orthopedists, who were concerned only with her bones.

I felt awful for her and angry at myself. When we'd first tried to address her condition she was at Spence School in New York, where she and the other girls in the Lower School had to walk up and down nine flights of stairs several times a day. What agony it must have been for her, but I didn't know about it because she never complained. Her suffering only increased when I moved the children to Cloudwalk, our house in Connecticut, when she was in the fifth grade, and the school there stressed athletics. Tatiana struggled and struggled, thinking her disability was all in her head—one doctor had told her flat out there was nothing wrong with her—but still, she didn't complain. Like my mother, Tatiana refused to think of herself as a victim.

I will never forgive myself for not realizing or understanding the scope of her disability, how it made her feel different from the other children and was a source of great physical and emotional pain. We have since had many long, long conversations about it, and I discovered that, just as I hadn't wanted to upset my mother, she didn't want to worry me when she was growing up. She saw the pressure and stress I was under with my business (she and Alexandre always called my business my "third child") and she didn't want to add any more pressure on me.

In 2014, Tatiana learned she does not have myotonia, but rather Brody disease, also a genetic condition that affects the muscles, including the muscle of the heart, which further explains her difficulty to keep pace with others. It brought home again how difficult it has been for her all her life. I wish she had told me. But maybe she did and I just did not hear it. I have kept a little note from her that she wrote to me as a very small child. It is on the bulletin board in my office in Cloudwalk. I cherished that note because I thought it was so sweet. It said "Mommy, you really know nothing about me." How awful I feel today when I look at this note that I thought was so sweet, and neither she nor I understood that it was a cry for help.

Tatiana may not be able to move as fast as everyone else, but her intelligence, her imagination, her heart, and her talent are so immense that she will continue to realize all of her dreams.

Tatiana always got the best grades in school—she was summa cum laude at her school in Connecticut—and did so well that she skipped the seventh grade. She always did her brother's homework as well as her own and held it over him for years, constantly reminding Alexandre: "I did your homework for you. I did your applications for you and I did your thesis for you," but she also admits that now she's getting paid back by Alexandre through his financial skills.

Tatiana never much liked the schools she went to so she just kept on jumping— from day school in Connecticut, to a year at boarding school in Switzerland, another in England, and then to Brown University at the age of sixteen. She graduated in just over three years. I was so very, very proud of her. I went to her graduation along with my mother and Mila, my housekeeper from France who had been very close to Tatiana, and was touched beyond measure when she presented me with a bouquet of flowers in gratitude for all I'd done for her. But even better than the flowers, I loved watching her huge smile and incredible beauty on that victorious day. Alexandre went to Brown, too, and graduated a year after Tatiana (though he is a year older) so both my children are better educated than I am.

I feel more and more connected to both children as the years go by. I can usually feel when something is wrong and when they need me. For me it is always "us," never "I." And that will never change. I look at them now, and love them, respect them, and admire them. Alex, an exceptional father, lover of life, and brilliant businessman and asset manager. Tatiana, a wonderful mother, a certified teacher and therapist, and a successful screenwriter and director. Her first feature film, *Tanner Hall*, which she cowrote, directed, and produced with her friend Francesca Gregorini, was the winner of the 2011 GENART Film Festival Audience Award, and launched Rooney Mara from her first starring role to a Best Actress Oscar nomination for *The Girl with the Dragon Tattoo*.

I like to joke that the children are my best samples, but those samples are definitely not for sale. As I look at them as adults and almost-beginning-to-age adults, it is possible for me to claim both success and failure in the kind of mother I was. I couldn't do that at the beginning of their lives, and certainly not during their teenage years when my constant prayer was to get them through it alive. But now I can enjoy the harvest from the seeds planted so many years ago and relax a little—though not too much.

The greatest thing about becoming a grandparent is watching your children being parents. For the first time you realize that they actually heard the things you told them throughout their childhoods. I see it in the way they make their children independent, the way they give them freedom, push them to make their own decisions, love and support them.

Just as my mother annoyed me with endless advice, I am sure I annoyed my children passing on that advice and a lot of my own, but it has paid off with my grandchildren. Alexandre's oldest child, Talita, the firstborn and now a teenager, is very much like her father, so I have a tendency to be both demanding and to take her for granted. She is beautiful and very bright, a great debater, a talented painter, and has an old soul. We love to talk about everything—the business of DVF, my mother's experience during the war, politics—everything. When she was nine I took her with me to Florence where I was preparing a fashion show in the private garden of a beautiful mansion. "Do you want to come with me and be my assistant?" I asked her. "I'm going to be working so you will have to work, too." "Yes, yes," she said, and she took part in all the magic of preparing a fashion show—watching the sets being made, casting the models, doing the fittings, choosing the final looks. We had a delightful and unforgettable week, stealing time out during the day to go to museums and at night to watch romantic comedies set in Europe like *Funny Face* and *Sabrina* from the Audrey Hepburn collection I had brought along.

When Talita's younger brother Tassilo was ten, Barry and I took him to the 2012 Olympics in London. At first I was a bit concerned what I would do alone with a little boy, but we ended up having a great time watching basketball and volleyball and laughing all the way. Tassilo is named for Egon's father, Prince Tassilo Egon Maximilian—and he was born very much a little prince, a little American prince. I don't really know what I mean by that, but that's the way we all look at him. He is cool, cute, and very kind, an excellent athlete and a good student. "I like to chill" is the way he describes himself.

Antonia, Tatiana's daughter, is a star. I think of her as the militant in the family, the political person, an A student, compassionate, a good painter, a born performer, and an amazing musician. She can hear a song and immediately play it on the piano. She impressed everyone at one of the DVF Christmas talent shows when, at the age of eleven, she performed an Adele song, not as a child but as a true artist. She is also wonderfully strong and centered. I got an indignant email from her after I sent a "Happy International Women's Day" email. "Shouldn't it be women's and girls' day?" she emailed me. "Aren't we women, too?"

Antonia, who, like me and her mother, went to boarding school in England, is great company. I have spent wonderful days alone with her in New York, London, Paris, and Shanghai, where we stole a day to visit the small towns outside the city known for their gorgeous gardens.

Barry and I spend every Christmas and New Year's holiday with the grandchildren, sometimes on our boat, other times on a land adventure. Since my birthday is on New Year's Eve, I always get a surprise from them: a collage, a song they have written, or a birthday cake in bed, as I remember from a wonderful New Year's holiday in Patagonia, Chile. And letters. We always exchange New Year's letters full of love and good wishes.

All grandparents think their grandchildren are amazing and I am biased, no doubt. As I write, I am recently blessed with a fourth grandchild, Leon (named for my father). It is Alexandre's third child and his first with AK, as we call his beautiful love and life companion, Alison Kay. I look forward to having a special relationship with little Leon as I have with the others.

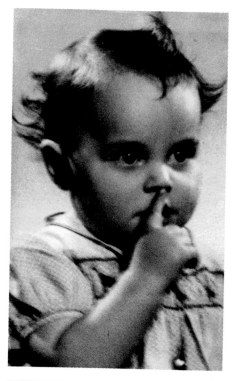

As a toddler,
curious already.

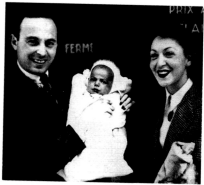

As a baby with
my parents.

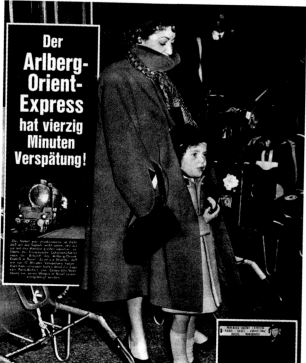

My mother and
I waiting for the
Orient Express,
the first time I
had my photo
in a magazine.

Unless otherwise noted, all photographs courtesy of the author.

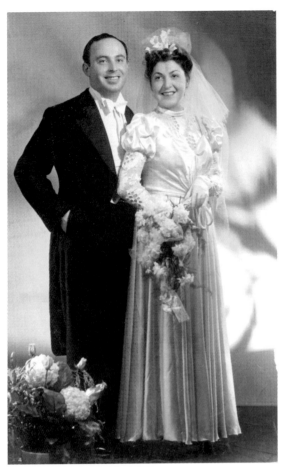

My parents on
their wedding day,
November 29, 1945.

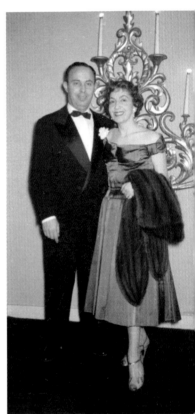

With my
baby brother,
Philippe, in
1953.

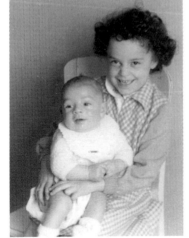

My parents going to
a party, 1958.

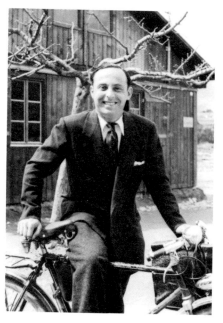

My young father on his bicycle.

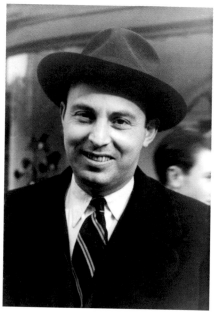

My father, Leon.

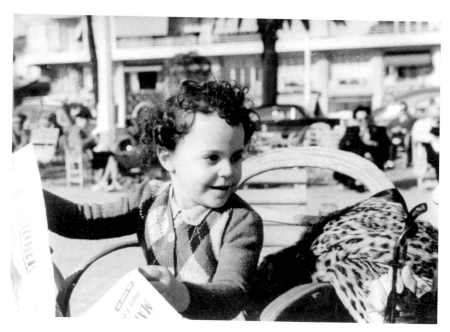

Age three, pretending to read the newspaper.

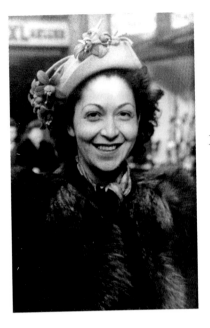

My mother, Lily.

One of the two notes tossed
by my mother en route to the
prison camp in Malines.

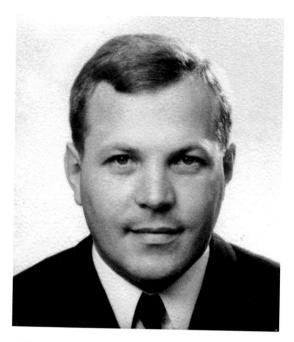

Hans Muller, my mother's longtime companion.

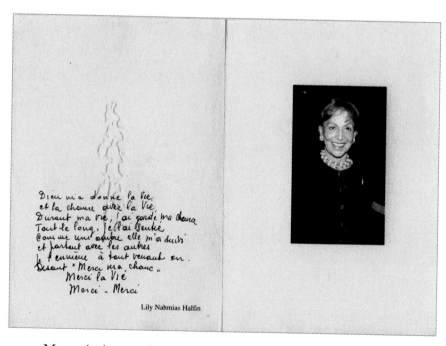

My mother's remembrance card featuring a note she wrote to herself.

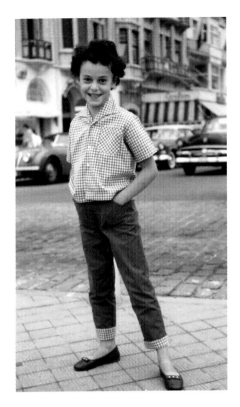

Age nine, in the Belgian resort of Knokke le Zoute.

As a preteen on vacation at the North Sea.

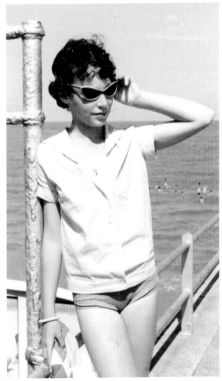

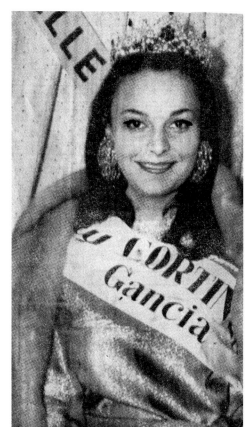

Lady Cortina, my first and
only beauty contest, 1967.

At age fifteen, flying solo.

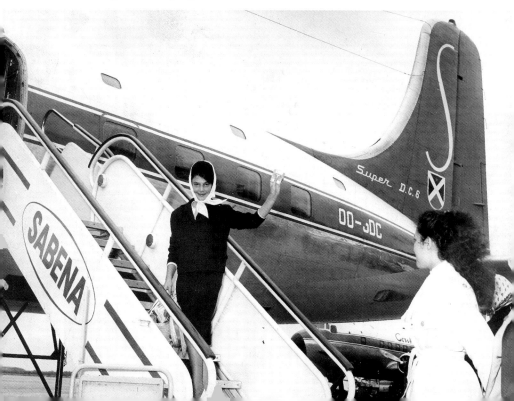

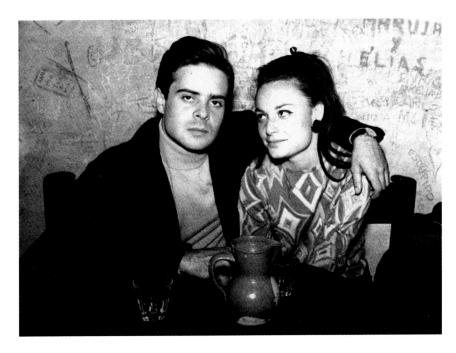

With Lucio, my Italian boyfriend, 1966.

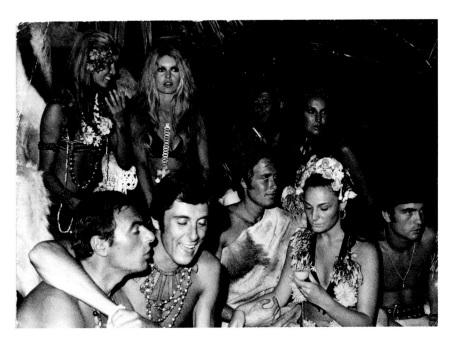

At a pirate-themed party at Brigitte Bardot's in St. Tropez.

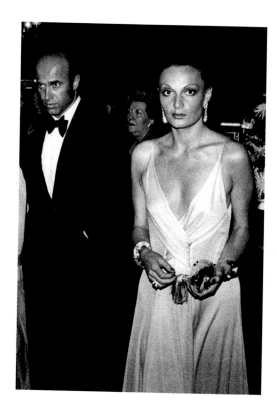

With Jas Gawronski
at a party in 1975.
(Ron Galella, Getty image)

With Alain Elkann in
New York, 1986. *(Ron
Galella, Getty image)*

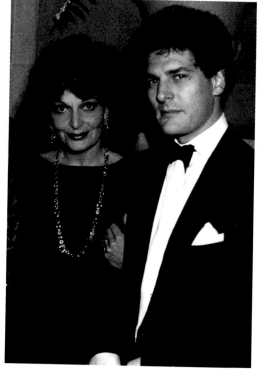

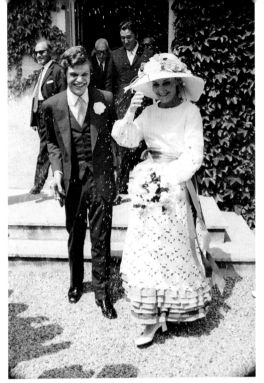

On my wedding day with
Prince Eduard Egon von
und zu Fürstenberg in
Montfort-l'Amaury, near
Paris, on July 16, 1969.
(Berry Berenson Perkins)

Egon and I in our Park Avenue
apartment in the early 70s.
(Horst, Condé Nast, Corbis Image)

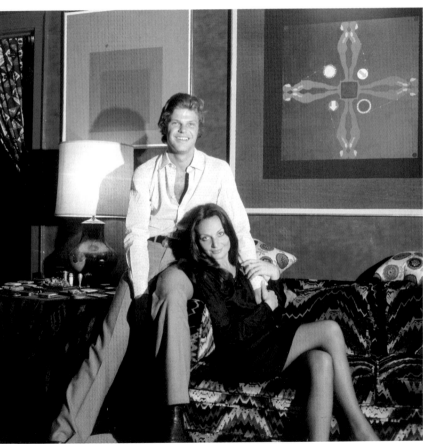

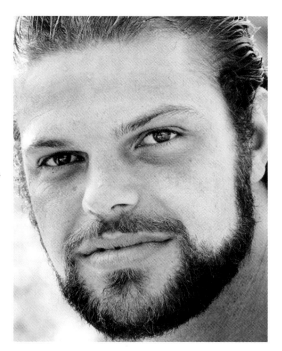

Egon in 1972.

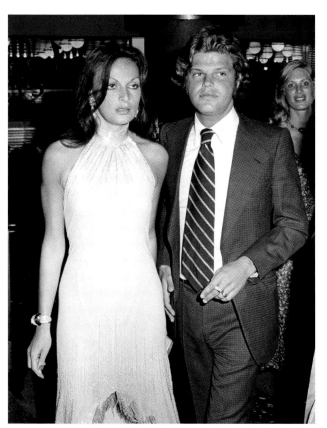

Egon and I at a party in New York 1970. *(Ron Galella, Getty image)*

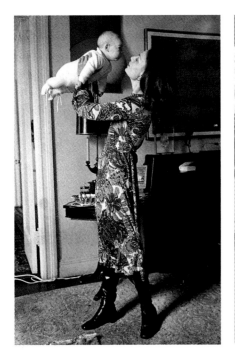

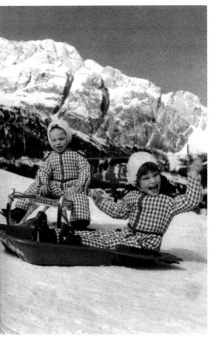

With my baby son, Alexandre, 1970.

Alexandre and Tatiana during winter
vacation in Cortina d'Ampezzo.

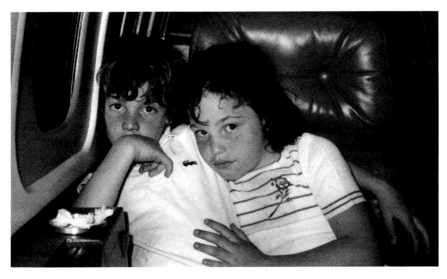

Alexandre and Tatiana on our way to vacation, 1977.

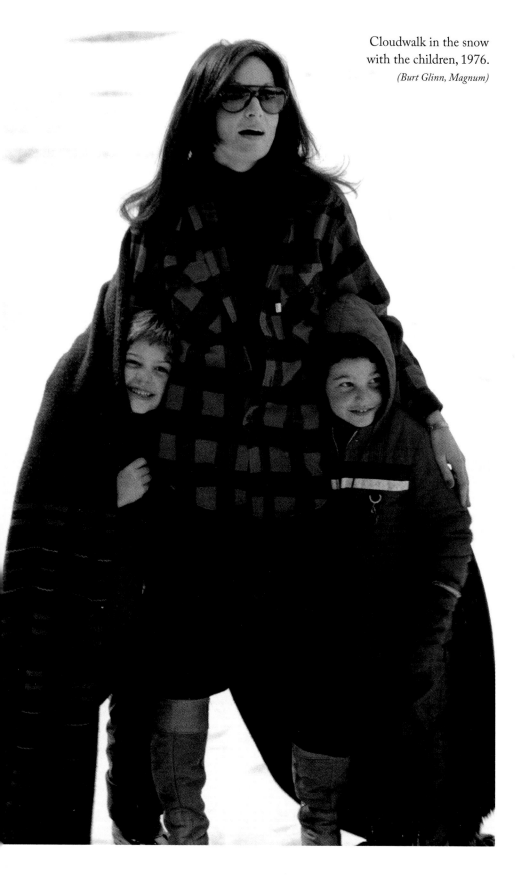

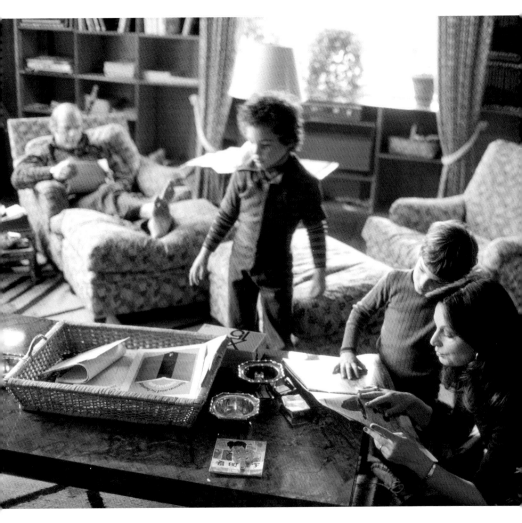

Cloudwalk living room in 1976 with Barry and the children. *(Burt Glinn, Magnum)*

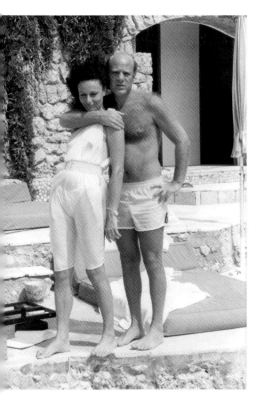

With Barry in
Santo Domingo,
1977.

At the premiere of the
movie *Grease*, 1978.

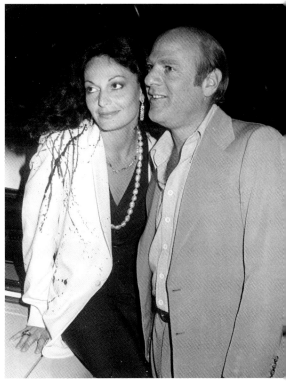

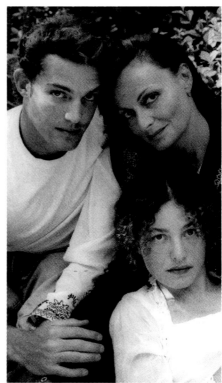

With the grown-up children, 1992. *(Wayne Maser, courtesy of the artist)*

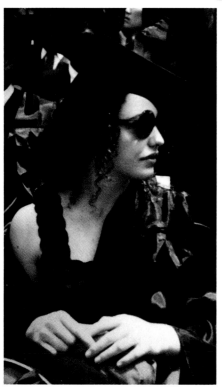

Tatiana graduates from Brown University at nineteen!

I have loved a lot and have been in love many, many times. Perhaps I've been in love so often because I asked little in return or maybe because I was just in love with being in love. For me, falling in love wasn't a need—it was an adventure. My father so filled me with love that I didn't think I needed, or wanted, much back. That emotional independence made some men feel insecure and frustrated, and others relieved. Not that I was never like every girl, dependent or jealous at times, waiting for "the" phone call or behaving stupidly. Of course I did, many, many times.

The first time I remember being in love was with a boy in Brussels who had absolutely no interest in me. His name was Charlie Bouchonville. I would see him in the NR4 tramway coming home from school. He had green eyes and a beauty spot at the end of his left eye, wore a suede jacket, and was very stylish. I was still a little girl, flat chested and all. I don't think he ever knew I existed, but I fantasized about him for a long time, and when I went to boarding school I boasted about a relationship with him that had never existed.

The first boy I kissed was Italian. His name was Vanni, short for Giovanni, and we kissed in the tearoom of the Hotel Rouge in Milano Marittima where my mother, brother, and I were spending a holiday on the Adriatic coast of Italy. I was fourteen. Vanni was a very, very sexy boy, who must have been more than eighteen because he was proudly driving a little yellow Alfa Romeo. We would meet after lunch in the tearoom of the hotel and kiss. My mother would send Philippe as a spy and he would just sit there. Philippe and I were sharing a bedroom and one night Vanni snuck up to our room while my brother was sleeping. I felt very grown up in the midst of our whispers and tiptoeing around the room, but I disappointed Vanni. He wanted to do more than I was willing to do, so our lovely flirtation stayed pretty much at the kissing level. We wrote letters to each other for a while afterward, which was perfect for my Italian. I learned Italian writing love letters.

My first serious boyfriend was called Sohrab. He was born in Iran and was studying architecture in Oxford. He had a beautiful smile, drove a turquoise Volkswagen, and was very nice to me. I had just arrived at Stroud Court, a boarding school for girls outside Oxford. School had not started but I had come early, as had Danae, a Greek girl from Athens who became my best friend that year. Danae and I went to see an exhibition of Henry Moore sculptures at the Ashmolean Museum, and afterward we went for tea across the street at the Randolph Hotel. There we met these two cute Persian boys, Sohrab and Shidan, and we immediately became great friends.

Our school allowed us to go out on Wednesday afternoons, all day Saturday, and Sunday afternoons. The next Wednesday, Sohrab took me to the movies to see *Dr. No,* the first James Bond. I could hardly follow the dialogue because my English was not very good, but I had a wonderful afternoon. Sohrab was kind and thoughtful. My parents were going through an unpleasant divorce, and the letters I received from home made me feel powerless and sad. Sohrab consoled me and took me to eat Indian food. I had never been in a restaurant with a boy before and it felt very special.

Later we would go to his room on Banbury Road. All he had was a large desk by the window and a big bed. It was very cold and humid and every hour he would put a sixpence coin into the heater to keep it going. His bed was cozy and so was he. We kissed a lot. I was a virgin and was still wearing little girl cotton underwear, which I felt embarrassed about. I wanted to pretend I was older and sophisticated but I did not really want to have sex. We broke up for a while and then started seeing each other again. By then I had bought silk underwear. I was sixteen. He became my first lover, kind and attentive. He made me happy. Many, many years later I found out that I, too, was his first lover. He was twenty-one.

The following summer, I was on holiday in Riccione, Italy, with my father and brother. Sohrab and Shidan drove from England to see me on their way to Iran, where they were going to sell the little turquoise Volkswagen for a profit before going back to Oxford. They did not stay long, barely an afternoon. To this day, my brother, who was still a child, remembers and doesn't understand what happened next. One day I was clearly in love with Sohrab, keeping his framed photo by my bed in my hotel room. The next day, I met Lucio on the beach. He became my next boyfriend.

Lucio was a very handsome twenty-two-year-old who looked like the Italian actor Marcello Mastroianni. We fell in love. He was passionate and experienced. He would hold my arm firmly and take me into the pine forest behind the beach. He would make love to me endlessly, making me feel like a real woman. During the day I was a normal seventeen-year-old girl having a nice holiday with her father and brother, but at night I had a secret life, a grown-up woman having a very sexy love affair. Lucio was very much in love and so was I.

We kept up a passionate correspondence for a long time and every now and then would manage to meet. Once, in Milan, where I had accompanied my father on a business trip, we locked ourselves in a hotel room near the railroad station for the entire day. Another time I went to Crevalcore near Bologna where he lived. Taking advantage of the fact that my mother was on a trip with Hans, I left boarding school early and took a detour to Italy on the way home to Geneva. I met his family, who had a small handbag factory. They organized a dinner for me in a local restaurant and I slept in a tiny hotel near his home. Later on he came twice to visit me while I was studying in Spain. Our passionate encounters remain a wild memory.

Two years ago I received a sad letter from Lucio's wife. He had died and she had found letters from me and some photographs. Would I like to have them? "Of course," I said, and to my delight I received a huge box with hundreds of love letters I had sent him as well as photos, menus, and train tickets. He had kept them all.

In England after the holiday I became infatuated with a French girl at my school. Her name was Deanna. She was very shy and masculine and she intrigued me. We became very close. We went on together to the University of Madrid where there were so many anti-Franco riots and so many strikes that we hardly ever went to class as the university was almost always closed. We shared a grim little room in a pensione for girls on the Calle de la Libertad in the center of Madrid. To get into our pensione at night, we had to clap and the Serrano, who held the keys for the block, would open our building's door and let us in. We made friends at the Facultad de Filosofía y Letras where we took Estudios Hispánicos classes. We watched flamencos at night and went to bullfights on Sundays. Madrid was a repressed city at the time, still wounded from the civil war. The mood was dark and I was bored.

My life took a different turn during the Christmas holiday that year. My mother, Hans, his son Martin, my brother, and I went to celebrate the holidays in Gstaad in the Swiss Alps. We were staying at the Hôtel du Parc having a dull time when suddenly, one afternoon in the village, I bumped into my best friend from Pensionnat Cuche, my boarding school in Lausanne. Isabel was from Venezuela, a bit older than I, beautiful and sophisticated. It was Isabel who had taught me how to French-kiss, practicing on mirrors. She lived with her mother and sister in Paris; her father, Juan Liscano, was a famous writer and intellectual in Caracas.

The encounter with Isabel changed the course of my life because that night she took me to a party and I made my official entry into the jet set world. The party was at the chalet of the Shorto family, a Brazilian/English lady and her five gorgeous children. The music was loud, people were dancing samba, smoking, drinking, laughing, and speaking many languages at the same time. Everyone seemed to know each other. I had never experienced that atmosphere before. They took me in immediately. I became part of the group and stayed on with Isabel after my family went back home to Geneva.

In Gstaad I met an "older man" in his midthirties who took a liking to me and never left my side for a week. His name was Vlady Blatnik. He lived in Venezuela where he had a successful shoe business. Vlady took me to dinner parties and we went skiing together every day. For New Year's Eve, my birthday, he bought me a Pucci printed silk top with black silk pants and matching black silk boots. This was my first designer outfit. That night I turned nineteen and even though I did not feel as beautiful or glamorous as the other women in the room, I thought life had finally begun!

Going back to Madrid to complete the school year was a bit of a downer, but during spring break Deanna and I planned a trip through Andalusia. We discovered the beauty of the Alhambra in Grenada and the magic of Sevilla. That trip was the end of my stay in Spain. I decided to continue school in Geneva where my mother was living with Hans. Deanna moved to Andalusia, and we stayed friends for a bit then lost touch.

I called Deanna a few years ago to invite her to the opening of my new boutique in Honolulu where she now lives. We picked up where we left off, as childhood friends do. "Can you believe we are in our sixties?" I said. We laughed at the absurdity of it. I felt the same age I was when I last saw her.

I have always tried to stay in touch with the people that were important in my life and the people that I loved. Once I love, I love forever, and there is nothing more cozy and meaningful than old friends and lovers. I'm so fortunate to have had and have so much love in my life. Without it, I would never be who I am.

I find great happiness in my relationships with old friends, living mirrors that reflect histories of laughter and sorrow, triumphs and failures, births and deaths, on both sides.

My closest, oldest friend is Olivier Gelbsmann, who has known me since I was eighteen. He has followed every step of my life and when we are together we don't need to speak to know what the other thinks. Olivier worked with me very early on, worked with Egon afterward, and later became an interior decorator. We now work together on DVF décor and home products. Olivier was present when my children were born, and at every important moment of my life. He consoled each of my boyfriends when I left them. Olivier was friends with my mother, my daughter, and now my granddaughters. My friend the Greek artist Konstantin Kakanias, with whom I collaborated on an inspirational comic book, *Be the Wonder Woman You Can Be,* as well as other projects, has also been friends with four generations of women in my family.

I treasure the memories I share with friends like Olivier and Konstantin. Landscapes change, people come and go, but all the landscapes, all the experiences, all the people weave into your life's fabric. Love is not just about people you had affairs with. Love is about moments of intimacy, paying attention to others, connecting. As you learn that love is everywhere, you find it everywhere.

Just as I collect books and textiles, I collect memories and friends. I love to remember. It's not that I dwell in nostalgia, but that I love intimacy. It is the opposite of small talk. It is the closest thing to truth.

"Beauty is truth, truth beauty," as I learned in Oxford when I studied the English poet John Keats.

I have tried not to lie my whole life. Lies are toxic. They are the beginning of misunderstandings, complications, and unhappiness. To practice truth is not always easy, but as with all practices, it becomes a matter of habit. Truth is cathartic, a way of keeping the trees pruned. The truer you can be the better it is because it simplifies life and love.

———————

There are many degrees of love, of course. I know now that of all the so many times I've been in love, only two men were truly great loves. I married both of them, one toward the beginning of my life, the other much later.

Egon. I cannot begin to describe all I owe to my first husband, Prince Eduard Egon von und zu Fürstenberg. I will be forever thankful to him because he gave me so much. He gave me my children; he gave me his name; he gave me his trust and his encouragement as he believed in me; he shared everything, all of his knowledge and all of his connections as he gave me his love.

I met Egon at a birthday party in Lausanne. I remember his big smile, his childlike face, and his gapped teeth. He had just enrolled at the University of Geneva where I was taking courses. He had also just returned from a few months in a Catholic mission in Burundi, where he had taught children and taken care of leprosy patients. I was impressed. I remember what I was wearing the night I met him because he complimented me on it—pink palazzo pajama pants and an embroidered tunic I had borrowed from my mother's closet. We were both nineteen.

Egon was the perfect eligible bachelor, an Austro/German prince by his father, and a rich heir from his mother, Clara Agnelli, the eldest child of the Fiat motorcar family. Egon seemed interested in me, maybe because I had already made a lot of friends in Geneva, and he had just arrived. We went out a lot and one Sunday we drove to nearby Megève in the mountains for a day in the snow. The car broke down and Egon went to get help. I remember opening the glove compartment to check his passport. I had never met a prince before and I wanted to see if his title was written on it. (It was not). When Egon came back to the car with a mechanic, the engine started immediately. There was nothing wrong with the car. To this day I remember Egon's embarrassed face. It was his helplessness that seduced me.

Egon lived in a small, luxurious rental apartment near Lac Léman while I was living at home with my mother and Hans, but we were always together. My mother, who had never acknowledged a boyfriend of mine before, immediately adopted him. They would become very close. Egon had a lot of energy and a great sense of adventure. He was always planning trips and places to discover. He suggested a group of us join a package deal trip to the Far East. I managed to convince my mother to let me go with them only for her to discover when she brought me to the airport that the only passengers going were Egon and me. The others had dropped out. I panicked, worried she wouldn't let me go alone with Egon, but she did.

We had a great time. India, New Delhi, Agra, and the magnificent Taj Mahal, Thailand and its floating market, Burma and its hundred pagodas, Cambodia and the ruins of Angkor Wat, the making of clothes overnight in Hong Kong. We went sightseeing all day every day as perfect tourists, and at night, we were invited to dine with local people through Egon's Fiat connection. Egon was the most charming young man in the world. His charisma and enthusiasm were contagious and traveling with him was always full of surprises and serendipity.

In Bangkok we dined with Jim Thompson, a famous American who had settled in Thailand after the war and had organized all the independent silk weavers into the huge business he owned, the Thai Silk Company. Mr. Thompson was wearing a silk shirt and pants and embroidered velvet slippers. He lived in a magnificent old Thai house full of antiques. From the house, we could see the weavers working at night, lit by lanterns, all along the floating market. I remember him telling us he was leaving for a holiday the next day in the jungles of Malaysia. He was never to be seen again. Rumors say that he was a double, triple agent and had been killed.

Another night, in Thailand, I was so mad at Egon—I'd found him in our hotel room having a massage from a beautiful Thai girl—that I'd gone down to the bar. A rather gloomy American man bought me a very strong Thai beer, announced he worked for a defense contractor, then said, "Oh well, the Vietnam War will soon be finished, but it doesn't matter because there will be a new arms market now in the Middle East." (Two months later, the 1967 Six-Day War erupted in Israel, Jordan, and Syria.) I was shocked. I had never realized that wars actually meant business for some people. They use research, marketing, sales—everything a normal company does—but for the business of weapons and war. It was a jolt to learn that as soon as defense contractors hear there is a conflict somewhere, they send salesmen and open a new market.

Egon and I went everywhere and discovered everything together. I remember the first time he took me to Villa Bella, his mother's chalet in Cortina d'Ampezzo in the Italian Alps. I had never been in such an elegant, welcoming, unusual house before. All in wood, it looked like a glorified gingerbread house full of antiques, an unexpected mix of colorful fabrics and quantities of silver and Murano glass. There were many housemaids dressed in Tyrolean fashion and butlers in full gear, yet the household was not stiff. The young ones would go skiing all day and gather with all the others for dinner. Food was abundant and delicious, of course, and the conversation humorous and superficial.

Clara, Egon's mother, was there with Count Giovanni Nuvoletti, who was to become her second husband a few years later. Giovanni was a writer and a man of the salon. He was very eloquent and held court, while Clara was light and witty. We were a group of friends from university who had come to Villa Bella for the Christmas holidays, and I shared a room with a beautiful redheaded girl called Sandy. I celebrated my twentieth birthday there, still feeling slightly out of place. By the time I celebrated my twenty-first birthday in that same villa the following year, I had become more comfortable and at ease with the family, the milieu, the lifestyle in general.

Egon took me to the South of France to meet his glamorous uncle Gianni Agnelli on his yacht and to watch the Grand Prix of Monaco, the famous car race. He took me to the film festival at the Lido of Venice and the Volpi Ball on the Canale Grande. I met everyone that was anyone anywhere—aristocrats, courtesans, businesspeople, actors, painters, and all of the Café Society entourage. How would I ever remember all these names, places, all this information, I wondered, taken by the dizziness of it all. It all felt like what Hemingway so eloquently described as a "moveable feast."

But our experiences were not only about glamour and wealth. Egon was a real traveler, inquisitive, full of energy and curiosity, eager to meet all kinds of people in whatever country we were in, keen to eat into the adventure—sometimes literally. I remember a man he befriended in the old souks of Djerba, Tunisia, who invited us to his house for lunch. We followed him through the narrow twisting alleyways, turning to the left, to the right, and to the left again, having no idea where we were going. We finally arrived in what looked like an abandoned apartment building, climbed the stairs, and arrived in the man's house, filled with children, some of whom were obviously sick. Food was served and I couldn't touch it, I felt repulsed, but Egon downed it with grace as if we were at the most elegant home in Paris. I will always remember that day, the lesson it taught me. Egon had an incredible ease about him, which made all people feel good about themselves. He was a true prince.

I'd traveled a lot with my family as a child, but Egon brought it to a different level. He infused in me the same curiosity and sense of adventure, which I carry to this day. I'm always ready to go. I pack lightly. I travel lightly, leaving time for the unknown. Even as a child I loved to travel, through my Tintin books. It was with Tintin that I learned geography and discovered the world first—America, Egypt, Peru, China, the Congo. When I arrive somewhere I have never been before, I always think of Tintin.

But Egon's most important gift was our children, all the more because I was hesitant about having them, especially Alexandre. He was the unexpected result of a weekend I spent with Egon in Rome in May 1969. I was living in Italy then, working as an intern for a fashion industrialist, Angelo Ferretti. Egon was taking the summer off, having completed his training program at Chase Manhattan Bank in New York, and was on his way to India and the Far East with a friend from school, Marc Landeau, before starting another job at the investment bank Lazard Frères in New York. I was very excited to see him and he, evidently, me. He had organized a big dinner with friends at Tula, a fashionable restaurant off Via Condotti, and I went with him wearing an evening jumpsuit with a plunging décolleté we had bought on sale that afternoon on the Via Gregoriana.

I remember there were paparazzi outside in the streets, but what happened inside was brighter than all of their flashbulbs. Egon gave me a beautiful ring he had designed, a pale sapphire in a big gold setting. To my complete surprise, this dinner was an engagement party. I was very excited, even though I did not totally believe it. Yet that night, in the intimacy of our bedroom, I remember whispering to Egon: "I will give you a son." Did I really mean it? Or was I only trying to be seductive? In any event, after the weekend, Egon went to India and I went back to Ferretti's factory.

A few weekends later I went to Monaco with friends to watch the Grand Prix again. Ferretti was in Monaco, too, and offered me a ride back to Milan at the end of the weekend. He drove his Maserati very fast and I thought it was all the high-speed twists and turns in the road that were making me nauseated. I felt even more sick the next day and thought a sauna might make me feel better. It didn't. Instead I fainted in the middle of Piazza San Babila and remember hearing people saying "She's dead, she's dead" and all I could do was move a finger to show them "No, I'm not dead." What I was, of course, was pregnant. I couldn't believe my ears when the doctor told me the news.

Here I was, barely twenty-two, and what I wanted most was to be independent. Furthermore, Egon was one of the best "catches" in Europe. Who was going to believe that I had not done it on purpose? I went home to Geneva to see another doctor who told me he could help me end the pregnancy. I was torn.

I went to my mother for advice. She had taken Egon's gift of a ring more seriously than I had and was horrified at the thought that I could make such a decision on my own. "You are engaged," she said. "The least you can do is discuss the matter with your fiancé."

Reluctantly, I drafted a telegram to Egon, who was in Hong Kong, offering him the choice. I have kept the telegram of his wonderful reply in my scrapbook. He was clear and definite. "Only one option. Organize marriage in Paris July 15. I rejoice. Thinking of you. Love and kisses, Eduard Egon."

Suddenly my life was giving me vertigo, though it was a happy dizziness. No time to waste. All the wedding preparations: invitations to be printed, wedding dress to be made, ceremony and party to be arranged, trousseau to be bought. As usual, my mother was a great help. We visited Clara, Egon's mother, in Venice and planned it all together.

Clara was very supportive, but on Egon's father's side, the patriarch of the Furstenberg family was evidently not. Jewish blood in the family was unheard of and there was opposition. I also overheard a slight at the Agnelli house—something I interpreted as a clever, ambitious little bourgeois girl from Belgium getting what she wanted. I felt belittled and hurt and remember walking with a very determined stride around Clara's garden, caressing my pregnant stomach. It was then I had my first conversation with Alexandre. "We'll show them," I said out loud to my unborn child. "We'll show them who we are!"

The wedding took place on July 16, 1969, the same day that the first American astronauts were sent to the moon, in the countryside outside Paris, in Montfort l'Amaury. My three-month pregnancy did not show at all in the Christian Dior wedding dress its designer Mark Bohan had created for me. The mayor married us at the town hall and there was a huge luncheon reception afterward at the Auberge de la Moutière, a charming inn and restaurant managed by Maxim's.

The crowd was young, beautiful, and glamorous; the food exquisite; and the entertainment enthusiastic. My father had hired the entire company of fifty musicians and singers from the trendy Russian night-club Raspoutine. To my embarrassment, he took the microphone, sang in Russian with the Raspoutine musicians, and broke glasses. Every-one else loved it and the wedding party was a huge success. The only nonparticipant was Egon's father, Tassilo, who had been so pressured by the family's disapproving patriarch that he came to the ceremony but boycotted the reception, though it barely diminished the celebra-tion or our joy. Egon and I left the guests dancing and singing, and went back to the center of Paris, changed our clothes, and went walk-ing the streets and in an out of the shops of the Faubourg St-Honoré.

For our wedding present his mother gave us a beach house on Sardinia's beautiful Costa Smeralda, where for the whole month of August we packed a crowd of sixteen friends into three tiny bedrooms. We were all so young and had so much fun.

Our beautiful son, Alexandre Egon, was born six months later on January 25, 1970, in New York. Our equally beautiful daughter, Tatiana Desirée, followed just thirteen months later. Just as Egon in-sisted that we marry and have Alexandre, he was insistent that I have Tatiana. I'd gotten pregnant again just three months after the very difficult birth of Alexandre by emergency cesarean after sixteen hours of labor. The idea of starting all over again needed some encourage-ment. Lovely Tatiana was born on February 16, 1971, this time by a scheduled cesarean. There are no words to describe how grateful I am for Egon's enthusiasm and support. He played a bigger part in both my children being born than I did, though I played a bigger part afterward.

Life in New York was lots of fun in the early seventies. Real es-tate was cheap, so many diverse and creative people could live there.

Pop art in the galleries and nudity on Broadway made us feel that everything was new, allowed, and the freedom we felt had just been invented. Prince and Princess von Furstenberg (we had dropped the "und zu") were the "it" couple in town. Our youth, our looks, and our means put us on every invitation list and in social columns. On any given night, we went out to at least one cocktail party, a dinner, sometimes a ball, and always a stop at some gay bar at the end of the night. We lived on Park Avenue but still felt very European and continued to spend a lot of time there.

We hosted lots of parties for Europeans coming to town. I remember the big party we gave for Yves Saint Laurent and the last-minute dinner we gave for Bernardo Bertolucci, who had just opened *Last Tango in Paris*. The movie was quite racy and shocking and its talented and handsome director was the hit of New York. Everyone came to our parties—Andy Warhol and his entourage, actors, designers, journalists, and, of course, many Europeans. Life was fast, to say the least, too fast, finally, for me.

The marriage itself had its own stresses. Egon was my husband and my first true love, but our marriage became complicated. He loved to have fun and was very promiscuous, wanting to experiment as much as possible. I tried to embrace his behavior and accept an open marriage; I certainly did not want to judge him. I acted cool and hid my suffering, not wanting to be a victim. But I had two young children to take care of and was starting an equally demanding business. It finally became too hard to manage it all.

Strangely enough, what saved our relationship and preserved our love was the end of our marriage in 1973. The tipping point was a February cover story about us in *New York* magazine: "The Couple Who

Has Everything—Is Everything Enough?" The title was bannered over the ravishing photo of us posing in our tented living room.

The idea for the story came from the magazine's editor in chief, Clay Felker. Clay was traveling home from Europe when he saw a small photo of Egon and me at a charity ball in Texas in the newsmaker section of *Newsweek*. The ball had been designed by Cecil Beaton and dignitaries had been invited from all over the globe. Egon and I looked particularly glamorous. The young princess was wearing a beautiful, practically topless Roberto Capucci gown and the young prince was breathtakingly handsome in a perfectly cut tuxedo.

Clay, who was the creator of the weekly, decided to assign a pictorial cover story about this young, intriguing couple. A serious feminist writer, Linda Bird Francke, and a highly qualified photographer, Jill Krementz, were assigned the story. There were photos of Egon in the subway, me at the hairdresser, the babies in their nursery, the two of us walking the streets and at an art gallery with Egon's parents. The photos looked very good and the quotes were unusually candid and titillating. Egon teased about having an open bisexual relationship and I compared sex in a marriage to a left hand touching a right one. It sounded so blasé and cynical but we were very young, acting cool at all cost, and, ultimately, very naïve with the press.

The result was shocking and it destroyed our marriage. Reading the magazine and seeing our lives exposed under a magnifying glass, I realized that that couple was not who I was. I didn't want to be a European Park Avenue princess with a pretend decadent life. That woman was definitely not the woman I wanted to be. I had to leave the couple in order to be me. Egon moved out soon after that piece in *New York* magazine, but our friendship and shared family lasted forever.

Egon and I had an easier, deeper, more sincere and respectful relationship after we parted. Of course he was sad and resentful at first, but the breakup was absolutely the only right thing to do, so eventually he accepted it. Parting ways does not mean erasing entirely someone from your life. The relationship can evolve, and be nurtured, but in a different way. Not an easy task, but as anything meaningful, well worth it.

I didn't have to work at being nice to Egon. He was my first true love, the man I married, the one who gave me my children. I never judged him and always loved him; I just could not endorse us as a couple. We remained extremely close for the rest of his life. He was family. When Barry came into my life, we often traveled together with Egon and the children, and we always spent Christmas all together.

I was with Egon in Rome when he died of cirrhosis of the liver in June 2004, two weeks before his fifty-eighth birthday. He had had hepatitis C for a while. He had led a life of excess until his health finally failed him. He had been too ill to come to Cloudwalk and cold Connecticut for Christmas the previous December, so we went to him in Florida and celebrated the holiday with the children and grandchildren in a hotel suite in Miami. As usual, Barry was with us, as was Egon's second wife, Lynn Marshall. My mother was no longer with us, and between missing her and seeing Egon so weak, our reunion that year felt a bit sad. Nonetheless, we were still together, a loving and extended family.

Egon was back in Rome when he was first hospitalized. He was not the type to ever complain, but he started calling more and more frequently to express his worries. Should he, could he have a liver transplant? The children alternated in going to visit him. With Alex he went to a thermal spa hotel in Abano, where his mother, Clara, was already staying with her husband. Then Tatiana went to spend weeks with him at his home in Rome. With his brother, Sebastian, Egon attended his uncle Umberto's funeral. It was his last outing—he had to be rushed back into the hospital again.

Tatiana got to Rome first. Alex and I arrived on the morning of June 10, 2004. It was very hot. We bought fruits in the street and brought them to him. Egon took me aside and asked me to talk to the doctors. He was worried that they were not telling him the truth. I promised I would. We stayed in his room until dusk, talking and laughing a lot. His vision was blurred, but in his unique way of beautifying everything, he referred to the spots he was seeing as intricate embroideries on the wall. He insisted on telling us what restaurant we should go to for dinner, but we didn't want to go to a noisy restaurant. Instead, we hurried back to our tiny connecting rooms at the Hotel Hassler and ordered room service. The three of us wanted to be as close together as we could. We were very worried.

As Egon had asked, I spoke to the doctor and the news was not good. His lungs were filling with fluid, his heart was weak, and his kidneys were failing. I did not discuss it with the children. There was nothing to say. We all knew.

Egon called the next morning as we were having breakfast. He sounded weak and a little breathless. "You'd better come soon," he said, then added, "I hope you can stay a few days. You will have a lot to take care of."

We raced to the hospital, where we found his room filled with emergency staff and machines. Egon seemed agitated and in pain, and we were asked to leave the room. As I walked the corridor feeling helpless, I found myself looking toward the sky, begging, "Stop the suffering." Soon enough we were allowed in again. He had a small oxygen mask on his mouth and nose and was breathing heavily. Alex sat on a chair, sobbing. Tatiana was caressing Egon's head and I was holding his hand when the breathing stopped. He fell silent, empty and at peace. Gently, I closed his eyes. It felt natural, an act of love, of trust, of remembrance for all we had been to each other. I felt honored and privileged to be there.

My first instinct was to protect the children. I felt like a lioness and commanded them out of the room as the nurses came in and, after confirming the death, went about gathering his belongings, covering the body, and rushing him out of the room on a gurney. I followed it down the long corridors, and found myself in no time at all in a room with a man handing me something that looked like a menu. It had photos and prices. "I need your help," I heard myself pleading to the children as they joined me in what I realized was the morgue. "We have to choose the coffin."

At first it was all about arrangements. Egon's godmother and aunt Maria Sole appeared, and together we decided on the mass the next day at Egon's favorite church, the Chiesa degli Artisti on Piazza del Popolo. I asked a friend of the family, Father Pierre Riches, to lead the funeral mass. Maria Sole's daughter, Tiziana, put the announcements in the papers. Egon wanted to be buried in Strobl, Austria, with his father and ancestors. We needed to get the papers from the embassy. Susanna Agnelli, another of Egon's aunts, had been Italy's secretary of state, so her office handled that, and Sebastian, Egon's brother, made the preparations for the funeral in Austria for Monday. It was Friday. All went so fast. Egon was right. There were many things that had to be organized.

The whole family and hundreds of friends rushed to Rome for the funeral. Tatiana and I had chosen the flowers, white lilies, his favorites, and the church service was beautiful—except for the absence of music. I had simply forgotten to arrange for any music. I did, however, arrange a drink at Egon's apartment for his friends after the service, committing apparently a major mistake by bringing the body back home after church. At sunset, a fleet of three cars with handsome, elegant drivers drove Egon to Austria.

Egon's burial was scheduled for Monday. We flew to Salzburg on Barry's plane. Ira, Egon's sister, and her son Hubertus were with us. When we got to Strobl, Egon's coffin was waiting in the library of Hubertushof, the family house on the Wolfgangsee near Salzburg. It is a huge old hunting lodge, which has been passed down from male to male in the Furstenberg line and now belongs to Alexandre. There were flowers everywhere. There, I finally had time to sit by Egon and properly say good-bye.

We had known each other since we were eighteen. We had grown up together, played together, pretended we were adults together, became parents together. Since we had met, our relationship had evolved and changed but we never stopped loving each other. Now he was gone.

I went for a walk alone in the garden, came back, sat at the desk in the library, and wrote him a letter. I had picked a very light paper so I could fold it many times into a small square and I put it on my heart under my bodysuit. Family and friends arrived, drinks and light food were served. At twelve o'clock Egon's casket was put on a carriage pulled by horses. A band accompanied us as we walked slowly from the house to the little church in the center of the village. The sun was shining on the lake.

The service was moving, with music this time, organs. Tatiana read a beautiful speech she had written, so beautiful I had it printed later as a remembrance. Then everyone walked behind the casket to the little churchyard where Egon joined his ancestors in the family graveyard. His burial marked the end of a long tradition. He was the last Furstenberg to be buried there because there is no more room in the vault. I took the letter that was still on my heart and tossed it on the casket when my turn came to throw the dirt. Egon had always loved and kept my letters to him; this one would be with him forever.

For all that it had been my idea to separate from Egon those many years before, I had felt unsettled as most women do when a meaningful relationship ends. I was only twenty-six. Jas Gawronski was in his midthirties, an Italian newsman of Polish origins who reported from New York every night on Italian television. He was very handsome, and the best friend of Egon's uncle Gianni Agnelli. My friendship and love affair with Jas gave me the assurance I craved after the separation from Egon. Our affair was secret at first. One summer, when the children were with their grandmothers, he took me to the little island of Ponza where he had a house. Every day at sunset we used to walk to the top of the mountain and along the whole island to the lighthouse. That is where I discovered the joy of hiking, and to this day, when we sail to Ponza, I always take Barry and the whole family on that same gorgeous hike.

It was Jas who was with me the first night I spent at Cloudwalk, New Year's Eve 1973, when we cooked lamb chops and drank champagne to celebrate the New Year, my new house, and a new life. It was Jas who started to prune the pine trees around the house and it was with him that I went on my first long walk there. Jas was well educated and very kind. He was married but lived apart from his wife. He did not want to commit; nor did I, really. It was a healing period, pleasant and light. My children at home and my dresses at work occupied most of my time. Jas was my personal, private garden even though he and the children did get along fine.

At work I could smell the growing success. The wrap dress was born and selling very well. I was traveling all around America and had become a household name. At home in New York, I lived with my children and my mother. I would dine with them and go out after they went to bed. I felt free and empowered; it wasn't easy managing it all and I was often under huge stress, but it was my choice and well worth it. I felt light traveling with a tiny bag full of jersey dresses and perched on my high heels. It was my turn to feel free and experiment. On a business trip to Los Angeles, I flirted with Warren Beatty and Ryan O'Neal on the same weekend. I was truly living my fantasy of having a man's life in a woman's body. Life was fun if you were young, pretty, and successful in the seventies.

And then I met Barry Diller.

I was twenty-eight when Barry exploded into my life and into our family. I had no idea that this mysterious, successful thirty-three-year-old studio head would become so important to me and my children. We were both young tycoons then: he, the very young chairman of Paramount Pictures; I, the young runaway fashion success. I had read about Barry but I had no inkling of the passion that would overtake us both after we met at a party I gave in my apartment in New York for the powerhouse Hollywood agent Sue Mengers. I remember him coming to my crowded apartment, I remember Sue introducing us, I remember his deep, authoritative voice, and I remember thinking he could be an interesting friend to have. He did not stay long but called me the next morning. He asked me out to dinner that night but when he came to pick me up, I surprised him with a dinner

I'd prepared at home. We ate, sat around briefly. We were both nervous. He left quickly.

I went to Paris the next day. He called me every day, his voice was seductive and, after a few days, he abruptly said, "Why don't you come to Los Angeles for the weekend?" Why not, I thought, intrigued and excited by his commanding tone. Adventure was calling. The flight from Paris to Los Angeles stopped in Montreal. I remember looking for a phone booth to call Jas. I told him I was flying to LA to visit someone I had just met. Looking back, I see how cruel I was, but my total need for honesty just made me do it and I felt freer once I had.

I was so excited to get to Los Angeles I don't think I needed an airplane to fly. Once over Arizona, I disappeared into the bathroom and stayed there until we were about to land. I did my hair, my makeup, changed my clothes, and arrived fresh and looking sassy in a skinny little pin-striped pantsuit with very high platform boots. Barry was at the gate. He had arranged a car for my luggage and I joined him in the yellow E-type Jaguar that he drove. It was a very glamorous welcome; I was in Hollywood and it felt like a movie. He offered me the choice of stopping for drinks at the home of his friend, the legendary producer Ray Stark, or going home. We went home.

That home turned out to be a beautiful hideaway, a California Mediterranean-style house at the end of a long driveway in Coldwater Canyon. An English butler showed me the guestroom where a colorful bouquet of flowers welcomed me. I did not need to freshen up; I was superfresh. I assume we had dinner. I don't remember. What I do remember was cuddling close to him on the living room sofa. Just as abruptly as he had commanded me to come to LA, he said, "Let's go to bed." We were both very nervous, lying frozen in his bed under the blanket. We were actually shaking. We each took a Valium and went to sleep.

The next day he went to work and I went exploring the house. What a mysterious man he was. I knew nothing of his life and I was so curious. The drawers were empty, and the books on the bookshelves did not reveal much either. What I did not know and soon found out is that he had just moved into the house and all of the furniture belonged to Paramount's props department. He came home at midday, we had lunch and hung around the pool. Sexual tension was rising. When we finally succumbed, it was major passion and from the first moment our bodies met he surrendered to me in a way that no one had ever done before. He had certainly never opened himself like that before either, he confessed to me later. Something very special and major had happened and we loved each other passionately from that moment on.

His friends were incredulous. No one had known him with a woman before. That made me feel that I was the most special woman in the world.

Barry was in my life forever after. He was to love me unconditionally, guessing my desires and needs and always impressing me with his unquestioning trust. When I went back to New York after this extraordinary weekend, our lives had changed completely. Barry divided his work and his time between LA and New York, where he lived at the Hampshire House on Central Park South. I would visit him there and he would come to me on Park Avenue. I remember the first time he came to Cloudwalk. The children had gone up the night before with the babysitter and I was to join them with Barry on Saturday. He was terribly anxious about meeting the children. He kept delaying the departure, insisting we first visit his tailor, where he ordered some suits. He kept telling me over and over that he didn't know any children. Finally, in the early afternoon, we arrived.

The minute he got there, he became totally at ease, sinking into the coziest chair by the phone in the living room, where he still sits today. Alexandre and Tatiana were as cool as they always were meeting my friends and his nervousness disappeared instantly. I remember him telling me that left alone with him in the room, four-year-old Tatiana smiled at him, and trying to figure him out, asked, "Who are your friends?" Neither of us remembers his answer but we will never forget her question.

From that moment on, he cherished weekends with us in Connecticut, as we still do decades later. One afternoon, as we were driving back to New York, we saw an old couple crossing Lexington Avenue. As Barry slowed the car down to let the couple, holding on to each other, cross the street, we both had the same thought and the same wish: One day we would be that old couple helping each other to cross the street. We both remember that image vividly although he believes it was Madison Avenue and I am sure it was Lexington.

Barry landed in our family life with a wonderful "everything is possible" attitude.

For Mother's Day, 1976, Barry bought me a tiny little speedboat so the kids could learn to water-ski on Lake Candlewood near Cloudwalk. We had a festive Fourth of July party that year. Mike Nichols came with Candice Bergen, Louis Malle came alone (they were to marry a few years later), director Miloš Forman and writer Jerzy Kosinski were there, and my closest neighbor, socialite Slim Keith, brought her houseguest, the old 1930s and '40s movie actress Claudette Colbert. "Oh, I'd love to go on your yacht," Claudette said to Barry when we told her we had spent the day on our boat. We all had a good laugh over the fact that she had imagined our small speedboat was a yacht. But Claudette must have been clairvoyant, because Barry's taste for boats never went away. The boats just got bigger and bigger.

Barry spoiled us all. He brought the children paraphernalia from his show *Happy Days,* and took us to the Dominican Republic and Disneyland. His house in Los Angeles was a favorite with its pool and his collies, Arrow and Ranger, and he invited the children to the Paramount set where they were shooting *Bad News Bears.* On New Year's Eve, for my twenty-ninth birthday, he took me to a party at Woody Allen's where he gave me twenty-nine loose diamonds in a Band-Aid box.

In March 1976 I was on the cover of *Newsweek.* The same Linda Bird Francke who had done the *New York* magazine article that had ended my marriage with Egon wrote a wonderful seven-page article on my business success. Barry was very proud. That Monday he had a photographer take photos of the magazine on all the newsstands in all the different neighborhoods of New York and made an album for me. I teased him that he left out all the foreign newsstands; my cover ran on every continent. Here we were, two young tycoons, twenty-nine and thirty-four, living a fast life on top of the world!

On the drive to Cloudwalk we often stopped at theaters along the way to study people's reactions at his sneak previews. The first preview we went to was *Won Ton Ton: The Dog Who Saved Hollywood.* Not a big hit. Thankfully, after that, Barry had many blockbusters, such as *Marathon Man, Saturday Night Fever, Grease,* and *Urban Cowboy.* I also remember how anxious he was on Sunday mornings tallying the movie numbers that were called in by his VPs of sales. The ashtray beside our bed would fill quickly as the numbers came in from around the country.

The summer of '77 we decided to take the children on a cross-country drive. We flew to Denver and started out in a rented RV with Barry at the wheel. We were hardly out of the airport and there he was, on the side of the highway, changing a flat tire. We spent four days or so in that camper, which we had named Fantasy 1. We drove from Pike's Peak to Durango in Colorado and visited Monument

Valley on our long way to Lake Powell in Utah, where we'd rented a houseboat that we named *Fantasy 2*. I was in charge of the food, Barry and Alex were in charge of getting us to the right places, and Tatiana was in charge of making the beds, but after two nights in the RV, we opted to sleep in motels along the way instead.

The houseboat had its own challenges. Barry was stressed because he was afraid that the boat would slip its mooring and go by itself over the dam and down the waterfall, so he stayed wide awake all night. As soon as I heard about the dam, I started having a fit because I thought the dam had something to do with nuclear power. I drove Barry crazy about the nuclear fears I was having while Alexandre and Tatiana amused themselves by killing flies, hundreds of which were swarming in the boat. Lake Powell is beautiful, though, and we managed to have lots of fun during the day.

The last leg of the trip was rafting down the Colorado River, but Barry gave up—driving the RV and the houseboat had worn him out—so he left and took shelter in a hotel in Las Vegas while Tatiana, Alexandre, and I ended up going down the river alone with the two boatmen, brothers, and camping out on the shore. We had a wonderful time on the river all day and sleeping under the stars at night, as I expect the boatmen did, too, with the large supply of booze they had taken along. At the end of the rafting trip, Barry picked us up by helicopter at the Grand Canyon and we all flew home exhausted, dirty, and happy.

At the end of 1977, for my thirtieth birthday, I bought myself a beautiful apartment on the twelfth floor of 1060 Fifth Avenue. It was a very large apartment that had belonged to Rodman Rockefeller and had an amazing view over the reservoir of Central Park, where every night we could watch the most extraordinary sunset. My good friend Oscar de la Renta's first wife, Françoise, helped me to decorate it in a style that was both lavish and somewhat bohemian. Huge comfortable velvet sofas, upholstered silk fuchsia walls, leopard carpet, and rose print walls for the master bedroom. Barry moved in with us and I built him his own bathroom and dressing room off our bedroom. He was in LA half the time but we all lived very happily together when he came to New York. We gave huge fun parties to celebrate the movies he produced. The children loved Barry and he loved them in return, though like any reasonable person, he cursed at them when they were naughty. Egon appreciated Barry's involvement and used to joke that the children had "two fathers."

Barry and I went out a lot when he was in New York, and I would go out alone when he was not there. Sometimes I flirted with other men or boys. It was that time in New York; we were very free. Barry did not ask questions, nor did I for that matter. Our relationship was above that. We loved being together and we loved being apart.

I had a little fling with Richard Gere, who had just finished *American Gigolo*. Hard to resist. His agent, Ed Limato, was upset with him and told him that seeing me was not a good move for his career as Paramount distributed the film. Barry never said anything but I know he was not happy. Barry was always cool, above anything and anyone. He knew it would pass.

Studio 54 had opened, and was the final stop for any evening in New York. Sometimes, when Barry was in LA, late at night I would put on my cowboy boots, take my car, park in the garage, walk into 54, meet my friends, have a drink, and dance. What I loved best was going in alone, the long entrance, the disco music. I felt like a cowboy walking into a saloon. But the idea of being able to go to 54 alone is what thrilled me the most: again, a man's life in a woman's body! It was fun. We all felt very free as we did not know yet about AIDS. I never stayed too late though. I had my children and my mother at home and had to wake up early to go to work.

I kept going back and forth to the factories in Italy and would sometimes stop in Paris on the way, to shop and act like a rich American tourist. I remember having tea in the lobby of the Plaza Athénée with my friend, the tall, flamboyant André Leon Talley, who was the *Women's Wear Daily* Paris correspondent at the time. I used to force him to pretend he was an African king.

I had become the woman I wanted to be and I absolutely loved my life. I had two beautiful, healthy children; a wildly successful fashion business; a lot of fun and a wonderful man with whom I shared so much. In 1980, Barry rented a sailboat called *Julie Mother* and he and I sailed the Caribbean. I was reading a fascinating book *The Third Wave* by the futurist writer Alvin Toffler. The book predicted that soon we would communicate through computers, that we would have ways to connect to information and in turn send that information around the world. It sounded wild, like science fiction. I was amazed, underlining paragraphs and taking a lot of notes. I remember my fountain pen had turquoise ink, the color of the sea, on which we were sailing . . . I had a feeling the world would change. It did.

The night we came back, I got the call from Hans Muller. My mother was in bad shape. He needed me to come to Switzerland immediately. I jumped on a plane. After spending a few very difficult weeks in the mental ward of the hospital taking care of my mother and watching her fight her demons, I returned to New York, but things had changed. I felt out of place in my own gilded, easy life. Barry was as loving as ever, but I felt off balance. To see my mother so bad, to relive with her the horrors of her past, took a toll on me. I had to escape the excess of my fast-moving life. I took the children and went as far away as I could: the island of Bali.

———————

"Do your work, then step back. The only path to serenity," wrote the Chinese philosopher Lao Tzu in the sixth century BC. I took that big step back in the summer of 1980 as I walked five miles along a beautiful, peaceful Balinese beach and watched the sun come up on my first day there. New York, Barry, Richard, success—I had run away from it all. That morning, at five a.m., I chanced upon Paulo, a handsome bearded Brazilian with long, curly hair who lived in a bamboo house on the beach and hadn't worn shoes in ten years. I felt so far away and my life took yet another turn. Paulo smelled delicious, a mixture of the frangipani flowers that decorated his house and cloves from the Gudam Garang cigarettes he smoked. He collected and sold textiles, spoke Bahasa Indonesia, and took me and the children to discover all the temples and mysteries of the island. At first it was a vacation affair, a way to forget the terrible weeks of my mother's illness . . . another escape. In retrospect, it should have stayed that way, but it didn't.

I was completely and absolutely infatuated with everything in Bali, including Paulo. I did not think of or wish for a future with him, but I was captivated by the adventure of the unknown. When I returned to New York, there was Barry, looking at me lovingly, searching into my eyes and my heart, being sad. He knew something had changed. I felt terrible, but my rush of emotions was overruling my reason.

My children were not happy with me when Barry moved out and Paulo joined us in New York. Nor was my mother. What was I doing? Was I really in love with that "jungle man"? Was I going to give up

Barry's unconditional love? Everyone was incredulous. I was defiant. More than being in love with Paulo, I was in love with the disruption that love can cause.

Paulo made his official appearance on the New York scene at a dinner I gave in my Fifth Avenue apartment for Diana Vreeland and her book *Allure*. He appeared barefoot, wearing a silk shirt over an ikat sarong from the island of Kupang. Eyebrows were raised, but I didn't care. In fact, I enjoyed it. I was on a mission to be provocative, and craved the adventure of it all.

Paulo was also a constant reminder of Bali, that magical island which had so inspired me with its beauty, its fabrics, and its colors. I created a whole makeup line called Sunset Goddess. I was living the fantasy of being a goddess myself and dedicated a perfume, Volcan d'Amour (Volcano of Love), to my new man. Cloudwalk was soon filled with Indonesian textiles and artifacts and I planted colorful ceremonial flags along the river that are there to this day.

Change followed change when I took the children out of school in New York, moving them permanently to Cloudwalk. I felt a sense of danger in the city. John Lennon had been killed by a deranged fan at the doorway of his building in December 1980, and I was haunted by the kidnapping of Calvin Klein's eleven-year-old daughter, Marci, for ransom. Thankfully she had been released unharmed, but my anxiety persisted. Alexandre and Tatiana were eleven and ten, too old to be taken to school and young enough to be swayed by the temptations of city life and the pseudosophistication of some of their city friends. I wanted them to connect with nature, to do without the constant activities in New York, and develop their own resources and imaginations. With some amazement, I realized there had been value to my periods of childhood boredom in Belgium.

I also made the move because of me. I was less interested in being a tycooness with a fast life than I was in being a more present mother and a more devoted partner to a man. It was a phase, but it was real. I went to New York on Tuesday mornings and was back at Cloudwalk on Thursday nights. Paulo spent his days building a new barn and the children went to Rumsey Hall, a nearby private school.

My makeover extended to my clothes. I gave up wearing my own dresses, which were then being designed by licensees anyway, and wore only sarongs, then replaced my sexy high heels with sandals in the summer and boots in the winter. I wore exotic jewelry and let my hair go very curly, often with a fresh flower in it. Paulo and I traveled back to Bali and his bamboo house on the beach whenever we could. Often the children came along.

Looking back, I smile at the ways I tailored my personality to merge with those of different men at different times in my life. I think most women consciously change their stripes or at least modify them in their relationships with men, especially during the delicious period of seduction. They become instant football lovers or sailing enthusiasts or political junkies, then taper back to their own personalities when the relationship is either cemented or over. No one I know, however, went to the lengths I did.

My relationship with Paulo lasted four years, as did my wardrobe of sarongs. "Why don't you wear real clothes?" my mother kept asking. But even she couldn't envision my next metamorphosis when I left Paulo to become the muse to a writer in Paris.

The summer of 1984, after I sold my cosmetics business to the English pharmaceutical company Beecham, I chartered a sailboat to sail around the Greek islands. The children were young teenagers, their relationship with Paulo was not good, and the mood on board was heavy and unpleasant. My close Brazilian friend Hugo Jereissati, who had first led me to discover Bali, was with us. I remember telling Hugo while we were sunbathing, "My life is going to change again." It did.

Wool skirts. Buttoned-up sweaters. Flat shoes. They would dominate my wardrobe for the next five years. Alain Elkann, an Italian novelist and journalist, didn't like the sexy clothes I had just started designing, so, yet again, I changed my stripes for love. My new image startled me every time I looked in the mirror.

I'd met Alain in New York at a fourteenth-birthday party Bianca Jagger was giving for her daughter, my goddaughter Jade. Tatiana and Alex were both home from boarding school, she from England and he from Massachusetts, and we were all in New York that weekend.

Alain was very attractive and we knew a lot of people in common as he had been married to Margherita Agnelli, Egon's first cousin. "Come with me to Paris," Alain said soon after we met. I didn't hesitate. The children were away at school and I couldn't bear another day in New York. Just as I had found Paulo during my introspection after my mother's collapse, I found Alain in 1984 during my disenchantment with New York. Life in New York had become all about money—*Dynasty* and *Dallas* were the hits on television—and after four years cloistered at Cloudwalk with Paulo, Paris intellectual life was very appealing to me. My work wasn't really interesting anymore. Though I was working on starting a new business, my heart wasn't really in it.

What was in my heart was Alain. And Paris. Paulo was very angry and moved to his native Brazil; I moved to a beautiful apartment I rented on rue de Seine between a courtyard and a garden. My friend François Catroux, an interior decorator, helped me to set up a chic and bohemian interior filled with Empire furniture and the pre-Raphaelite paintings from my recently sold Fifth Avenue apartment.

Alain and I entertained a lot: writers, artists, and designers, even though fashion was no longer my priority. Alain had a day job at Mondadori, the publishing house, and wrote novels after work. My all-time favorite writer, Alberto Moravia, stayed with us for weeks at a time. He would write in the morning, and in the afternoons he and I would go to museums, movies, or to Café de Flore for hot chocolate. I could not believe we had become such close friends.

In my new Parisian life I rediscovered my first love, literature, and was living yet another fantasy—having a literary salon and founding a small publishing house, Salvy, where we published in French the great writers Vita Sackville-West, Gregor von Rezzori, and Bret Easton Ellis, among others.

Alain and I also had a lively, loving family life during holidays. He had three children with Margherita Agnelli: John ("Jaki"), Lapo, and Ginevra. Maybe because they were related to my own children, we immediately became a family. We only had the five children on vacations and occasional weekends, but took full advantage of the time. We skied together in Gstaad, swam in Capri where Alain and I rented a small apartment, and sailed up the Nile to discover ancient Egypt. The rest of the time I was with Alain, the perfect writer's muse, listening to his writings and following his many moods. I ran a perfect intellectual stylish home, with abundant food and fresh flowers at all times. I had long known that writers may live the bohemian life, but they love luxury. I set up a small office on the attic floor and talked to my very reduced New York office daily.

For all that I loved my life in Paris, being with Alain was sometimes difficult. Though I shared his life and interests entirely, he did not share mine. In 1986, I was one of eighty-seven immigrants chosen to receive a Mayor's Liberty Award for my contribution to the city of New York and the United States. I was very proud and wanted to go to New York for the ceremony and receive my award from Mayor Ed Koch, but Alain did not want me to go, so I didn't. My mother went for me.

Looking back, I realize how many things I let go for my relationship with Alain. He wanted me to give up my personality and my success and I actually did it with enthusiasm. No one had ever asked me that before. I traded my passion for independence to be "the woman of." My children were astonished. "Mommy has zero personality," they used to say, and I smiled. I knew deep down it wasn't really true, but I was seduced by the role I was embracing of the devoted artist's woman.

All probably would have continued except I came to realize that Alain was having an affair with my good friend Loulou de la Falaise, muse of Yves Saint Laurent. Loulou was all the things I had given up: glamour, work, success. I was shocked, very sad, and upset at first, but I grew to understand on some level that it was, at least partially, my fault. By altering my personality, I had lost what had attracted Alain to me in the first place. I had become the docile, passive person I thought he wanted only to have him stray toward the same sort of person I had been. I am not one to accept humiliation, however, and instead, I turned the betrayal into a determination to win. By staying cool when I confronted them and exposed the affair, I trusted my calm attitude would diminish the lure of the "forbidden fruit" and eventually destroy it. I was right. The affair soon lost its appeal and ended. Alain and I stayed together a bit more, but I knew it would soon be time to move on.

In retrospect, I would not give up those years in Paris with Alain or the years with Paulo in and out of Bali for anything in the world. No one goes through life with one rigid personality. We are far more complex with various needs and desires that present themselves at different stages of our lives. Because I worked for and achieved financial independence so early in life, I had the unusual luxury of fully living those fantasies, and also having the ability to leave them when the time was right.

Paulo gave me the serenity I needed to heal from my mother's collapse and a refuge from the frenetic pace of my life in New York. Alain gave me my return to Europe and the world of culture and ideas I craved after closeting myself at Cloudwalk. Alain also gave me three wonderful stepchildren whom I love and have stayed close to. Jaki is now the respected John Elkann who runs Fiat motor company and its subsidiaries, Lapo is a very successful designer and a marketing genius, and Ginevra is a princess, mother of three, film producer, and president of Pinacoteca Giovanni e Marella Agnelli. All three are siblings to Alex and Tatiana and we are a family.

I've often asked myself what sort of woman I'd be today if I hadn't experimented with such greatly different lifestyles with Paulo and Alain. Would I have been ready all those years ago to stay with Barry? Part of me wishes I had instead of hurting him and losing the years we could have spent together. But another part of me is glad. I'm probably a better wife and partner to Barry now because of it. I needed to try on different versions of myself to see which one fit me best. And after Alain I still wasn't through.

My personal life was in limbo when I left Paris in 1989 and returned to New York. As usual, Barry was there to listen to me and reassure me, but to some degree we had lost each other and I did not want to hurt him again. I had to find myself first and that was not easy. I divided my time between Cloudwalk, the Carlyle Hotel in New York where I took an apartment, and the Bahamas where I helped my mother to settle into her little white house with blue shutters on the pink sand beach of Harbour Island.

I also renewed old friendships, and had some flirtations, but I really was not happy with myself. As much as I loved Barry's company—we went everywhere together—I still wasn't ready to commit. One of the reasons was that I had started a secret relationship with a handsome, mysterious, talented man, the only man who would, in the end, leave me.

I didn't mean to fall in love with Mark Peploe, nor he, I'm sure, with me. Mark had been a friend for a long time and had written the screenplay for Bernardo Bertolucci's *The Last Emperor* in the guest room when I lived with Alain in Paris. (It won nine Academy Awards in 1988, including Best Adapted Screenplay.) Mark also was "taken"—he lived with a woman I knew and their twelve-year-old daughter in London. It never occurred to me to have an affair with him until he called me one day in New York after I'd returned from Paris—and sparks flew.

It was the stuff of fantasy. Literally. When I was a young girl, I used to write poetry and short stories about love and always thought that stolen moments, the untold, the unasked, the secrecy, defined the most exciting and romantic relationships. And our affair was exactly that. Mark and I had a great relationship; I respected his intellect, he was one of the most handsome men I'd ever met, and he was a great traveling companion. Soon after our affair began he asked me to join him in Sri Lanka where he was scouting sites for *Victory,* a movie he was going to direct. I barely knew where Sri Lanka was, or that it was the new name for Ceylon. I immediately booked a flight.

I will never forget driving around the island of Serendib, the magical island that gave us the word "serendipity," with Mark, discovering the rubber and tea plantations, the reclining Buddha, the house of the author Paul Bowles, and the streets of Colombo. We were so far from everything. I was in awe of this elegant, handsome man who knew so much . . . our conversations were endless. They continued in all different landscapes—the streets and cafés of Paris, the trattorias of Rome, the streets of Lisbon, the souks and the harem of Topkapi in Istanbul, the Byzantine caves of Cappadocia, the Sufi mosque of Konya, the Vermillion Cliffs in Utah, and in discovering the artist Mantegna in Mantova. All through these landscapes, we talked and talked about everything. When traveling by car, I would read aloud the traveling adventures of the Polish journalist Ryszard Kapuscinski, or the passions of the Austrian writer Stefan Zweig. Those were our stolen moments, stolen from our everyday lives in anonymous hotels, airports, and rented cars.

Barry knew about Mark and Mark knew about Barry, although I avoided talking much about one to the other. I now realize that Barry was already like my husband and Mark was my secret lover. I could not give up one for the other. I must have been cruel to both, but I did not think I was at the time. Barry was waiting patiently, secure of the outcome. What was really in Mark's mind, I never knew. I loved our "unspoken relationship," and wanted it to go on and on, but it didn't.

I felt great pain when Mark left me for yet another woman, not the mother of his child. I thought he enjoyed the fantasy of our secret relationship as much as I did, but perhaps he'd wanted a more permanent and visible relationship. He never explained, I never asked.

In retrospect, I know that Barry's existence and my feelings for him had everything to do with my reluctance to commit fully to Mark,

Alain, or Paulo. After Mark and I parted, Barry began taking up more and more space in my life, in my bed, and in my heart, and we found a new serenity.

Sailing the oceans, we found a way to design our lives together. Barry had had a love affair with boats ever since I'd taken him with me on *Atlantis,* the elder Stavros Niarchos's sublime yacht, when the children were very small and spending the summer with Egon. That time we'd cruised the Amalfi Coast all the way to Greece. It was a revelation for Barry, the beginning of a dream to one day build his own yacht. We took many wonderful trips after that on chartered boats to the Mediterranean, the Caribbean, the Ionian Coast. I had always loved to travel to adventurous places, he needed his luxury and to be connected to his work. On those sailing trips we could do both ... go on adventurous inland hikes, visit small villages, and yet come back to our floating comfort and communications at night.

We had always talked about our future over the years and we both knew we would end up together. I loved Barry and knew he was absolutely the only one I could marry, but I fought the notion of marriage itself. People often refer to it as "settling down," and the words are so uninspiring to me. "Settle down" sounds like giving up your spontaneity and independence and that was not what I, or Barry for that matter, were about.

I began to soften when he started talking about marriage out of concern for the children. He wanted to be able to provide for them, he said, and marriage would make it much easier. When Alexandre married Alexandra Miller in 1995 (thus becoming Alex and Alex), Barry gave him a jar of earth as a wedding present to represent a sum of money for the down payment on a house. He was so sincere about caring for my children, I was moved.

My journals in 1999 tracked various family milestones. The birth of Talita, my first grandchild, was, of course, a major milestone. Another was that Tatiana was pregnant. She had wanted a baby so badly that when we went together to visit little Talita, she had gone outside and cried in a phone booth fearing she would never have one. The very next day she met Russell Steinberg, a loving, life-happy comedian. Antonia Steinberg was born one year and twenty-two days after Talita's birth, the exact same length of time between Tatiana and Alexandre. My diary notes another milestone: I finally paid off my mortgage on Cloudwalk. The last entry was not yet a milestone: "Talking marriage with Barry," I wrote.

It didn't happen in 1999. It didn't happen in 2000, but Barry did not give up hope. "Today, for my birthday Barry gave me a pearl ring that belonged to Marie Bonaparte and a card with a wish to marry," I wrote in my journal. Another entry was sad. "Lily not well," I noted, as my mother's health continued to slip away. Alexandre was in Australia, but the rest of the family, including my brother, Philippe, all gathered at her house in Harbour Island for Easter. Remarkably, she managed to hang on and pull together what strength she had left to fly with me to Los Angeles to be there with Tatiana for the birth of baby Antonia. It was during that flight that I told her I was thinking of maybe marrying Barry, to which she gloriously replied: "He deserves you."

How I loved my mother for saying that! She did not say I deserved him, she said he deserved me. In those three words was everything—how she valued me, the person I had become, and how she valued him for deserving me. I will never forget that. Not only had she given me her approval for marrying Barry, she was telling me how proud she was of me. She died a few weeks later.

I needed another approval—Egon's. I called him and said I was considering marrying Barry. "I want your blessing," I said to him. "You have it, but keep my name," he answered, laughing.

A week before Barry's fifty-ninth birthday, as I was looking for a present to give him, I decided to give him myself. "Why don't we get married on your birthday?" I casually said over the phone. "Let me see if I can arrange it," he answered with no hesitation. "Let me see if I can arrange it" is something he'd taken on from the minute we met . . . and always delivered. Sure enough, he arranged for us to marry at City Hall a week later.

I called the children, I called my brother in Belgium, and I called my friend, the world-famous portrait photographer Annie Leibovitz, to ask her if she could come and take the photos. Philippe flew into New York with his wife, Greta, and daughters, Kelly and Sarah. Tatiana flew in from Los Angeles with Russell and little eight-month-old Antonia strapped to his chest in a baby carrier. Alexandre and his pregnant wife, Alexandra, and twenty-month-old Talita were already in New York. We all met up the morning of the wedding in my design studio, a carriage house on West Twelfth Street, before going down to City Hall. I hadn't thought about flowers but happened to have met a florist a few nights before who offered to make me a wedding bouquet. I chose lilies of the valley to honor my mother. I made myself a cream jersey dress. I did not feel particularly pretty that day, but I was so happy.

As we left the studio, the DVF girls were screaming good wishes. We were met at City Hall by Annie Leibovitz, who, with great generosity, had answered my call and agreed to act as paparazzi. There were, of course, also real paparazzi, but they were not allowed to come with us into City Hall. We were all laughing, my little family and I. It all felt perfectly natural. Barry had arranged a lunch at some obscure restaurant near City Hall. The restaurant was a bit stiff and gloomy, so we did not stay long, but laughed the whole time, though we all missed my mother.

Long before we decided to marry that day, I had planned a big Aquarius party for that night at the studio on Twelfth Street because my three loves, Barry, Tatiana, and Alex, were all born under the sign of Aquarius. The hundreds of friends who joined us for that Aquarius party were startled and overjoyed to discover that it had turned into a wedding celebration! As a present, Barry gave me twenty-six wedding bands with diamonds . . . "Why twenty-six?" I asked. "For the twenty-six years we were not married," he answered.

It took me a while to accept that we were married. When I drove out to the country the next day I saw that someone had put a sign in my car that said "Just Married." I stopped in the middle of the road and turned it over. There was still that rebelliousness in me, and yet when I got to Cloudwalk I was so happy to see Barry already there waiting for me. It was not until quite recently that I actually started referring to Barry as "my husband," but now I do, and I do it with pride and much love. We so love being together. What we like best is to be quiet and alone. We are definitely soul mates and I am forever thankful to Sue Mengers for introducing me to this glamorous young tycoon thirty-nine years ago and to have seduced him forever.

How can I explain my relationship with Barry? The fullness of it all? It is simply true love. His openness to me, his unconditional acceptance, his deep desire for my happiness and that of the children brings tears to my eyes to think about. Barry has a reputation for being tough, yet he is the gentlest, most loving person I have ever met. We have been in each other's lives for decades, as lovers, as friends, and now as husband and wife. It is true that, as I did with my father, I took his love for granted. It is true that, as I did to my father, I sometimes rejected him. But it is also true, as it was with my father, that I love him totally and am there for him unconditionally. Love is life is love is Barry.

We spend at least three months a year on *Eos*, the dream boat Barry finally built. Named for the Greek goddess of dawn, *Eos* took more than three years to build, three years during which Barry spent at least two hours a day going over every detail, talking to the engineers, talking to the construction people in Germany, involving himself in the outside design, inside decoration, and every detail of everything on board. Launched in 2006, *Eos* is the most wonderfully comfortable yacht you can imagine, with a dream crew that creates extraordinary itineraries and always finds the best places for us to hike, and a young, talented chef, Jane Coxwell, who I encouraged to write a cookbook that all of my friends love.

We asked our friend, the artist Anh Duong, to do a sculpture for the figurehead of the boat and she asked me to pose for it. So, there I am in front of *Eos*, sailing the world, literally. With *Eos*, we've been to the Mediterranean and the Red Sea, to Egypt and Jordan. We've been to Oman, the Maldives and Borneo, Thailand and Vietnam. We've spent weeks in Indonesia and discovered the Pacific islands of Vanuatu, Fiji, and Papua New Guinea. Every morning we take a long swim in a new sea, and every afternoon we hike a new path. We have traveled thousands and thousands of miles this way. And we still keep going, exploring new horizons with our dog, Shannon. I take hundreds of pictures that I download at night on my computer. It is bliss to be on *Eos*, our floating home.

Traveling the world with the children and the grandchildren is our happiest time: holidays on the sea, the Galapagos or Tahiti, or on land on safari in Africa or skiing. Sometimes we only take the grandchildren. We forget they are grandchildren and we think they are our children. Years have passed and yet it feels the same as our first trip to Colorado and Lake Powell.

The most important thing Barry and I have in common is that we are both self-reliant. The presence in each other's lives was never a necessity, and therefore always felt like a huge luxury. Barry's generosity warmed me from the minute I met him and that feeling continues to evolve. He is generous with his heart, with his protection, with everything. "We," to us, is home, cozy and reassuring. Our love is our home. We are slowly becoming the old couple that crossed Lexington Avenue, guarding each other. "We" is also our family: the children aging, the grandchildren growing—Love is life is love is life.

Recently, as Barry was remodeling our house in Beverly Hills, he sent me this note:

"I'm in the plane after meeting at the house with the construction team. The house is going to be uniquely dazzling. We're going to have a slate roof and all glass bronze doors and we made your mezzanine room with full glass skylights, and glass sides—a little tree house garden in the sky.

"Hopefully, we'll add another place to grow old gloriously and glamorously. And in the meantime I'm so proud of what you accomplish every day in building your brand and your legacy . . .

"I love you, my honey."

And I love you, Barry.

3

BEAUTY

I am at a birthday party in Brussels for my best friend, Mireille, who is turning ten. As if it were yesterday, I remember us children around the dining room table at her elegant Avenue Louise apartment. The large, fancy cake is about to appear when we hear the hurried click click of a woman's heels in the hallway. Mireille's mother makes her entrance, dressed smartly in a pin-striped suit, her narrow skirt forcing her to take small steps, her makeup and auburn hair perfectly arranged. She is so glamorous and in charge. *"Joyeux anniversaire, ma chérie*—happy birthday, darling," she says to Mireille, kissing her on both cheeks while adjusting her hair. She blows kisses to all of us. The heart-shaped cake is brought in and she watches Mireille blow out the candles, directs the cake cutting, has a piece herself for good luck, talks briefly to each of us, admires our presents, and then, as we go back to Mireille's room to play, she click clicks back down the hall and out the front door.

I am awed. Though it may have been upsetting to Mireille to have her mother be too busy in her life outside the home to spend but the barest time inside, even for her daughter's birthday party, I am filled with wonderment at this glamorous, confident, engaged woman. I know vaguely that Mireille's mother, Tinou Dutry, is a leading businesswoman in Brussels. What I am totally sure of is that I want to be like her when I grow up. Decades later, I realize that my best friend's mother, a proud pioneer who created Belgium's organization for women entrepreneurs and who had been a resistance fighter during the war, was one of my early inspirations for the woman I wanted to be.

I felt the same admiration watching my mother get dressed to go out, whether at night to a party with my father, or by herself during the day. She took great care in what she wore, and her outfit was often punctuated by a hat. Her hair, her makeup, her perfume . . . she looked at herself in the mirror with a smile of complicity and confidence. She had a great figure and wore very tight skirts and dresses. Her heels clicked, too. Where is she going? I wondered. How does she know how to put herself together so well and always look so chic? I couldn't get enough of it, watching all the shine, the allure, the glamour that was my mother. She, too, was the woman I hoped to be.

I did not like my reflection in my mother's mirror. I saw a square, pale face. Brown eyes. And short brown, very, very, very densely curled hair made even more so by the humidity and incessant rain in Brussels. Almost all the girls in my class, including Mireille, had straight, blond hair, which they could have cut with big straight bangs. Not me. I felt alien. I looked like someone who'd snuck out of the forest. No one else looked like that.

I obsessed over my curly hair, which even my skillful mother couldn't deal with. When I returned from two weeks at a summer camp, she got frustrated spending the longest time untangling my hair. She finally succeeded in pulling it into a neat ponytail, braided it, and asked me for my hair clip. I had lost it at camp. After all her effort she got so irritated that she took a pair of scissors and cut the ponytail off. This did not improve what I saw in the mirror. I was miserable and full of shame.

What I did not know until I was told quite recently was that one boy in my kindergarten class loved me *because* of my hair. He, in fact, so adored my brown curls and my brown eyes that he asked me to marry him—and I evidently accepted! How embarrassing to have forgotten my five-year-old first husband, but I had until a few years ago, when I was invited to Belgium to speak to a group of businesswomen. After my talk, which included my childhood and probably a mention of my frustrations with my loathsome hair, Bea Ercolini, the editor of the Belgian edition of *Elle* magazine, asked me what school I had gone to, what years, et cetera, and then she connected the dots. "I think I live with the man you 'married' in kindergarten," she told me, smiling.

"What is the name of this gentleman?" I asked skeptically. "Didier van Bruyssel," she answered. Suddenly, it all started to come back to me. Some of it, anyway. I didn't remember Didier specifically, but I did remember the sound of his name and how, as a child, I had carefully practiced writing my signature with our combined names, Diane van Bruyssel, over and over. I was astonished that Bea had figured out that I was the little girl her partner had told her about. It showed how much she loved him, how carefully she had listened to his childhood stories. It also showed what an unexpected impact I had had on this five-year-old boy in kindergarten.

The point of all this is not to document my first seduction, but how wrong I was to be sad about not having straight blond hair. While I had been desperate to look the same as the other girls, Didier loved me because I was different. When finally we met after five decades, he told me that he had had no idea that "la petite Diane" with the curly hair had become Diane von Furstenberg, but as a little girl I had such an impact on him that he'd continued to look for Mediterranean-looking women with wavy hair. While I'd thought I was such an odd duck, he personified the familiar idiom "Beauty is in the eye of the beholder."

I wrestled with my curls for years and years, watching the weather and seeing humidity as the enemy, wearing scarves, falls, and straightening my hair with all kinds of tools. I ironed it on an ironing board at times, and had it blown out by hairdressers all over the world, convinced that straight hair was the key to beauty and happiness.

It was not until I was almost thirty that I discovered my curls could be an asset. The realization came about after my friend Ara Gallant, a very talented makeup artist/hair stylist turned photographer, was hired to photograph me for the cover of *Interview* in March 1976. Ara was a creature of the night, so it was no surprise that we shot in a studio well after midnight. Ara knew how to make anyone look sexy. He took scissors and made jagged cuts in the black bodysuit I was wearing. After shooting a few rolls, he started to spray my long and very straight hair with water. I was horrified! "Don't worry," he said. "We already have the cover, but I want to photograph you with wet hair." He shot me as my hair was drying into its true curls. A few days later, when I saw the two options for the cover, there was no question as to which one was better . . . The next day I let my hair dry naturally and it was the first time I wore my curls with pride and enjoyed being me. My "new" look was confirmed at a birthday party at Studio 54 for Mick Jagger's then wife, Bianca, who rode around the stage on a white horse at midnight as we all sang happy birthday. "You look like Hedy

Lamarr," the dashing designer Halston told me, referring to a movie star of the 1930s. I was not sure at the time who Hedy Lamarr was, but I knew it was a compliment. My curly hair had become an asset. I felt confident and free.

That confidence didn't stay with me all the time. My hair became a barometer for my self-esteem, and in the early nineties I started to straighten my hair again. Those were not great years. I was yet again in search of myself and was a bit insecure. As I regained confidence, I let the curls come back. I learned how to master them, how to use them and let them be a part of the true me. I even started to welcome humidity because it adds so much volume to curly hair.

It might seem trivial to give that much importance to hair, but I know all women with curls will identify with this struggle. So will some curly-haired men, I recently discovered. During a vacation last year on the boat of a friend, entertainment mogul David Geffen, I was having a conversation about hair with the women on board when Bruce Springsteen the macho, superhero rock star chimed in. He, too, used to hate his Italian curls when he was fifteen and starting out, he confessed, and so did his teenage band mates, The Castiles. They all wished they could switch their Mediterranean curls for straight bangs like the Beatles. So, at night, they would go secretly to a beauty parlor for black women in Freehold, New Jersey, to have their hair straightened! Bruce said he would also sneak into his mother's bathroom, steal some of her long hair pins, comb his hair all on one side, anchor it with the pins, and sleep on that same side to keep it flattened and straight. However, he never managed to achieve the cherubic, pageboy style of John, Paul, George, and Ringo.

My mother had no patience with my dissatisfaction with my appearance and my obsession with my hair. She dressed me in nice clothes and made sure I was always presentable, but beauty was not a worthwhile subject of conversation. She was much more interested in teaching me literature, history, and most of all, to be independent. Indeed, not considering myself beautiful as a young girl turned out to be a plus. Yes, I envied the blond, straight-haired girls, especially Mireille, who was striking to more than just me and would go on, at age seventeen, to marry Prince Christian von Hanover, twenty-seven years her senior. But being too beautiful as a child, I realized as I grew older, can be a curse. Counting too much on your appearance limits one's growth. Looks are fleeting and cannot be your only asset.

Early on I decided that if I could not be a pretty blonde like the other girls, I would accept being different, develop my own personality, and become popular by being funny and daring. I made lots of friends in boarding school as I did later in Geneva, where I lived with my mother and Hans Muller. I was considered "the fun girl," always ready to go and do anything, and people sought me out for that, including Egon, who arrived in Geneva a year after I did. Looking at pictures of those years, I realize that I did have a slim and agile body, long legs, good skin and was, in fact, quite pretty, but I didn't feel it, so my priority was developing a personality.

Though I believed personality, authenticity, and charm were what made a person attractive, along the way I did have many moments of awkwardness and insecurity. I remember my first visit to the Agnellis' house in Cortina d'Ampezzo over the Christmas holidays when I was turning twenty. The Agnellis were the leading family in Cortina and Egon and his younger brother, Sebastian, were the hottest, most eligible boys in the Alpine town. On my last night there, we went to a party where, to my great surprise, I was voted Lady Cortina. Although elegant enough in a lamé dress in rainbow colors, I remember feeling embarrassed and inadequate as I accepted my beauty award. Clearly it was not for my looks, but because I was Egon's girlfriend. They placed a silly rhinestone tiara on top of the hairpiece that was giving my straightened hair more volume and draped me with a Lady Cortina band. I felt foolish and that was visible in my photo on the front page of the local paper the next morning.

I was better prepared the next year when once again I arrived in Cortina on Egon's arm. By then I had lost some of the baby fat on my face, was a bit more polished, and much more at ease with Egon's Italian aristocratic friends. My transformation did not go unnoticed. Years later, Mimmo, a close friend of Sebastian and the son of Angelo Ferretti, my future mentor, reminded me how I'd gone from looking pudgy and awkward one year to looking beautiful and sexy the next. The pictures of those two holidays prove that confidence and ease can make the same person look quite different.

Egon was my guide and my Pygmalion in his world of beautiful, sophisticated people, all of whom seemed to live magical lives drifting from the Alps in the winter to the South of France in the summer and going to party after party in between.

I will never forget the costume ball he took me to in Venice given by Countess Marina Cicogna during the film festival. That weekend was a crash course in glamour. Marina Cicogna was a very successful producer of Italian cinema at the time, working with directors like Fellini, Pasolini, and Antonioni. There were many movie stars at the party: Liz Taylor and Richard Burton; Jane Fonda and Roger Vadim; Audrey Hepburn and her Italian husband, Andrea Dotti; Catherine Deneuve and David Bailey; the gorgeous model Capucine, who had been in *The Return of the Pink Panther*; and the young actor Helmut Berger with director Lucchino Visconti. I remember meeting

Gualtiero Jacopetti, the director of the very provocative new genre documentary, *Mondo Cane*. Gualtiero was a lot older, but very handsome and seductive. We talked all night and I felt beautiful because he paid me so much attention. I was to find out later that he specialized in courting young girls.

I was barely twenty, and only beginning to feel comfortable in Egon's world. I did not smile as easily as he did and he reprimanded me for appearing cold and detached. Slowly, as I felt more comfortable, I warmed up and began to stand on my own. For that party, the most glamorous, fun party I've ever been to, I dressed like a page boy in black midknee velvet pants and a matching jacket with white satin lapels, inspired by Yves Saint Laurent who had just created the tuxedo for women. Mine was definitely not a Saint Laurent; I don't remember where I found the jacket, but I'd had the pants made to my specifications. I wore black tights and thick-heeled shoes with rhinestones. I felt very stylish.

Egon's cousins, the counts Brandolini, and all their aristocratic friends dressed as hippies, all of that being new and daring in a Venetian palace. We danced all night, ate spaghetti at dawn, and watched the sun come up from the cafés of Piazza San Marco holding our shoes in our hands. The next day, the crowd met at the Lido, under the elegant striped cabanas where the parade of gorgeous women in beach attire spent the day under the critical scrutiny of the powerful doyenne of Venice, the Countess Lily Volpi. Exotic Brazilian star Florinda Bolkan and Yul Brynner's beautiful wife, Doris, were there along with all the other beauties, an endless inventory of what appeared to be effortless elegance and class. I was new to the scene and in awe of so much glamour, style, and allure. I wanted to be one of these stylish women in their thirties and could not wait to get older. I wanted to become one of those women across the room who look so poised and seductive.

I am always asked who the women are whose beauty and style inspired me. My favorite compliment as a young girl was being told that I looked like the French actress Anouk Aimée. Sophisticated, incredibly seductive with a deep sexy voice, always playing with her hair and crossing and uncrossing her legs, she was who I wanted to be. Her most famous movie, *Un homme et une femme* (*A Man and a Woman*) had a big impact on me. Anouk and I later became friends. She and I felt enormous simpatico and I often call her when I go to Paris. She lives in Montmartre with her many dogs and cats, the voice on her answering machine is as sexy as ever, and she has many admirers. Once a femme fatale, always a femme fatale!

The epitome of femme fatale will always be Marlene Dietrich, the most glamorous woman of all time. She had the best legs, an extraordinary voice, and a personal style and elegance as no one else. Her strength, courage, and independence were imposing. I never met her but so wished I had especially after I read her memoir, *Nehmt nur mein Leben* (*Just Take My Life*). She had been very brave during World War II, turning her back on the entreaties of the Nazi government in her native Germany and instead promoting US War Bonds and entertaining the Allied troops on the front lines in Algeria, Italy, France, and England. She laughed, sang, drank, cooked, cared little for convention, and had sexual liaisons with men and women into her seventies. She was a free spirit and an inspiration to me. I did try to channel her a few times, especially the two occasions I posed for Horst, the photographer who had captured and immortalized her beauty so many times.

As much as I was drawn to Dietrich's toughness, I've always found Marilyn Monroe's vulnerability touching and her beauty irresistible. She never manifested strength and independence so I did not want to be like her, but her appearance was so desirable and genuine. I was just a young teenager in 1962 when she died of a drug overdose. I have collected portraits of Marilyn ever since.

Jackie Kennedy Onassis inspired me with her elegance, her beauty, and her incredible style. Style has so much to do with the way one handles oneself and I always admired Jackie's dignity at all moments of her tragic life. She never acted as a victim and always looked impeccable, even with bloodstains on the pink wool suit she refused to change out of the day her husband was killed. I was at boarding school in England then, and my mother had come to visit for the weekend. We watched the tragedy unfold on TV, sitting on our bed at the Hilton Hotel in London.

I remember meeting Jackie when Egon and I had dinner with her and her then husband, Greek tycoon Aristotle Onassis, at El Morocco in New York. She was as charming as he was rough. I hated the way he belittled her but I liked her enormously. I loved it when later, after he died, Jackie decided to have a private, ordinary life for herself and her kids in New York. She became an editor at the publishing house Doubleday. I remember the paparazzi photos of her walking the New York streets in her camel-colored pants and a sweater, with her trademark large, incognito sunglasses.

We lived one block from each other on Fifth Avenue where we were each raising two children on our own, a boy and a girl, although mine were much younger. My perfume Tatiana was her favorite. Later, one of her granddaughters would be named Tatiana. We shared the same hairdresser, Edgar. I identified with her in many ways, including our respective battles with cancer. Of all the women I admire, Jacqueline Bouvier Kennedy Onassis will truly remain the model of style, beauty, and courage.

Angelina Jolie is another woman I find both ravishing and interesting. I was attracted first by her free spirit and her unconventional life. I thought her desire to create a large family, adopting children from all sides of the world, was commendable. But it was when I saw the movie she wrote and directed about Bosnia, *In the Land of Blood and Honey*, that I began to truly admire her. I went to see the film on a rainy afternoon in Paris. Sitting by me were two Bosnian women, weeping. Angelina is continuing to address the huge issue of sexual violence in conflict and brought great attention to the cause. What makes Angelina uniquely beautiful is her substance and her wanting to give voice to those who have none.

Madonna was not what you would call a striking beauty when she appeared at a party in my apartment in the early eighties. She was nineteen years old and hiding under a huge dark felt hat. The only person who noticed her that night was my mother, with whom she talked for hours. What Madonna did have was personality, courage, ambition, and talent. She knew who she wanted to be. Her passion, her hard work, her constant desire to learn and improve, turned her into a great beauty, a superwoman, superstar, and role model, breaking boundaries and appealing to many generations. Madonna's personality created Madonna.

I had hoped to meet Mother Teresa in the 1970s when she came to New York and visited with Mayor Ed Koch. I found her strikingly beautiful and elegant in her white-and-blue-striped robe, full of humility, strength, love, and compassion. I was told she also had a lively sense of humor.

Another woman who personifies beauty, strength, and dignity is Oprah Winfrey. Oprah is simply the most formidable woman I've ever met. As a little girl, she knew she wanted a special life, so she defeated the huge obstacles she faced, worked incredibly hard, and became one of the world's most influential women. Oprah is bigger than life; she is life, all the good and purity of it. The strength of her desire to improve the world is a true example of beauty. I love her, respect her, and admire her, and feel so privileged to call her my friend.

I have been in awe of Gloria Steinem, who led the women's movement and improved our lives forever, since the moment I met her. Feminist and feminine, doer and dreamer, graceful, strong, and beautiful, her impact on the lives of all women is immeasurable. It is because of Gloria that I gave up using the title of princess and opted for Ms. It felt more glamorous at the time. Ms. meant freedom.

Character. Intelligence. Strength. Style. That makes beauty. All these attributes form beauty, and personality, that elusive state of being that is not necessarily perfect. "Beauty is perfect in its imperfections." It is our imperfections that make us different. Personality, not traditional beauty, is always what I've looked for in my models.

I was at a party in New York in 1970 when I saw this amazing-looking girl who was part of the court of Andy Warhol. She was very, very pale with an unusual face that looked like a mixture of Greta Garbo and a moonchild. She'd plucked off the ends of each of her eyebrows, which gave her a startled, almost comic expression—some said she looked like an exotic bug. She was about five foot six or so and weighed less than a hundred pounds—and looked different from everyone else.

I had just taken a showroom, my first, at the Gotham Hotel in New York for fashion week in April 1971 when I approached this seventeen-year-old. "Would you be interested in modeling my clothes to show buyers for a week?" I asked. "Sure," she said. And so Jane Forth became my first of many, many models.

I didn't know that I'd started a pattern that continues to this day: finding interesting-looking girls with personality at the very beginning of their lives and careers, girls I noticed because they were different. I'd found Jane just before she became famous—two months after fashion week, *Life* magazine did a four-page color spread of her titled "Just Plain Jane" that described her as "a new now face in the awesome tradition of Twiggy and Penelope Tree" and she starred in Andy's film *L'Amour*, which he wrote for her. I cannot claim that I discovered Jane or any of the other models who have worked for me over the years, but I do notice them very early on.

The models I hired for my second fashion show at the Pierre Hotel all became stars, as did the dress I was introducing for the first time—the wrap dress. The legends were born on an April afternoon, their names a future Who's Who of superstar models—Jerry Hall, Pat Cleveland, Apollonia. They also became my friends.

Apollonia was skinny, skinny, and tall as a beanstalk when she appeared for a go-see for the show. I'd never seen anyone so narrow and with such long legs. On top of that long body was a tiny head with a smiley, naughty face, and she spoke with a very strong Dutch accent (her last name was van Ravenstein). I liked her immediately. She had an amazing personality, kind and very funny and we became good friends. She worked for me many times on her way to becoming a top model in the seventies.

Pat Cleveland was a striking model, too, already well known by the time I started. She was a favorite of Stephen Burrows and Halston, the queen of the Halstonettes. Part black, part Cherokee, part Irish, Pat was unique and wonderfully flamboyant. She danced down the runway, moving her arms, her legs, and her derriere, living the clothes, embracing the music and taking the audience with her like a snake charmer. Pat also loved to sing, or was it lip-synching? I don't remember. What I do remember is that I always thought she was meant to play Josephine Baker, the spectacular black American performer who left America in the 1920s to establish herself as a megastar in France. Like Josephine, Pat was a real woman, bubbling with personality, and they looked very much alike. I tried to convince Barry to make a movie of Josephine Baker's life starring Pat, but it never went any further than my imagination.

At the same time I met Apollonia and Pat, Jerry Hall appeared on the New York scene and I used her as well for the show that launched the wrap dress. She, too, was very tall and very narrow; her six-foot frame seemed to be all legs. Jerry had huge blue eyes, flawless skin, and a cascade of long golden hair that she threw to one side like Rita Hayworth in the film *Gilda*. She was only seventeen, always accompanied by one of her many sisters. She laughed loudly and spoke with a very exotic Texas accent. She quickly became a major model and appeared on forty magazine covers in no time at all. She seduced the world and Mick Jagger, whom she subsequently married, and together they have four children.

Funny to think that so much stardom started on that April afternoon at the Cotillion Room of the Pierre Hotel . . . Jerry Hall, Pat Cleveland, Apollonia, and last but not least, the wrap dress!

I was doing a personal appearance at Lord & Taylor in New York in 1975 when I first saw this incredible Somali goddess coming up the escalator. "Who are you?" I asked, incredulous at such beauty and grace. She answered with a deep and secure voice: "My name is Iman, I've just arrived in New York and I am a model." When I asked for her phone number, she squatted on the floor to reach into the large basket she was carrying, looking for a pen and paper. Her magnificent body language and elegance were astounding. Squatting like that on the floor of a department store with her legs opened she could have been in a market in Mogadishu or a queen in a palace of a *Thousand and One Nights*. I was entranced.

Like many of the models I used, Iman was, and is, a strong, intelligent woman. She speaks five languages and went on to found a successful cosmetics and fashion company, establishing her own global brand. After one daughter and a divorce, she met and married the rock star David Bowie, with whom she shares another daughter and her life in New York. Iman has never forgotten her roots. She does important work for Raise Hope for Congo, UNICEF, Save the Children, and the Dr. Hawa Abdi Foundation.

Not all models have happy endings. I will always love Gia, whom I met at the Mudd Club in 1978. Dressed like a biker in a studded black leather jacket and cowboy boots, with no makeup, she was simply the most beautiful girl I'd ever seen. She was seventeen and doing a little modeling, she told me, having just arrived in New York from Pennsylvania. I was with Ara Gallant that night, and we both fell in love with her. To the best of my knowledge, I was the first to use her in an ad.

Gia was sassy and in your face—she loved to act as a bad boy, never wore makeup, and dressed often in men's clothes. Francesco Scavullo hired her to do *Cosmopolitan* covers, and later she worked with Richard Avedon, Arthur Elgort, and Chris von Wangenheim, the top photographers of the era.

She and I had a wonderful time together in 1979, when I hired her to do a campaign called "On the Eve of a New Decade." It incorporated all my products—clothes, perfume, intimate apparel, jeans. Chris von Wangenheim and I directed the whole shoot and I felt on top of the world. My business was booming. Gia was gorgeous. We laughed a lot and I adored her.

One weekend I invited her to come and join me in the Pines on Fire Island where Calvin Klein had loaned me his beach house with a striking black swimming pool. I was excited to see Gia. I had a girl's crush on her. She arrived, late, on a Saturday afternoon. I remember coming home after a long walk on the beach to find her inexplicably sitting on the floor of the bedroom closet. She became agitated and embarrassed when she saw me. I did not understand what was going on then, but looking back, I think she was probably shooting up; I found out later she had become a serious heroin addict.

A few months after that weekend, Gia came to my office in dirty clothes looking gaunt. She needed cash. Even though I knew what she "needed" it for, I could not refuse her and gave her what was in my wallet. I never saw her again. It was probably from a dirty needle that she contracted AIDS and died in 1986 at the age of twenty-six.

A very young Angelina Jolie starred in the HBO film of Gia's troubled life. For years I couldn't watch it. Recently I did and was astounded by how accurate and real the movie was.

Years after Gia's death, I was asked to be part of a documentary about her. I went to some studio on the West Side to do the interview. It was important to me that people know what a lovely, generous woman Gia was. As I was about to leave the studio, I met Gia's mother, herself a very beautiful woman, who had also come to be interviewed. I hugged her and felt close to her. She surprised me by telling me that after her daughter's death, she had found a sealed letter from Gia addressed to me. When I smiled, she immediately added, "I opened it, read it, but will never give it to you." I was hurt and confused by that comment, and I wish I knew what Gia had written.

There were so many other wonderful models that I worked with along the way. Cindy Crawford, who looked like Gia, though she turned her beauty into a happy, healthy family life. Patti Hansen, the rock'n'roll girl who ended up marrying bad boy genius Keith Richards and had two hip, rock 'n' roll daughters with him; French beauty Inès de la Fressange whom I used in 1982 before she became a muse for Karl Lagerfeld at Chanel; Rene Russo, who became a movie star. I then stopped working for a while, and never used any of the supermodels who appeared on the scene and who I admired from afar . . . Linda Evangelista, Claudia Schiffer, Christy Turlington, Stella Tennant, and Stephanie Seymour.

Though I did not have a runway for her to walk down at the time, I couldn't resist meeting Naomi Campbell. By then Barry had taken over QVC, the TV home shopping network, and I was acting as a talent recruiter. I wanted Naomi to go on it. I remember inviting her to lunch at the Four Seasons in New York. Everyone stared at her as she walked into the front, "power" room. She looked like a goddess. We talked about everything but TV shopping. I never brought it up. She was too fresh, too good for it. We stayed friends and worked together a few times and she showed up for me big time with her powerful Russian then fiancé when I had my first exhibition in Moscow years later. She came through again, a huge surprise, on the runway for my Spring 2014 collection. The crowd burst into cheers as the incomparable supermodel appeared to close the show.

I never worked with the biggest model of the decade, Kate Moss, but she is my kind of girl: true to herself, independent, and in charge of her own life. When I met her at a photography opening in London, she told me, "I want to grow up to be you." I answered promptly, "You already are, my dear!" We were both flattered.

Natalia Vodianova caught my attention immediately when she first came to New York in 2001 at the age of nineteen. I was drawn to her freshness and determination and felt her strength and her character as soon as I met her. She opened and closed my show. It was her first, I think, in New York. Soon after that she became a top international model and a close friend. Her strength, I learned, had been born out of hardship. Her father had left her mother when she was a toddler, and they were impoverished. She was only nine when she started selling fruit with her mother on the street in Gorky to help support her two half sisters, one of whom was born with cerebral palsy and deeply autistic.

I was in my office in September 2004 when Natalia came to me in tears. Masked terrorists had taken an entire school in Beslan, Russia, and held everyone hostage. Three hundred and thirty-four people were killed, among them at least 186 children. The children who survived suffered emotional trauma, burns, and other injuries.

"We've got to do something for the children," Natalia said. "Help me to raise money." We gave a fund-raising party in my studio on West Twelfth Street. She was so young then, so inexperienced, yet within days she had orchestrated the entire event: an ice palace décor, a vodka sponsorship, celebrities and paparazzi and a full charity auction that raised hundreds of thousands of dollars.

She created her own foundation, Naked Heart, that has built over a hundred play parks in areas of Russia where there were none so children can have a place to be safe. Now her organization has expanded its work to provide support to families raising children with special needs throughout Russia.

In February 2008, I had the wild idea to put her together with my longtime friend, French writer, photographer, and artist François-Marie Banier, to create an ad campaign. I had always admired François-Marie, first for his novels and plays in the seventies, and recently for his extraordinary photographs. I called him in Paris and arranged for him to meet Natalia. A few weeks later they came to New York.

"Make magic," I told them, and magic happened. They walked the streets of the Meatpacking District and he photographed her with wet hair and no makeup in front of walls covered with colorful graffiti, then painted on the photos and decorated them with endless stream-of-consciousness writings. It was quite a rebellious campaign. You could not see the clothes at all, just a beautiful woman tattooed with splashes of color and writings. It was art and the only thing that indicated they were ads was the logo, DVF. I'm not sure those images were commercially understood, but I was thrilled when, at a party in Paris, Karl Lagerfeld congratulated me on the boldness of the campaign. I was very proud that the "magic" collaboration I'd thought of was later published by Steidl in a beautiful art book.

Because I know how to bring out a woman's strength and make her feel confident, and because I have become skilled at photography, I have, along the way, taken memorable photos of women. I photographed the ravishing, exotic, French/Italian/Egyptian Elisa Sednaoui for *V* magazine; the Colombian politician, activist, and FARC prisoner of seven years, Ingrid Betancourt, for the art magazine *Egoïste*; and did a full fashion story for the French magazine *CRASH*. I enjoyed making those women feel the strongest and the most desirable they had ever felt. Last but not least, I loved that process with our family's own gorgeous Alison Kay, mother of my fourth grandchild, Leon. We did two DVF advertising campaigns together. She is as beautiful outside as I know her to be inside.

Casting for a fashion show is very different from choosing a model to advertise your brand. Each time we cast a show, we hire a stylist and a casting agent. They know all the best girls and call a "go-see." I am often amazed how plain and unassuming some of the new top girls look in real life, and how you need a special eye to recognize a strange face that can become beautiful, an unusual bone structure that catches the light, an oddness that becomes magical. Every casting takes me back to an episode decades ago, in Geneva, Switzerland, when I was briefly a receptionist at IOS, the "Fund of Funds" company created by financier Bernard Cornfeld.

Bernie was a friend of Jerry Ford, the founder, with his wife, Eileen, of the Ford model agency in New York, and Jerry was visiting the IOS office. As he was waiting in the reception area, he went by the desk of the other receptionist and handed her his card. "If you ever want to model," he said, "let me know. You have potential." I was shocked and offended. Why her and not me? I certainly thought I was more interesting than that pale, tall, very plain skinny girl, but it turned out that it was precisely because she was that white canvas of a woman that he thought she could make an interesting model. I have thought about it at every one of my castings since.

Runway models don't move the way they used to. Unlike Pat Cleveland who danced down the runway, they are taught to march like soldiers without a smile. I always surprise my own models when just before the show I tell them, "Smile, seduce, and be you. Be the woman you want to be!" I believe I am one of the very few designers who ask their models to smile. Joie de vivre is very much on brand at DVF.

My definition of beauty is strength and personality. Strength is captivating: the women I've seen in India working the fields in their orange saris, their arms covered with colorful glass bangles; the women working in construction in Indonesia, carrying heavy bricks on their heads; the women carrying their children to bush hospitals in Africa.

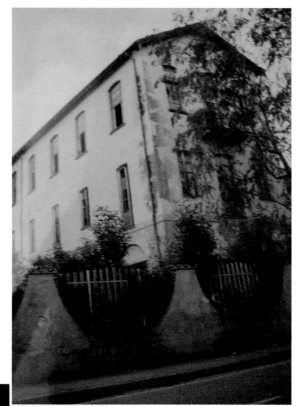

Manifattura Tessile
Ferretti in Parè, Como.

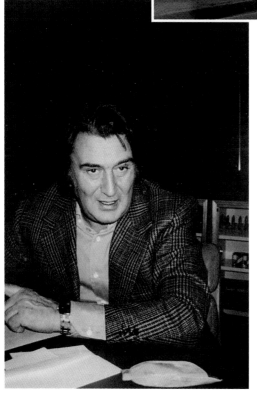

My friend and mentor
Angelo Ferretti.

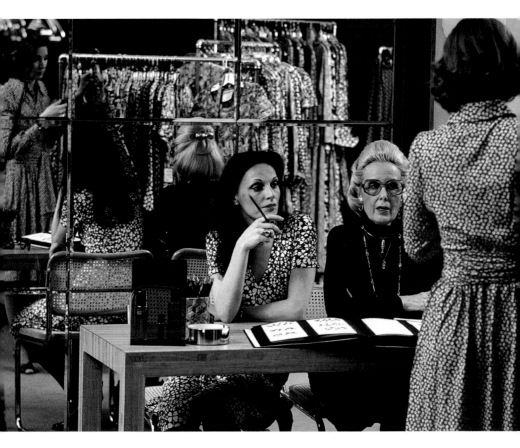

In my 7th Avenue showroom in 1976. *(Burt Glinn, Magnum)*

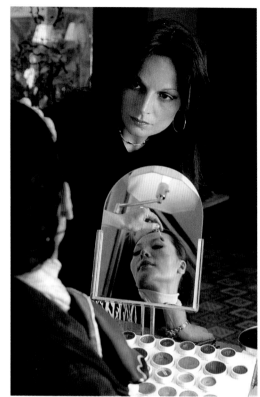

Applying makeup on a customer. *(Burt Glinn, Magnum)*

Working on Tatiana fragrance products, 1976.
(Elliot Erwitt, Magnum)

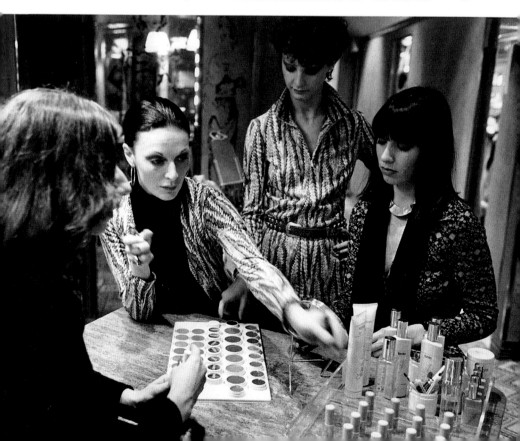

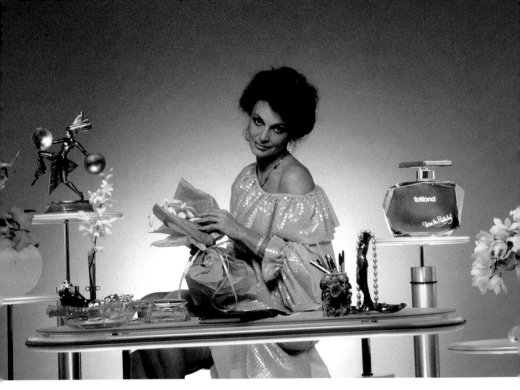

TV commercial for Tatiana
fragrance, 1982. *(Albert Watson)*

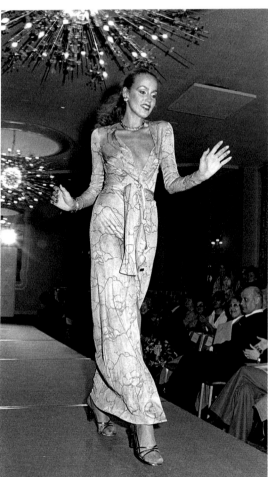

A teenage Jerry Hall
on the runway at the
Pierre hotel in 1975.
*(Nick Machalaba, Corbis
Image)*

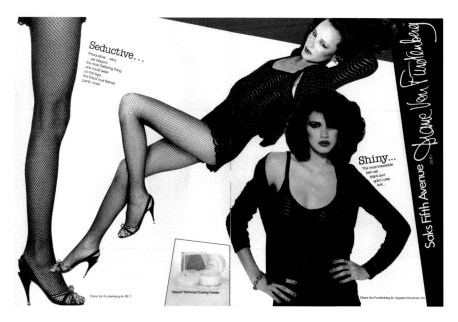

Gia Carangi for Diane von Furstenberg ad campaign, 1979. *(Chris von Wangenheim)*

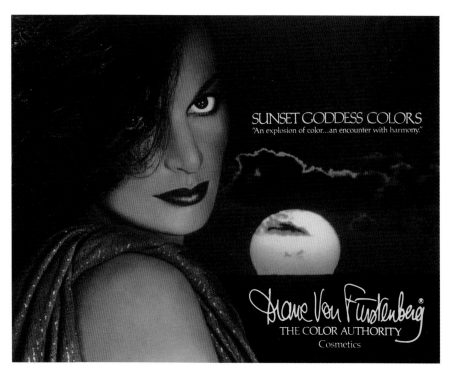

Ad campaign for the Color Authority cosmetics line in 1982. *(Albert Watson)*

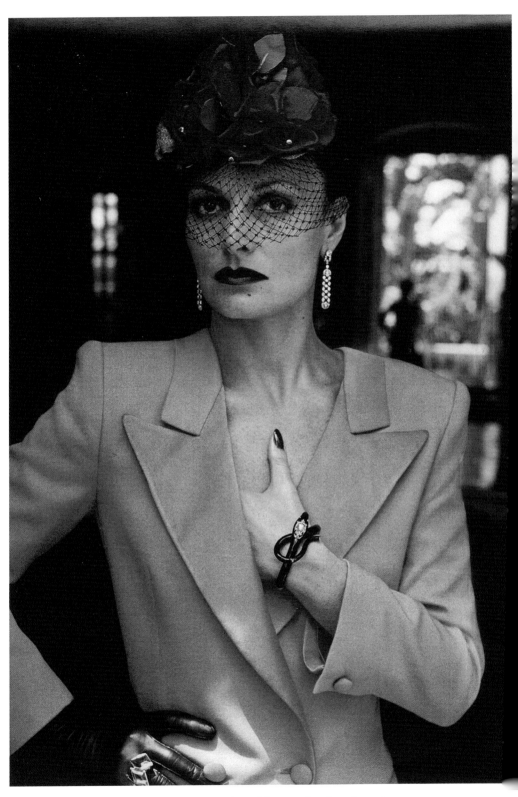

Photographed by Helmut Newton for the advertising
campaign for the couture line. *(© The Helmut Newton Estate)*

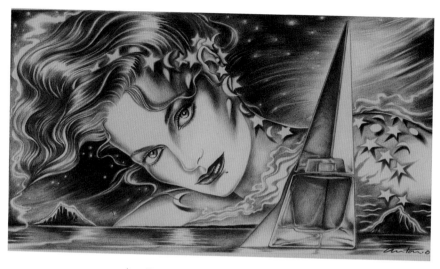

An illustration by Antonio Lopez for
Volcan d'Amour perfume. *(Artwork by Antonio Lopez)*

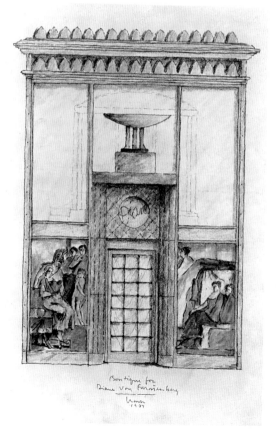

Architect Michael Graves's
sketch for the Diane
couture boutique at the
Sherry-Netherland hotel.
*(Drawing by Michael Graves,
courtesy of Michael Graves &
Associates)*

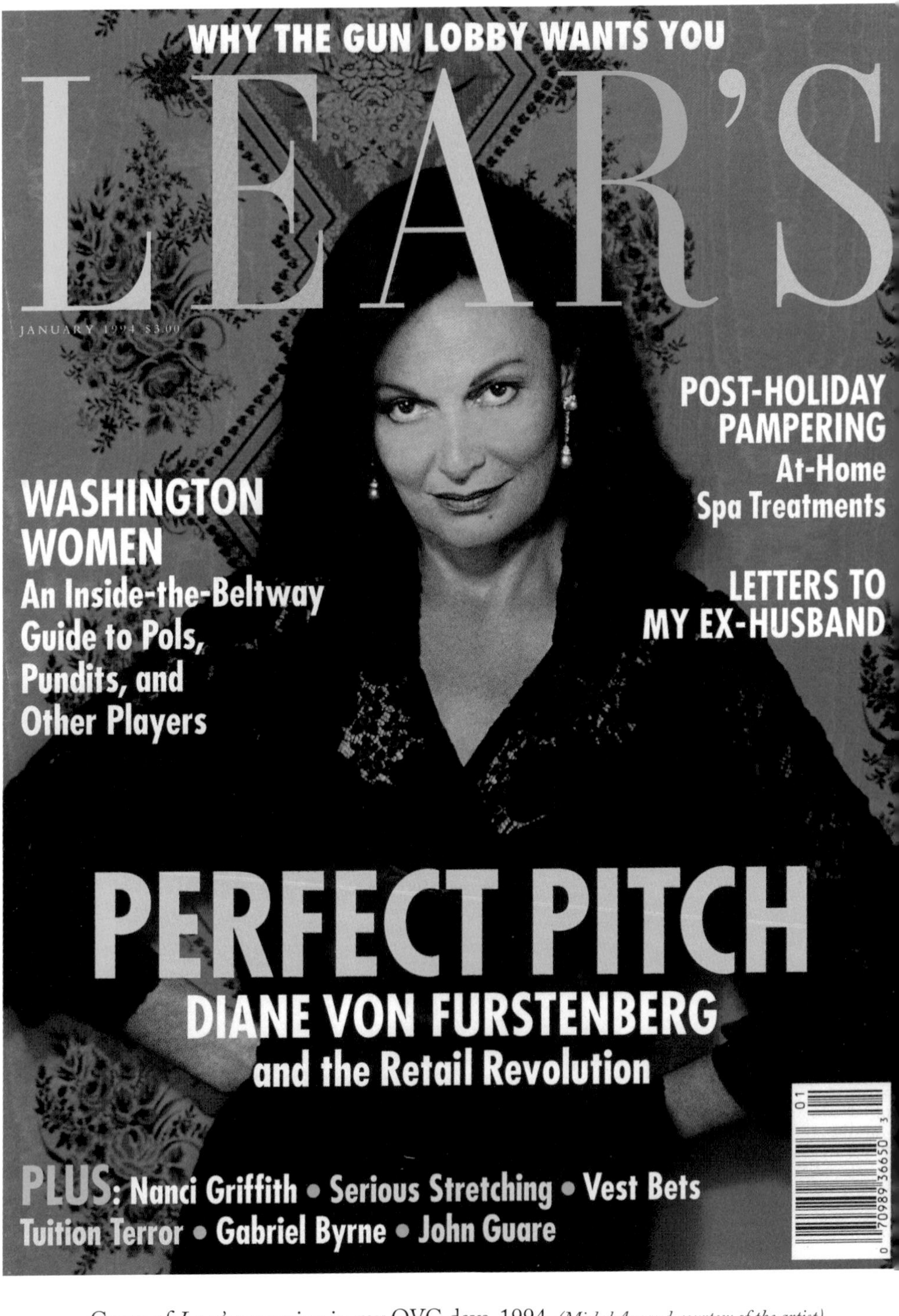

WHY THE GUN LOBBY WANTS YOU

LEAR'S

JANUARY 1994 $3.00

POST-HOLIDAY PAMPERING
At-Home
Spa Treatments

WASHINGTON WOMEN
An Inside-the-Beltway
Guide to Pols,
Pundits, and
Other Players

LETTERS TO MY EX-HUSBAND

PERFECT PITCH
DIANE VON FURSTENBERG
and the Retail Revolution

PLUS: Nanci Griffith • Serious Stretching • Vest Bets
Tuition Terror • Gabriel Byrne • John Guare

Cover of *Lear's* magazine in my QVC days, 1994. *(Michel Arnaud, courtesy of the artist)*

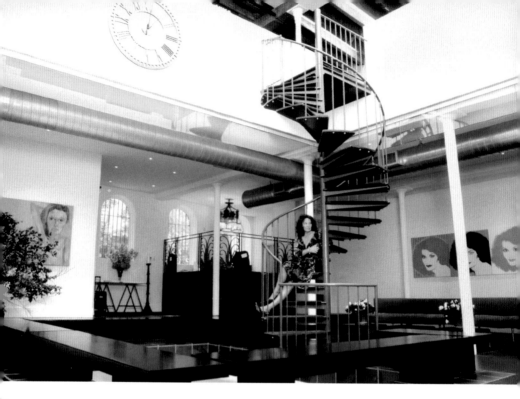

Inside of DVF Studio
on West 12th Street.
*(Emanuele Scorcelletti,
courtesy of the artist)*

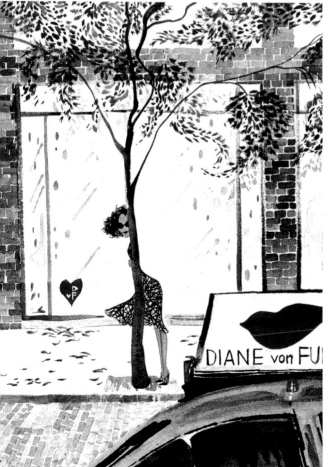

Ruben Toledo's
illustration of the
first shop on West
12th Street. *(Artwork
by Ruben Toledo)*

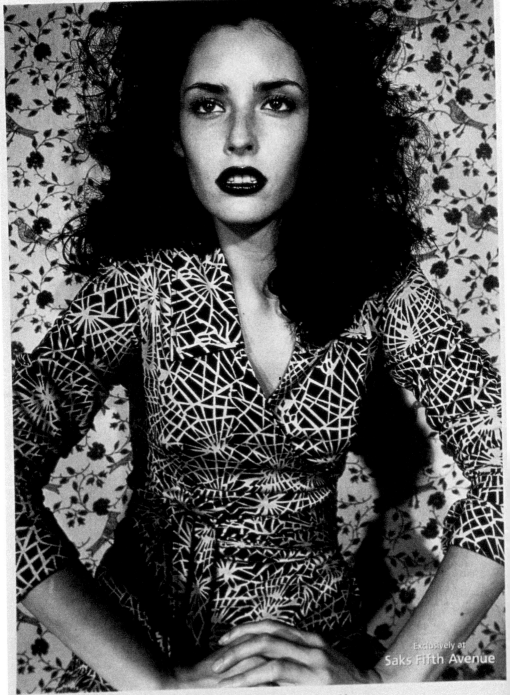

Exclusively at
Saks Fifth Avenue

He stared at me all night. Then he said...

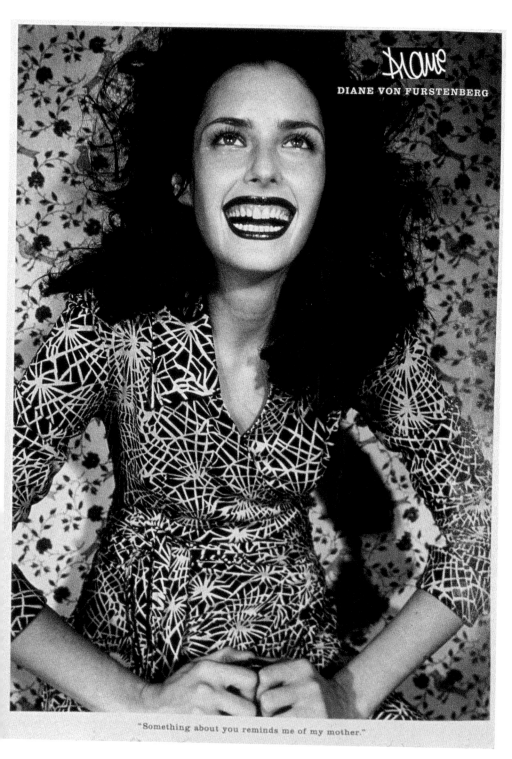

Model Daniela photographed by Bettina Rheims for the wrap dress relaunch, 1997. *(Bettina Rheims, courtesy of the artist)*

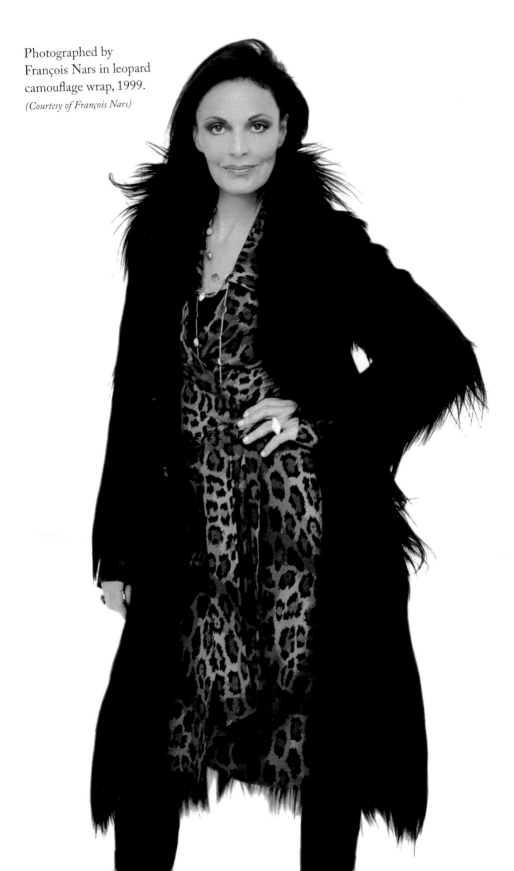

Photographed by
François Nars in leopard
camouflage wrap, 1999.

(Courtesy of François Nars)

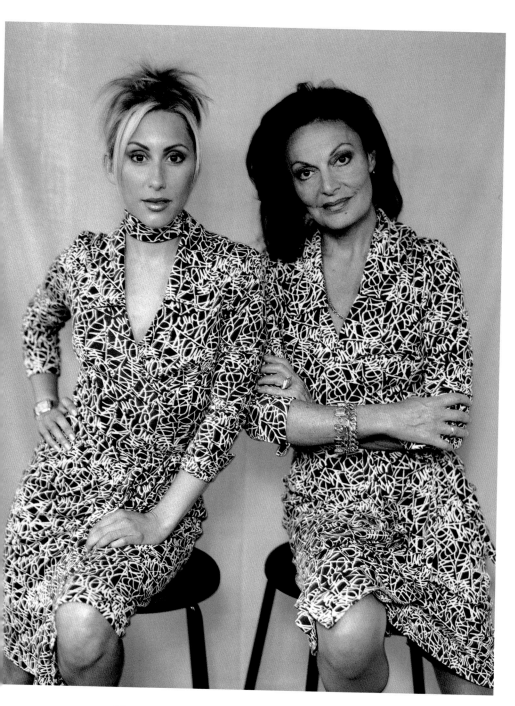

Wrap for a new generation. With daughter-in-law,
Alexandra, in 1998. *(Steffen Thalemann)*

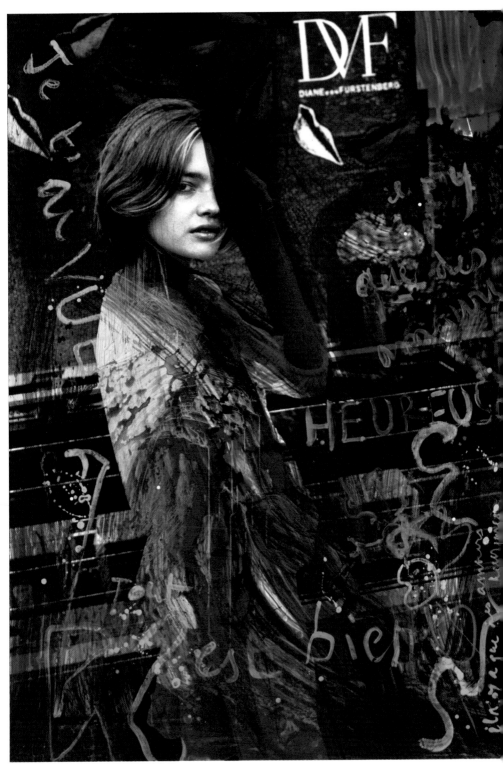

Natalia Vodianova photographed and painted by François-Marie Banier, 2008.

(François-Marie Banier, courtesy of the artist)

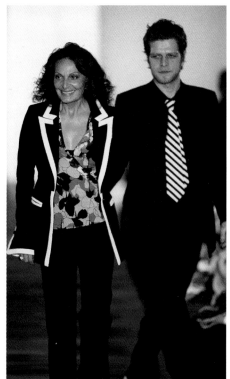

Walking the runway with creative director Nathan Jenden, 2002.

(Dan Lecca)

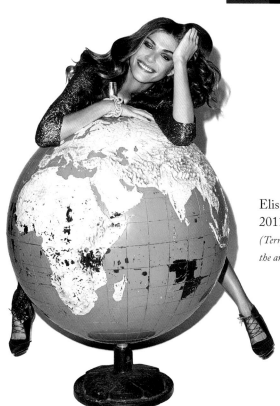

Elisa Sednaoui for the 2011 DVF campaign.

(Terry Richardson, courtesy of the artist)

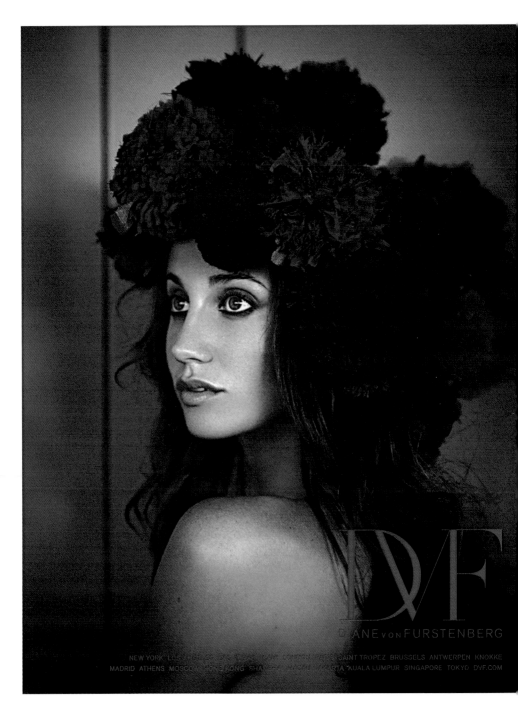

Ali Kay photographed by me for the 2010 DVF campaign.

The dignity of these women with their innate elegance is a true inspiration of beauty.

Some of the strongest women I know are the women of Vital Voices, a global nonprofit originally founded by Hillary Clinton when she was First Lady, on whose board I sit. Vital Voices identifies women leaders from around the world and helps them to increase their leadership potential. I've been both humbled and inspired by these women who not only have survived their own misery, but are committed to helping others in their communities.

Women like tiny, four-foot-six Sunitha Krishnan, who was gang-raped by eight men at fifteen and went on to form an organization in India called Prajwala that rescues and rehabilitates girls from brothels and sex traffickers. Sunitha has been beaten up and regularly receives death threats, but perseveres, harnessing what she calls "the power of pain." You barely notice Sunitha, she is so small, but once she starts speaking, she becomes so beautiful and majestic.

And Dr. Kakenya Ntaiya, a Kenyan who was engaged to be married at five and later bartered with her father to be circumcised in return for the opportunity to go to high school. Kakenya went on to college and graduate school in the US and returned to her Masai village to establish a girls' boarding school that changed the direction of education in her country.

And Chouchou Namegabe, a young journalist from the Democratic Republic of Congo who recorded the stories of hundreds of voiceless rape victims and played them on the radio to try to shame the government into taking action, then testified on behalf of the women at the International Court in the Hague.

These are but a few of the many women I've met through Vital Voices who have left me almost breathless with their courage and determination. "My God," I think to myself. "I've done nothing." Though

I've dedicated myself to empowering women through my work in fashion, mentoring, and philanthropy, *I* am empowered, mentored, and filled with riches from these women. It is they, and many others like them, who inspire me with their strength and beauty.

One day, after hearing me talk so much about Vital Voices, my children had an idea: "You are always talking about these Vital Voices women. You're so inspired by them; you should give them awards. The family foundation can sponsor them—we can help finance their work."

That idea stayed in the back of my mind, but it was unresolved until my friend Tina Brown, editor then of The Daily Beast, asked me to join her in organizing the first Women in the World Summit: three days of the most powerful women meeting, talking, and coming up with solutions for global challenges. I was so excited to be involved in this conference and it felt natural to turn one evening into a big dinner at the United Nations, and give awards, each with a $50,000 grant.

And that is how the DVF Awards were established in 2010 by the Diller–von Furstenberg Family Foundation to honor and support extraordinary women who have had the courage to fight, the power to survive, and the leadership to inspire; women who have transformed the lives of others through their commitment, resources, and visibility. Since 2010, we have honored so many inspiring and truly beautiful women, among them women from the Vital Voices network. We have also honored Hillary Clinton; Oprah Winfrey; Robin Roberts, anchor of ABC's *Good Morning America*; and Gloria Steinem with Lifetime Leadership Awards. Ingrid Betancourt, Elizabeth Smart, and Jaycee Dugard have received Inspiration Awards. What these three women have in common is that they were all kidnapped and, like my mother, held in harrowing captivity, and, like her, refuse to think of themselves as victims. "My hope is to be remembered for what I do, and not what happened to me," said Jaycee, who was held for eighteen years and has since founded the JAYC Foundation, which helps families recover from abduction and other trauma.

We also established a People's Voice Award, chosen by popular vote from four nominees who are working within the United States. They are women who all start in a small grassroots way. As my mother told me, if you save one life, it begins a dynasty. The life you save can save another, so one life is never too small.

Bravery and determination: that is also beauty.

Beauty is health and health is beauty. That is the reminder I email, as president of the Council of Fashion Designers of America to designers every season before their shows. When I was elected president of the trade organization in 2006, there was a lot in the press about the causes of anorexia and its prevalence in young girls. I had no personal experience with eating disorders for myself or my daughter or anyone close to me. So I was puzzled at first when I was told that the fashion industry was complicit in the rise in eating disorders.

I was naïve, perhaps. Many top models have become celebrities so it would be natural for young girls to want to emulate them. Still, starving themselves was not the answer. Long, thin bodies are genetic, not engineered. Models watch what they eat, of course, but for the most part, their bodies are predisposed to be thin. This can be difficult for young girls to accept.

Though becoming a model is a dream for many all over the world, the truth is it is not an easy job. More often than not it is about being rejected, about feeling bad about yourself. Most of the top agencies mean well and are caring for the girls—some are even outstandingly protective—but there are pseudoagencies and there is trafficking and prostitution that happens "in the name of fashion." I cannot warn girls enough to be vigilant. Don't dream of becoming a model unless it is genuinely possible. Look for other doors. The business of beauty can often be anything but beautiful.

In fact, I plead with young girls, except the very few genetically exceptional ones, not to try and become models. "Use your brains, your common sense and do not become an object," I told one graduating high school class. "The way you look is important, but who you are and how you project it is eventually who you will become and how you will appear."

I became convinced that the CFDA had to take the initiative to promote health as beauty. We established industry standards in 2007, working in partnership with medical experts, modeling agencies, and *Vogue* editor in chief Anna Wintour. These standards include commonsense recommendations to protect the girls; workshops for designers, models, and their families on how to recognize the signs of eating disorders; and encouraging models with eating disorders to seek professional help.

Next we addressed age. Youth is a huge factor in the business of fashion and the age issue is a stubborn and long-standing one—for many, the younger the better. It is a hard battle because many designers think clothes look better on very tall, extremely skinny girls, and the younger they are, the less formed they are. Those designers influence the bookers and force the model agencies to supply girls who are younger and younger. We had to stop that downward spiral, or at least slow it down. Every member of the CFDA—the top 450 designers in America—is now required to check a runway model's ID to ensure that she is at least sixteen and that those under eighteen are not kept at work past midnight at fittings or photo shoots. Health is beauty. Beauty is health.

I was diagnosed with cancer in 1994, at the age of forty-seven. One minute I was fine, the next I was undergoing radiation at the base of my tongue and soft palette. It started at a lunch with Ralph Lauren at the famous midtown New York restaurant La Grenouille. It was supposed to be a business lunch but we talked about everything, including love and the fragility of life. He had recently had a benign tumor removed from his brain, he said. "How did you find out you had the tumor?" I asked. "I kept hearing some noise in my left ear." As he said those words I heard a noise in my left ear. The following day it was still there. Could it be my imagination? I made an appointment with an ear doctor.

"There is nothing wrong with your ear," the doctor told me, but he found a swollen gland on the right side of my neck. He didn't seem concerned and gave me antibiotics. The noise disappeared but the swelling did not. I then had a biopsy and nothing bad came out. "It is a benign cyst, don't worry," I was told. I did not like the idea of having a cyst, so I scheduled a surgical procedure to have it removed the following week, on Friday, May 13. The unlucky date proved prophetic. As I woke up groggy from the anesthesia with Tatiana and my mother by my side, the doctor told us the news. When they removed the cyst, they had cut it in half and found tiny, tiny bad squamous cancerous cells that had already metastasized. Tatiana was shocked. My mother thought she'd misunderstood what she'd heard so she turned to Tatiana and kept insisting, "Translate for me! Tell me in French!"

The following days were terrifying, going for all kinds of tests and fearing the worst. An operation that would cut most of my neck away? Chemotherapy? Everything sounded scary. It did not help when I went home the night of my diagnosis and turned on the news to hear that Jackie Kennedy Onassis had died of cancer that day.

At first I felt in the dark and very worried, but little by little, as I understood better what the doctors were explaining to me, I regained my strength and pushed away the fear. I had to accept that I had cancer and deal with it. Seven weeks of radiation. An unexpected summer was suddenly laid out in front of me. It was going to be a time of treatment and healing. I had no choice but to accept it, take time for myself, and focus on my health. I had to get well, kill the bad cells forever, and never, ever let them come back. I repeated that sentence over and over to myself so often that it became a little victory song in French.

My mother stayed by me. She did not act worried, which gave me strength. Alexandre returned from Hong Kong where he had been working at a bank; Tatiana was nearby. Barry was hit hard by the news. My doctor told me he saw him walking to his car the day I was diagnosed and never had he seen someone's posture reveal so much distress.

On my first weekend in Connecticut after the diagnosis, my friend, producer, and agent Sandy Gallin, gave me a life-changing gift. He sent Deepak Chopra, the famous Indian New Age doctor and author, to visit me at Cloudwalk. We sat together as he taught me how to meditate. His way of explaining things reached me, reassured me, and turned out to be extremely helpful. He invited me to the Chopra Center for Wellbeing in La Jolla, California, and I went before starting the radiation. Tatiana took me there and spent the first two days with me, but I needed to be alone. I meditated and repeated the sutras Deepak gave me: Peace, Harmony, Laughter, Love, Creativity, Affluence,

Abundance, Discrimination, Integration, Freedom, Truth, Knowledge, Infinity, Immortality, Enlightenment, Holiness. I walked on the beach for hours, swam hundreds of laps in the pool, and had long conversations with myself and God. All of that plus the Ayurveda treatments of diet, herbs, and massage, along with the calmness around me, helped prepare me for this unexpected battle.

Back in New York, Alexandre took me to an appointment where they made measurements for a mask and put tiny tattoos on my face to ensure the rays would aim precisely. Years later my doctor told me Alexandre had returned to him after walking me out to ask him to take special care of me, "Remember: it's my mother you're dealing with."

I took a photo of my face in the bathroom mirror before I went to my first radiation session. I wanted to remember me as I was, not knowing if I'd be changed forever. And then the routine began. Every day I walked to Sloan Kettering and put on the mask that was attached to the table. For thirty seconds, the rays targeted each side of my neck and the middle. I would then start walking home to the Carlyle Hotel, stop to have wheat grass juice at the health food store (it was nauseating, but I believed in its natural healing powers), and then walk on singing my little French victory song to kill the bad cells. At home, I meditated for hours, had a daily massage to stimulate the immune system, and gargled with sesame oil. On the weekend, when there were no treatments, I went to Cloudwalk and enjoyed the beauty of nature—the forest, the flowers, the deer among the apple trees. Nature had never felt more beautiful, more peaceful, and more reassuring.

Deepak called every day. So did Egon from Italy, Mark Peploe from London, and my friends from all over the world. I felt loved without being pitied and serene from the strength that comes from love. Barry started to talk about us living together, getting a house, and started inquiring about my relationship with Mark, which he'd never done before. I was vague. My future was uncertain; I did not know what I wanted except to get well.

In the middle of the treatment my friend Mort Zuckerman, the real estate tycoon, invited me to go to the White House for a state dinner the president and Mrs. Clinton were giving for the emperor and the empress of Japan. I was excited and accepted. The grand master fashion designer of the moment, John Galliano, happened to be doing his first personal appearance at Bergdorf Goodman across the street from my office, and I borrowed his most beautiful ball gown: pale pink and blue chiffon, with lots of ruffles and a long train that went on forever. In spite of the radiation burn shadings on each side of my face, which I managed to hide with makeup, I ended up looking beautiful as I walked into the tented Rose Garden. The dinner was a historic event and I really enjoyed being there. At my table were some important Japanese businesspeople who could not believe that they actually were in the same room as their emperor. In Japan, they would have had to be separated by a screen because no common subjects can be in the same room with his Excellency the Emperor!

For me it was a different kind of excitement. I loved my voluptuous dress, though I had to shuffle carefully with my long train that nonetheless was stepped on by everybody and ended up in shreds by the end of the evening. Feeling frivolous and beautiful in the middle of my painful treatment was a wink to myself. It felt great.

The news from Belgium, however, was not good. Philippe phoned me just before the Fourth of July. My father's health was failing; we had to get ready for the worst. The radiation center in New York was closed for a few days over the holiday weekend and Barry generously gave me his plane to visit my father. By then, I had lost all sense of taste, my throat was hurting, and my skin was very burned, but I had to see my father. His Alzheimer's had taken a bad turn and I knew he would no longer recognize me. Still, I wanted to kiss him and thank him for the love he had given me. Tatiana came with me. It was the last time we saw him.

On the way back from Belgium, we landed in Gander, Canada, to refuel. It had been raining and the plane sat between two complete rainbows. Tatiana told me to make a wish. I wished to be cured. There were another dozen daily treatments left to go, a dryer throat, and more burns. Deepak kept on calling, my mother, Barry, and the children were nearby, and I was counting the days. It was the year of the World Cup. Brazil won, and I did, too.

I went back to Deepak's center in California after the treatments to recuperate. That was the worst week of all. As my doctor had predicted, the discomfort increased. I was burned inside and out from the radiation and exhausted. The adrenaline that had sustained me during treatment was gone because I knew the treatments were over. I locked myself in my room and moaned. The only thing I forced myself to do was fifty laps in the pool, repeating my sutras.

At the end of the week, a call came in the middle of the night, morning in Brussels. My father had passed away. My brother and my mother were on the phone, crying. My eyes stayed dry; my father was gone forever and there was nothing I could do to change that. On the plane from La Jolla, I picked up Alexandre in Las Vegas and we flew to New York and then on to Belgium. Tatiana met us at the Brussels airport—she had come from Portugal. We went straight to my father's apartment, the apartment I grew up in. His room seemed smaller than I remembered; the coffin seemed small, too. I sat by it. On the side table there was a lit candle and photos of my father's parents and brother. I felt helpless but peaceful, thankful for the love my father had given me. We buried him in a lovely cemetery, surrounded by trees and stillness. The children left that afternoon. I needed a break. I decided to go to Berlin for a long weekend and meet Mark, who was there editing his movie *Victory*. My brother thought I was too weak to travel, but I wanted to feel life and love, so I went. I rested in my hotel room during the day while Mark was working, but at night we walked around the streets of the newly united Berlin and loved it.

A few days later, I went back to Brussels to tidy up my father's home. Like me, he had kept everything: diaries, letters, photographs ... memory lane in all its splendor. I missed his presence, his smell, but in the mirror I could see him—our features are so similar. Before leaving, I took his favorite watch, a gold Omega, his crocodile wallet, and his two Russian glasses with silver holders in which he drank his tea every day.

———————

Confronting my cancer was challenging, but enriching. I became more compassionate to the sufferings of others, appreciated the value of health, became more spiritual and understood both my fragility and my strength. I have been thankful ever since to God, the doctors, my family, my friends, and my own power. My little French song worked and I have been cancer-free ever since.

I became much more health conscious after my bout with cancer. I eat lightly and in moderation—fresh, organic vegetables and fruits, grains and beans, little meat—and I resist sugar as much as I'm able to, but I still love dark chocolate and an occasional glass of great red wine. I drink lots of water—lots—and cups of hot, fresh ginger tea with lemon and honey.

My legs are stronger than they were when I was thirty because of all the hikes I love to do. Uphill, the steeper the better. The Appalachian Trail winds through the hills near Cloudwalk on its way from Maine to Georgia, and Barry, Shannon, and I hike on sections of it every day we are there. In LA we meet the children between our homes, at the bottom of Franklin Canyon, and hike to the peak together. When we're on the boat, we hike on whatever island or coast we pull into. I lead the way because I am faster. We are silent going up. Hiking is a meditation of sorts to me and I use it as a time to go within myself and enjoy the effort of climbing and the beauty of nature. We linger at the top, enjoying our accomplishment, and Barry leads the way down. That's when we talk, often our best talks, because of the long silence of the climb and the space that nature has given our minds to get clearer. I love those moments.

When I'm in New York, I climb up and down the five flights of stairs at the DVF headquarters, sometimes taking the steps two at a time, even in high heels. I swim just as strenuously, whether in the sea, the pool at Cloudwalk, or any hotel I stay at around the world. It is also a meditation. Exercising and counting the lengths crowd all thoughts out of the brain and I'm alone with myself.

I stay supple by doing yoga a couple of times a week in the yoga studio I built in a room next to my office. The stretching and the twists make me aware of every part of my body and keep me very flexible. Deep breathing is an integral part of yoga and I practice the long inhale and slow exhale to ease stressful moments. I also have a facial once a week from an Englishwoman named Tracie Martyn who attaches something, I don't know what, to her fingertips, which channels low-voltage electricity to my face and helps fight gravity. (So does smiling, I learned from fashion photographer Mario Testino.) I've been going to Tracie for fifteen years now, and my office knows it's the only appointment that can't be canceled.

Most important, I have a massage at least once a week, especially when I'm traveling. I used to think massages were vain and indulgent, but I've learned that isn't true. Massage bolsters the body's defense system, aids circulation, and rids your body of toxins.

While I was undergoing the cancer treatments, I started a weekly Shiatsu session. (I also have deep-tissue massages from Andrey, an excellent Ukrainian masseur.) My wonderful Shiatsu practitioner, who unexpectedly died of a stroke last year, was a talented Japanese man named Eizo who also healed the radiation blisters in my mouth by giving me a powder from a rare mushroom. He worked on me for nineteen years, every Tuesday morning before Tracie Martyn, giving me a deep-tissue massage to correct disharmonies and walking up and down my back to crack me. I miss him dearly.

Another result of my encounter with cancer is Dr. Durrafourd, a homeopathic doctor in Paris that my friend actress Marisa Berenson introduced me to. I see him once a year. He does full blood work, calculates the results, and prescribes me all kinds of antioxidants—all plant-based and natural. I have a dozen little bottles of pills and some liquids, which I keep together in a bag that I carry with me around the world. Have they had a positive effect? I like to think so. I went through menopause easily, for example. One day I stopped having my period and that was it.

Marisa also introduced me to Bianca, a healer who was able to ease the discomfort of my burns. I still call her in moments of crisis. I am the godmother of her son, Julien.

What I have learned is that when you are sick, much of healing is in the hands of doctors and science, but part of it is finding and using your own power.

Aging is out of your control. How you handle it, though, is in your hands.

When I was a girl, I always wanted to be older than I was. Instead of sitting, I knelt next to my father in the car so that people would think I was a grown-up. I pretended I had wrinkles and scratched my face with my nails because I wanted to have a lived-in face like the French movie star Jeanne Moreau. When I turned twenty and my mother asked me, "How does it feel being twenty?" I said, "Well, I've been telling people I've been twenty for so long that it doesn't make a difference." I always looked older than my actual years, so much so that when *Newsweek* put me on the cover on March 22, 1976, the editors didn't believe I was twenty-nine and sent a reporter to the Brussels town hall to check my birth certificate.

I had started my adult life at twenty-two, had two children by the time I was twenty-four, and a successful financial life by thirty. Looking back, I realize I was pretty in my late twenties, but I didn't really think so. I knew how to enhance what I had, highlighting my eyes and cheekbones, playing with my hair and my legs and acting with confidence. I knew I was seductive, but I never thought I was beautiful.

My thirties were my best years. I was still young but felt grown up, lived an adventurous life, raised my two children, and ran a business. I was independent and felt very free. I had total complicity with myself and my looks and I felt in charge. I had become the woman I wanted to be.

The forties were harder. My children went off to boarding school and college, and I sold my business. I was not sure who I was or who I wanted to be anymore. I went in and out of looks and started to question my own style. When I lost my fashion business, I lost the way of expressing myself creatively. I also had my battle with cancer.

Things got better when I hit fifty. I went back to work, creating a new studio environment and repositioning my brand. I surrounded myself with a new generation of girls. I was again the woman I wanted to be ... engaged and engaging. I married Barry and became a grandmother. I embraced my age and my life. It was the beginning of the age of fulfillment, which continues. Now, in my sixties, I know I have less time ahead and want to enjoy, enjoy as much as possible.

———————

I'm grateful I never thought of myself as beautiful when I was young. We all fade somewhat as time goes on. Women who relied only on their beauty can feel invisible later in life. It's a pity, for I feel in the latter part of your life you should feel fulfilled, not defeated. My advice is that as a woman gets deep into her forties, she should start becoming a myth. To become a myth for whatever she does, even if it's making the best chocolate mousse or being the best flower arranger. She has to stand for something and she's got to stay relevant, to be active, to participate. That's why I think it's so important for women to have an identity outside the home.

And never, ever lie about your age. Who can lie with the Internet anyway? To embrace your age is to embrace your life. Lying about your age, or about anything for that matter, is the beginning of trouble; it is the beginning of lying about who you are. What is important is to live fully every single day of every period of every age so that no time gets wasted. Because the time goes by, faster and faster.

So much of physical beauty is youth, pure and simple. The skin is fresh and tight, the eyes clear and wide, the waist slimmer, the hair full and lush, even the teeth, white and unworn. I never understood that as a girl. When somebody told me that I looked fresh, I hated it and found it unappealing. It's only when you stop being fresh that you appreciate it.

Youth is wonderful; it's exciting because it is the beginning of life. Everything is ahead and there is nothing more thrilling than beginnings when everything is possible and you can dream big dreams. But every day is a beginning. Living and enjoying the present moment to its fullest is the best way, the only way, to approach life. It is essential to learn from the past and look into the future without resentment. Resentments are toxic and can only pollute the future.

The best thing about aging, I have come to understand, is that you have a past. No one can take that away, so you'd better like it. That is why it is so important to waste no time. By living fully every day, you create your life and that becomes your past, a rich past.

When I was very young, I was arrogant and used to boast that I'd retire at thirty. As I got older, I continued to be arrogant about my age, but in a different way. I defied it. I would be dismissive and say, "Oh, age means nothing."

Today my energy has yet to let me down and I am more engaged than ever. But I am not as dismissive about it as I realize that aging can make you feel vulnerable. Perhaps it was a ski accident I had at the start of 2011 that made me more humble. One minute I'd been skiing happily with Barry in Aspen, Colorado; the next minute I was flat on my back in the snow with my face bleeding.

It had been a spectacular, sunny day on the mountain and I was skiing well and carefully between my ski instructor and Barry, and avoiding all of the aggressive snowboarders. My friend the actress Natasha Richardson had died the year before in a freak ski accident and she was very much on my mind when suddenly, out of nowhere, came an out-of-control first-time skier. I was standing still, waiting for Barry, when he hit me! He barreled into me with such force that he left my face bloody and numb.

After an X-ray in Aspen showed my ribs were fractured and my nose was broken, we flew to LA to have an MRI of my face to make sure the eye orbit bones were not broken as well, which would have required immediate surgery. In the plane I kept touching my cheekbones, terrified they were broken; they are my face's best asset. Luckily there were only hairline fractures around my eyes that would heal and the cheekbones were fine, but my mangled face set off alarms when we got to the hospital. I felt that everyone I saw in the corridors thought I was a victim of domestic abuse. It is amazing how quickly you can feel like a victim and I felt that I had to justify my bruised face to everyone who passed by. "Ski accident," I kept repeating. "Ski accident."

The timing of the accident couldn't have been worse. I had a couple of big months coming up—a photo shoot that week, the acceptance of a huge award at a gala benefit for amFAR (Foundation for AIDS Research) in New York, my Fall runway show during fashion week, and a high-profile trip to China in the spring where an extensive retrospective of my life and work was being installed in Beijing's prestigious Pace Gallery. It was because of that very busy schedule ahead of me that Barry had rented a house in Aspen for just the two of us for a few days.

Immediately after the MRI, the doctor mentioned surgery. I was not quite sure what he had in mind, but I said no. I wanted my face to heal completely first and then see what needed to be done. From that moment on, it was all about ice and arnica, arnica and ice. Very slowly the swelling went down to reveal dark blue bruises that spread downward, creating a devastating expression. Arnica and more arnica slowly lightened the color from dark purple to a lighter shade of purple, lavender, and eventually, weeks later, yellow. I recorded the progress daily on my iPhone; I had taken the first photo immediately after the fall and sent it to all of my friends. I continued to document the map of my face every day for the next two months. "This is what I look like," I would say to myself, "and it is not pretty."

I was still so bruised two weeks later that I considered passing up the amFAR benefit where I was going to be honored together with President Bill Clinton. I dreaded showing my face publicly, but then I felt ashamed for being so frivolous. "What are a few bruises compared to AIDS?" I scolded myself. "Of course you have to go."

Still, to partially cover my face, I asked my art department to make me a little fan. They made it heart-shaped, inscribed with my motto: "Love is life is love is life." I hid behind it at the beginning of the evening, but as soon as I went up onstage to accept the award, I put it down and simply said, "Excuse my appearance, I had a ski accident."

I didn't hide my face again. I wore sunglasses to my fashion show, and that was all. I also kept my long-standing appointment to be photographed by Chuck Close for *Harper's Bazaar*. Having your photograph taken by Chuck Close is like having an X-ray. There is nothing between you and him, no filter, no makeup, no flattering lights, and practically no space because he takes his photos close up and head on. "How am I going to do this?" I thought at first, then surrendered, "I'm just going to." The result was raw, very raw: My recovering face looked droopy and was laced with black smudges. I should have really hated the photo, but I kind of liked it because it was real. So did *Harper's Bazaar*, which ran it as a full page and it hung very large on one wall at the Pace Gallery in Beijing, and even more prominently at my exhibition in Los Angeles in 2014.

The Chuck Close shoot wasn't the last that made me hesitate. The hardest thing for me now is to be photographed; I've never really liked it, but at my age, it's twice as hard. Two shoots I've done recently with Terry Richardson have taught me a lot about the nature of beauty. I've known Terry since he was a toddler, when I was working for the photo agent Albert Koski, who represented his father, Bob Richardson. The first time Terry photographed me was for *Purple*, Olivier Zahm's very edgy fashion magazine. Olivier called me and asked if I would be the model for the collections in their spring/summer 2009 issue. "Are you insane? I'm sixty-two years old!" I told him. But he was so persistent that finally I laughed and told him, "OK, I'll do it, but only if you put me on the cover." "I can't promise you that," Olivier told me, "but I will try." Their last cover model had been Kate Moss.

The day of the shoot arrived, and the last thing I wanted to do was have my picture taken. My eyes were swollen. I was tired. I was supposed to model half the collections, and a young, professional model would do the other half. I desperately wanted to back out, but there was no way. After hours of dreading, I said to myself. "I will just do this as fast as possible." I couldn't let them see how unhappy I was, so I affected confidence, and exaggerated all of my movements. With Terry, it's quite easy to do that—he likes exaggerated movement. So I laughed, I was silly, and threw my arms out triumphantly. I ended up on the cover of *Purple* magazine at the age of sixty-two in only my stockings, my bodysuit, and a Maison Martin Margiela jacket made of blond hair.

For the fortieth anniversary of the wrap dress, *Harper's Bazaar* asked if I would be photographed by Terry again, this time as "the original wrapper" with the famous American rap star Wale. It was a wild idea and my team was enthusiastic about it, so I reluctantly agreed. When the day arrived, once again I woke up looking exhausted. It was a Friday, and it had been a busy week; I'd met with the mayor at seven a.m. on Monday, and it had been nonstop after that with design and merchandising meetings, interviews and speeches. Barry and I had had a dinner or a gala every night. I wanted to be alone in my car, driving to Cloudwalk, not in front of a camera, surrounded by young makeup artists and photographer's assistants, all staring at my tired face. But I put on the wrap dress they had chosen for me and told Terry, "Let's do it." Again I laughed, I posed, I exaggerated. And in the end, I loved the photo of me with my hand on my hip and my leg on Wale's knee. You can't tell my face is swollen when it's lifted by a huge smile. Clearly confidence is everything.

Confidence makes us beautiful, and it comes from accepting yourself. The moment you accept yourself, it makes everything better. I saw this in Nona Summers, who has been one of my best friends since we met at university in Geneva. Nona is this wild, glamorous, redheaded woman who was the inspiration for *Absolutely Fabulous*. She had been wild all her life . . . until the day she was diagnosed with retinitis pigmentosa, which meant she will eventually go blind. We were all very shocked at the news, but Nona took complete charge at the very moment she could have surrendered. That day she decided to get sober. To accept yourself, to be true to who you are, is the only solution to being fulfilled.

Zakia is another strong illustration of self-acceptance and its power. I met her at the 2012 *Glamour* Women of the Year Awards at Carnegie Hall when I was asked to give an award to Pakistani filmmaker Sharmeen Obaid-Chinoy for her Oscar-wining documentary on Zakia, an acid attack survivor. Zakia was asked to join us onstage, and her strength and quiet confidence moved the entire audience. After we left the stage, the three of us went downstairs to do some interviews. When I step into an elevator, I always check my makeup and adjust my hair, but in respect for what had happened to Zakia's face, I turned my back to the mirror. To my surprise, when Zakia stepped into the elevator, she faced it, gazing at her scarred image. I was awed watching her looking at herself, and embracing her image. Two operations and a skillful makeup job helped, but it was her dignity that made her very beautiful.

I certainly don't like to see my face aging in photographs, but I know if I wait ten years I will love those pictures. So I accept my image as who I am. What I found amusing about my ski accident was the number of people who said, "What a great opportunity for you to have a face-lift." Some did think I had had a face-lift and was just faking a ski accident. The truth is, I've never wished for my old face more than I did in the month or so following the accident. I didn't want surgery. I didn't want a new face. I wanted my old face back.

I know that people look at me and wonder why I have not succumbed to the progress of technology. Why have I not frozen or filled in the lines of my forehead. Why I have not clipped the bits of surplus skin on my eyelids. I am not sure, but probably because I am afraid of freezing time, of not recognizing myself in the mirror, the image I have been so friendly with. Losing the complicity with myself is something I would not like to happen, the wink in the bathroom mirror as I pass it in the middle of the night, the straight-on look that I recognize. My image is who I am and even if I don't always love it, I am intrigued by it and I find the changes interesting. I don't like the freckles and age spots that I have all over, but they are there, so I joke and say I have a printed skin like one of my favorite leopard-printed dresses. Even staring at the small wrinkles that curl around my lips can be interesting. They just appear one day at a time.

In my older face, I see my life. Every wrinkle, every smile line, every age spot. My life is written on my face. There is a saying that with age, you look outside what you are inside. If you are someone who never smiles your face gets saggy. If you're a person who smiles a lot, you will have more smile lines. Your wrinkles reflect the roads you have taken; they form the map of your life. My face reflects the wind and sun and rain and dust from the trips I've taken. My curiosity and love of life have filled me with colors and experiences and I wear them all with gratitude and pride. My face carries all my memories. Why would I erase them?

I don't judge those who choose to have cosmetic procedures. I sometimes contemplate the idea, ask around, get a phone number of a doctor, and then forget. I may one day, out of the blue, decide to do something myself, but until now I have chosen not to. I cannot pretend that I am younger than I am, and truly I feel that I have lived so fully that I should be twice my age. It is no longer about looking beautiful, but about feeling beautiful and fulfilled.

The other day I was struck by a bouquet of garden roses that was on my night table near my bed in Paris. There was one particularly lovely rose in this fragrant bouquet. Days went by, and slowly the rose began to fade. Even fading, it maintained its beauty. Some of the petals dried, curled, and had little brown spots on them, giving it a special beauty that was different from the beauty it had when it was fresh and new. I felt connected to that rose. Every time I see a new imperfection appear on my face, I think of that rose and how beautiful it was. I want to grow to be that rose.

Because of my work, I'm fortunate to be surrounded by youth and beauty—the models, the young women who work in my studio. They are a tonic for me. They make me feel young.

My surroundings are beautiful, too, which is very important to me. The six-story DVF headquarters at 440 West Fourteenth Street in the old Meatpacking District is filled with light. The building is a model of "green" technology, of which I am very proud. It has three geothermal wells that heat and cool it. The interior is lit by a "stair-delier," a broad light shaft of a stairwell that runs all the way up from the ground floor to the "diamond" prism glass penthouse on the roof, where I sleep when in New York. There are mirrors and crystals along the central stairs to direct the natural light into all the interior spaces. The garden outside my glass aerie on the roof is planted with wild grasses, which, even though it's in a working environment in a busy neighborhood, makes it an oasis of beauty and peace.

I love sleeping on the roof. My glass bedroom feels like a tree house, a comfortable urban tree house. I look out at the New York skyline and the Empire State Building from my bed, which is nestled under a tent of linen panels. The freestanding bathtub is teak, re-minding me of Bali. When I was a young mother, I lived in an old, established building on Fifth Avenue and felt very grown up. Now a grandmother, I live like a bohemian and it keeps me feeling youth-ful. When in New York during the week, Barry and I sleep apart, he, uptown in his apartment in the Carlyle hotel, I on Fourteenth Street. I like our arrangement; it makes our weekends and vacations all the more special.

No place, however, is more beautiful than my home, Cloudwalk. However blessed I am with energy, I need quiet to preserve it. I find it in the beauty there—the apple orchards, the openness of the green lawns, the Balinese flags along the river, the basso profundo song of the frogs. I was fortunate to have bought what was then a fifty-eight-acre farm for $210,000 when I was only twenty-seven. I'd fallen in love with it without even getting out of the car and immediately handed the startled real estate agent a deposit check. I have spent every possible minute there ever since. The trees at Cloudwalk have been my friends for forty years. I'm sure if I were sawed in half, our rings would match.

Nothing makes me feel more thankful than Cloudwalk. Nothing is more peaceful and reassuring. My children, Barry's love, Cloudwalk, and my work have been the most consistent things in my life. All my memories, all my photos, letters, diaries, all my archives are stored there.

I can spend hours sitting in front of the fourteen-foot-long desk created by George Nakashima out of a single piece of wood, reading and working. Barry and I like to read and be silent. Our dogs are by us, Shannon, the old Jack Russell terrier that Barry found on a bicycle trip in Ireland; Evita, a new Jack Russell puppy; and two terriers we brought home from a recent trip to Chilean Patagonia.

But what brings me to Cloudwalk more is the beauty of nature. The older I get, the more important it is to me. The fact that we cannot control nature appeases me and somehow brings me back to a normal dimension. Whereas my size is magnified in the city where everything is man-made and every problem is mine to be fixed, when I go on a walk in the forest and climb the hills around Cloudwalk, I feel small and I like it.

Nature is never still. Things are growing, ripening, aging, fading, and then starting again. The trees are beautiful even when bare. I love every phase and I am endlessly fascinated by that life cycle moving on. Nature never stops. Sometimes it can be cruel, bringing droughts or floods. Sometimes it's scary, spawning tornadoes and hurricanes. It can be unpredictable. We were hit one recent autumn by an early snowstorm that killed many trees and left us without power for weeks. I was sad to lose those trees that have been my companions, but I think it's good to be reminded of how little we are, how vulnerable.

One of my favorite walks at Cloudwalk is through the white pine forest to a sunny open field, then on to the side of the hill where I've chosen to be buried. For years, every Saturday I would go on a walk around Cloudwalk trying to think where I wanted to be buried. First I thought it would be in the woods among the beautiful stand of cathedral white pines, but then a few years ago the farm next door was put up for sale and to save the eighty-six acres from being turned into a housing development, we bought it. My original choice suddenly seemed too close to the house, so we chose this new spot as a meditation garden and a future burial place. I asked my friend Louis Benech, the French landscape architect, to think about it and he did a beautiful, simple design of two half-circle walls set in the hill. Victor, who, with his wife, Lourdes, has cared impeccably for Cloudwalk for years, has now built those walls with local stones. It is a special, quiet spot. Visitors to Cloudwalk always make fun of me for taking them to visit my future burial ground, so for now, we call it the meditation garden.

I love Cloudwalk and its beauty. I love to watch the sun set from one of the little stone walls and look out at the gorgeous views. I feel I become that view, that blend of meadow, forest, and hills. I am privileged to have all this beauty in my life. I worked hard for it and I'm still working hard. It's satisfying to know that one day, as far away as possible, this perfect land will be the place of rest for the woman I set out to be fifty-seven years ago in Brussels at Mireille's tenth birthday party.

THE
BUSINESS
OF FASHION

I didn't dare call myself a designer for many years despite the overwhelming success of my wrap dress. Yves Saint Laurent was a designer. Madame Grès was a designer. Halston was a designer. Me, I came into fashion almost by accident in the hope of becoming financially independent. I never dreamed that the simple dress I launched in 1974, a dress that was easy, sexy, elegant, and affordable all at the same time, would catapult me into fashion history. Yes, I'd sold millions of dresses by 1978. That dress had been inducted into both the Metropolitan Museum of Art's Costume Institute and the Smithsonian Institution collection, though I'm embarrassed to say I didn't even know what the Smithsonian was at the time. At the age of twenty-nine I'd even made the cover of *Newsweek*, which identified me as "Dress Designer Diane von Furstenberg."

Still, I didn't dare call myself a designer then, any more than I dared call myself a good mother while my children were still growing. You cannot make these claims until you get much older, because you need to have the proof, and so it wasn't until after I discovered I did have a second act, that I could do it again and be relevant and be right that the first time was confirmed, that it wasn't an accident. Only after almost two decades since I'd created the wrap dress, did I call myself a designer.

Looking back, what has been a whirlwind life in fashion fits neatly into three distinct phases: The American Dream, The Comeback Kid, and now, The New Era. This third phase, which I'm just moving into now, promises to be the most fulfilling. The goal is ambitious: to capitalize on all that I have done before and create a legacy for the brand so it will last long beyond me. The process has been painful at times and stressful, but the result, I hope, will be worth it. For me, it already is. To still feel relevant and so engaged at my age is a wonderful adventure. In a lot of ways, I am doing the same thing I did the first time. But finally I can use my experience and my knowledge to form a long-term vision. My instinct remains the constant. Being impulsive is my most valuable quality, though it is also my biggest fault. I have to caution myself, but it is still the driving force behind the brand, and amazingly, forty years after its birth, the wrap dress and I are still here and kicking.

I owe everything to that little dress: my independence, Cloudwalk, my children's education, the trips we took, the donations I make, the Bentley I drive, my place in fashion history—it all comes from that one little dress. That one little dress has taught me everything I know about fashion, women, life, and confidence.

I did not think much of the little wrap dress when I created it, but I now appreciate its value and uniqueness.

Looking back, I can't help but think, what if? What if I'd never met Egon? Gotten pregnant? Felt driven to support myself after we married? What if I hadn't met Angelo Ferretti in Cortina or Diana Vreeland in New York or Halston or Giorgio Sant'Angelo? What if?

I've long believed that the "ifs" were the doors to my future, and I dared to open them, one by one, as they came along. I knew the kind of woman I wanted to be but I didn't know how I would become her. Opening those doors led me on a path to fashion, and that became the path to the woman I am today.

4

THE AMERICAN DREAM

The journey began after Egon and I left Geneva in 1968, he to New York to train at the Chase Manhattan Bank, I to Paris to look for a job. We were both twenty, too young to think seriously about a future together, so we each set off on our own adventures. It was in Paris that I discovered a world I didn't know, the glamorous world of fashion, which would seduce me forever.

I stumbled into it through my best friend in Paris, Florence Grinda. Florence was a vivacious socialite whom I'd met in Geneva but became close to at a party in St. Tropez. Her husband, the tennis champion and playboy Jean-Noël Grinda, had disappeared into the bushes with a Swedish model when I found her sitting alone and feeling sorry for herself. We started to talk, and to console her, I took her to the port for an ice cream. We became best friends, and when we returned to Paris, night after night I left my tiny ground-floor studio on avenue Georges Mandel in the 16th Arrondissement to go out with Florence and her husband. Through her I met exciting people and got invited to lots of parties. She got designers to lend me clothes, a common practice that was new to me. A fun new world was opening. However, what I desperately wanted was a job.

A friend of hers introduced me to the handsome and mysterious fashion photography agent Albert Koski, who represented all the best fashion photographers of the time: David Bailey, Bob Richardson, Art Kane, and Jean-Louis Sieff, among others. Koski hired me on the spot to be his assistant, his do-everything girl, from answering the phone in the little house in which he worked and lived in the 16th Arrondisse-ment to curating the photographers' books to send to advertising agencies and magazines. That house on rue Dufrenoy was a beehive of talent filled with cool photographers and young models, a hot spot of glamour, beauty, and fashion.

I was much younger and certainly greener than all the people com-ing in and out of the office and was a bit intimidated by it all, though I was determined not to show it. It was my first involvement with mod-els, many of whom came to rue Dufrenoy. The big models were Jean Shrimpton and Veruschka, probably the most beautiful women ever; Twiggy and Penelope Tree, the strangest ones; and, of course, Marisa Berenson who, along with Florence, was to become my best friend and godmother of my son, Alexandre. From Italy, there were Isa Stoppi, Albertina Tiburzi, Marina Schiano, and Elsa Peretti, who became the successful jewelry designer for Tiffany. There were also Americans, Cheryl Tiegs and Wallis, along with the timeless, forever magical Lau-ren Hutton. I did not meet every one of them then, but I dealt with their photographs all day. They were all Diana Vreeland's "girls." As editor in chief of American *Vogue,* she had invented them.

Working for Albert Koski was an invaluable indoctrination, though I didn't see it at the time. I was assimilating a lot of information without totally comprehending it, but assimilating it nonetheless. In years to come, I would often refer back to what I learned there. It's only in retrospect that you realize that all the little experiences add up to a whole. What I did know then was that the world of fashion was fun, glamorous, very cool and I loved it. It was 1968. Everyone felt free, acted laid-back, and projected an image of being bored, though we were anything but.

It was then that I realized that fashion was a huge industry, a long chain of professions linked together. It started from the fabric mills making fabrics to designers making clothes and models showing them. Editors would choose them, photographers and illustrators and writers captured them, and magazines printed them. That long chain of inspiration, talent, emotion, and ideas would end with the women buying and enjoying fashion.

I became aware of trends, the must-haves of the moment. Big, clunky costume jewelry was in, fueled by the antielitism era of counterculture youth. So were big belts and hippie clothes—Indian silks, Afghan embroidered coats—and long hair, furs, and jewelry for girls and boys. Hairpieces, fake eyelashes, hot pants, and platform shoes were in and I wore them all.

Marisa Berenson was the perfect "it" girl of the time. She had traveled to meet Maharishi in India with the Beatles and was on the cover of *Vogue* covered with bold turquoises and corals. She was the image of glamour. I met Marisa through Florence and we immediately became friends. We were barely twenty but Marisa was already a top model. She was tall, skinny, and very elegant, and, like a chameleon, could transform herself into many different creatures of beauty. I saw a lot of her then. On the weekends, we would do a marathon of movies, going from one movie theater to another, crying watching Vanessa

Redgrave in the tragic role of dancer Isadora Duncan and laughing at the Stanley Donen comedy *Bedazzled*. We would end up late at night at La Coupole in Montparnasse to eat oysters, meet friends, and go on to nightclubs.

Marisa lived with her grandmother, fashion designer Elsa Schiaparelli. At the time Schiap (as people called her) was no longer working. She was an old, ailing lady, retired in her *hôtel particulier*, a grand townhouse on rue de Berry. Although her terrifying presence could be felt throughout the corridors, I never met her. Marisa, who would go on to become an actress, working for director Luchino Visconti in *Death in Venice*, Stanley Kubrick in *Barry Lyndon*, and sharing the screen with Liza Minnelli in *Cabaret*, had her own side entrance through the garden.

I remember being at that house with Marisa one day when she received an invitation to go to Capri to a fashion weekend called "Mare Moda." She asked me to go with her, but I didn't have the money. When I told her, she plunged into her handbag and gave me a few five-hundred French franc notes to buy my ticket. I will never forget that generosity, nor will I forget that very glamorous fashion weekend on the Mediterranean island. We dressed up eccentrically, stayed out late, laughed a lot, and flirted with attractive young Italian playboys. Marisa was a top model, but, to my surprise, I managed to hold my own.

That weekend turned out to be more than just fun. It was there that I ran into Angelo Ferretti, the flamboyant industrial fashion tycoon whom I had met once before at Egon's house in Cortina with his lovely wife, Lena, and son, Mimmo, the best friend of Egon's younger brother, Sebastian. Ferretti and I had become friends in Cortina, and we were happy to meet again in Capri. After I told him about my work with Koski in Paris, he invited me to come to Como, visit his factories, and learn about his business. It was an intriguing and unexpected offer. Ferretti was on the other side of fashion, the manufacturing side.

He owned two factories in Pare, near Como, Italy: one, a printing plant where he printed intricate colorful scarves for Ferragamo, Gucci, and other large companies; the other, next door, where he produced knitted silk and high-quality mercerized cotton jersey fabric for shirts and T-shirts. A T-shirt seems like the most common thing now, but it was a novelty at the time. Until then, T-shirts were worn as an undergarment, mostly by sailors. But fashion T-shirts became the hot new trend in the late sixties when Brigitte Bardot started to wear those sold at Choses, a boutique in the port of St. Tropez. They came in a variety of colors and had an anchor with the words "St. Tropez" printed around it.

Ferretti was a pioneer in mass-producing his own upscale T-shirts, having converted old World War II silk stocking knitting machines to knit contemporary jersey fabric since silk stockings had been replaced by nylon panty hose. He also came up with the idea of printing on the jersey and using it to make new, bolder T-shirts. He was a genius really. He was also very much an Italian man: handsome, a serious gambler, a bit of a flirt, and great fun.

Ferretti's invitation to learn from him was tempting. "I'll think about it," I told him. Truth was, for all the glamour of Paris, I wanted to go somewhere else. Paris was a mess. The students had gone on strike in the spring of '68 and occupied the Sorbonne, soon followed by the workers who went on a general strike and shut down the airports and train stations. I was the age of the demonstrating students and I sympathized with them, but I must confess that my time crossing the barricades was mostly going to and from Régine's New Jimmy's nightclub on boulevard Montparnasse.

That summer I left Koski and took Ferretti up on his offer, moving in with my mother at her new apartment on rue Pergolèse and commuting back and forth to Italy to watch Ferretti operate and learn from him. Many years later, Koski would come back into my life, as he fell in love with my dear friend the screenwriter and director Danièle Thompson. Every summer, they spend time with Barry and me on our boat.

I see myself as if it were yesterday, sitting behind Ferretti in his printing factory as he is yelling at the colorist who made the yellow too bright or the pink too pale. I see myself sitting behind him at his fabric-knitting factory and he is yelling, yelling, at the engineer who has knitted the jersey fabric too tight or too loose. Always screaming, always passionate about the quality of his printing or the tightness of his jerseys, while I sit behind him watching and learning.

Como was the Italian center of silk and attracted a huge community of illustrators and artists who sold their artwork to the silk manufacturers. Through Ferretti's eyes I learned how certain designs can make good prints, how to create a repeat, and the difference between printing in application on greige or in discharge on a dyed fabric. I learned from his talented colorists how to create a harmonious palette and from him how to negotiate the prices of the designs. I realize today what a supertalent Ferretti was and how lucky I was to sit in with him creating patterns and watching the plain fabric going from screen to screen to screen to become colorful, precise prints.

He also taught me everything about jersey. He showed me how to evaluate the quality and density of the knitted fabric samples when they were brought to him, presentations that usually prompted the most yelling of all. I sat in on passionate meetings with the fiber engineers.

Jersey, I learned, can be knitted with many fibers, usually silk, rayon, cotton, or acrylic. "Mix is the magic, just like in cooking," he used to tell me. He was also a great cook, and his favorite dish was *bollito misto.*

I learned about dyeing and finishing techniques, about using imbibing agents to give the fabric breathability, and why, with certain fibers, the fabric gives or doesn't give. I learned all this and more just by sitting behind him in all the meetings with these talented, skillful technicians who had learned from their families for generations. I thought I was doing nothing, but every single thing I heard, I ended up later putting to use.

Soon after I'd started shadowing him, he bought a new factory near Florence, which was making fine, slinky nightgowns. The factory had excellent equipment and the perfect needles to work on jersey fabrics, and he converted it to manufacture his shirts and T-shirts. From that moment, Manifattura Tessile Ferretti became a vertical operation from fibers to knitting jersey to printing to finished clothes. The conversion of the new factory prompted more yelling, but I'd gotten so used to it I hardly paid any attention. What I did take in was the development of an amazing manufacturing company that would soon have a huge impact on my life.

Many of the things I still do today, I learned from that man. I had no idea that would happen, which is something I always tell young people. "Listen, always listen. Most people at the beginnings of their lives don't know what they want to be unless you have a real vocation, like a pianist or a doctor, so it is very important to listen. Sometimes there are doors that will open and you think it is not an important door and yet it is—so it's very important to be curious and pay attention, because sometimes you learn and you don't even know you're learning."

I spent almost a year with Ferretti, and learned so much, even though I was distracted. I was thinking about Egon and my heart was heavy. I knew Egon was coming home to Europe for the winter holidays and was taking his new Italian girlfriend, not me, to his family's house in Cortina. He was stopping first in Paris and he asked me to arrange a dinner at Maxim's with our Geneva University friends. Although it was a painful evening, I didn't show it. I made a huge effort to be cool, smooth, and funny so Egon wouldn't know how fast my heart was beating as he stared at me from across the table. I was even more depressed because of the fortune-teller I'd been to that afternoon who told me I would be married within a year and traveling far away. What nonsense, I thought. I was in love with Egon and knew I'd lost him.

For all my unhappiness, I refused to mope. I had a life to live, after all, with or without him, so after spending Christmas with my father and Philippe skiing in Crans-sur-Sierre, I went to St. Moritz to join Marisa for the New Year. The Palace Hotel had a habit then, and probably still does, of giving a very special rate to young, pretty girls, and Marisa and I had a fabulous time, skiing, dancing, and laughing day and night. After the New Year, which was also my twenty-second birthday, who showed up but Egon. Without the girlfriend. It took only one night for our love to be rekindled, and with it, an invitation to visit him in New York. My mother gave me the best twenty-second birthday present ever—the airplane ticket—and the journey began toward that little wrap dress.

I stayed in New York only two months but that short time changed my life. I loved the city, I discovered. The people were alive, creative, and ambitious. There were no boundaries; everyone was young, doing interesting things and free of all the suffocating traditions and class distinctions of Europe.

I wanted to stay but I had to find some way to support myself.

Egon suggested I try modeling, which seemed a possibility after I met the famous photographer Francesco Scavullo at a party one night. "Let me photograph you," he said. I remember how nervous I was the next day as Way Bandy, the infamous makeup artist of the time, lined my eyes and added rows of false eyelashes while François, the French hairstylist, piled three hairpieces on my head. I posed topless, the very long hairpieces hiding my breasts. I was astonished with the result. "Could that seductive creature be me?" I wondered. With no hesitation I went to show the photos to the famous, grande dame model agent, the German-born Wilhelmina, expecting her to marvel and invite me to join her beauty stable. Wilhelmina looked quickly at the pictures while inspecting me from head to toe from the corners of her eyes. She was just as quick to coldly announce that I could never be a professional model. At least it was confirmed: Beauty was not what I should pursue as a career.

The busy social life I had with Egon in New York proved to be an important fashion education. Because I was Egon's girlfriend and he was so visible as a young, attractive aristocrat, various designers in New York, like those in Paris, offered me their clothes to wear. I spent time discovering the back rooms of those designers and saw how different the fashion in America was from Europe. In England it was the time of Carnaby Street, Biba, and Ossie Clark, influenced by India and the hippie movement. In France, fashion was more serious with couture and dressmakers leading the way, although in 1966, Yves Saint Laurent had cleverly democratized fashion by creating the first designer ready-to-wear at his Rive Gauche boutiques.

In America, fashion was different because of its large distribution through hundreds of department stores across the country. Seventh Avenue firms were running the show, keeping their designers anonymous. But a clever publicist, Eleanor Lambert, had the idea of bringing those designers out of the back rooms and into the spotlight. She created the Council of Fashion Designers of America and Bill Blass, Anne Klein, Geoffrey Beene, and Oscar de la Renta became celebrities. I fell in love with the new breed of designers—Giorgio Sant'Angelo, Stephen Burrows, Halston—who used soft fabrics, jersey, and bright colors. All that inspired me no end and as I left New York to return to Ferretti, I was excited, hoping I could learn more and one day create some things on my own to sell in New York.

I looked at all of Ferretti's resources with a different set of eyes when I went back to Como. He was extremely successful at making tens of thousands of silk scarves and jersey tops, but I believed more could be done with the incredible infrastructure he had built. The innovative uses of jersey I had seen in designs from Giorgio Sant'Angelo and Stephen Burrows inspired me, and an idea began to percolate in my mind. I wanted to try and make some dresses in the Ferretti printed fabric. I was drawn to the opportunity of filling the void I had seen in New York between the high-fashion hippie clothes and the stale, double-knit dresses. Maybe I could fill it with an offering of colorfully printed sexy easy jersey dresses.

I started to spend lots of time at the factory outside Florence and became friends with Bruna, the patternmaker. Together we made my first dresses: a T-shirt dress, a shirtdress, a long tented dress, and a long tunic with pants. We used whatever printed fabric was leftover in her sample room. Then, on my days in the Como factory, I spent hours going through Ferretti's archival prints, choosing some and begging Rita, Ferretti's right hand, to print some sample yardage for me.

The family had adopted me and I felt very much at home with them. Ferretti's son, Mimmo, was around a lot and he helped me, too.

We had fun working together. The Tuscan countryside around the factory was lovely and Mimmo and I used to have some great meals in the neighboring villages. Ferretti was encouraging and allowed me to carve out a small corner for myself in their sample room. Even though I was cautious, I knew it was disruptive. I now realize he must have seen in me some potential I didn't yet see in myself. He also introduced me to his tailor in Milan, and with him I started to drape some fancy evening clothes, but I was more comfortable in the factory working with Bruna on simple little dresses.

I don't know what my future would have been without the generosity and support of Ferretti. I was still working at the factory when I got pregnant and my life changed drastically. With my accelerated marriage to Egon, the dream I had of a career in fashion also accelerated. The only person that could help make that dream come true was Ferretti.

"This is what's happening," I said to him on a short trip to the factory in the midst of the wedding preparations. "I am pregnant, I'm getting married to Egon, and I'm moving to America. Please allow me to complete all the samples I have been working on and let me try to sell them in New York." Ferretti smiled and his response was more than I could have dreamed: "Go ahead. I believe in you and I think you will be successful."

I put a sample line together, most of it made with Bruna in Ferretti's printed jersey, except a few velvet dresses made by the tailor in Milan. All the clothes had easy shapes, were sexy in their simplicity, and packable for sure. One hundred dresses folded in a single bag. I was at another door to my would-be career. I could only hope it would open.

Egon and I married on a beautiful, sunny day, three weeks after his twenty-third birthday. I love the photo of us laughing and smiling under a shower of rice as we exited the town hall in Montfort-l'Amaury. It was taken by Berry Berenson, a young photographer and Marisa's sister, who later married actor Tony Perkins and was tragically killed on 9/11 aboard the first plane that crashed into the World Trade Center. That exuberant photo reminds me not only of our wedding day and of beautiful Berry, but right behind us, out of the five hundred guests, is Ferretti! There, in one happy image, are the two most important men in my life at the time, though I didn't know yet just how important Ferretti would be.

After a short honeymoon sailing the fjords of Norway and a great month with our friends at Liscia di Vacca on Sardinia's Costa Smeralda, I picked up my samples from the factory in Tuscany.

As I boarded the Italian liner *Raffaello,* I carried all of my hopes with me: the baby in my womb, and that suitcase filled with dresses. Egon had gone by plane weeks before but I insisted on sailing. I wanted to take the time to visualize my new life and arrive slowly in New York Harbor, past the Statue of Liberty, like any immigrant with an American dream. I had no idea how quickly that dream would come true.

When young people eager to start their own lives and careers ask me for advice I smile and always say: "Passion and persistence are what matter. Dreams are achievable and you can make your fantasy come true, but there are no shortcuts. Nothing happens without hard work."

That advice is the essence of my journey with the little dresses when I arrived in New York. Egon would go off in the morning to his new job at the Lazard Frères investment bank and, greatly pregnant and with my dream in place, I'd struggle out of the apartment with my suitcase full of clothes to make the rounds of department stores and centralized buying offices. The people I met were amused and intrigued by the unorthodox presentation of little jersey dresses pulled out of a Vuitton suitcase by a young, pregnant European princess, but it did not materialize into anything. I persevered, though, especially after the birth of Alexandre.

The door that opened two months later, in March 1970, was the most critical one in New York: that of Diana Vreeland, the intimidating, all-powerful dragon lady editor in chief of *Vogue*. It seems amazing to me now that I had the audacity to enter her fashion shrine and show her such simple little dresses. I had the advantage, of course, of having social status, but my youthful confidence is what made me push open that door. Diana Vreeland? Why not? And that was the beginning.

It was Diana Vreeland who first understood and appreciated the simple uniqueness of the jersey fabric and the easy, flattering fit of the dresses. They may have looked like nothing on hangers, but the dresses looked strikingly sexy and feminine when she put them on two of her in-house models, Pat Cleveland and Loulou de la Falaise, both of whom later became my friends. "How incredibly clever of you, and how modern this is," Mrs. Vreeland told me, ending our brief meeting with "Terrific, terrific, terrific." And along with my suitcase I was back out that door and facing another.

I opened that one, too, with the assistance of Kezia Keeble, one of Diana Vreeland's young and beautiful fashion editors. I had no idea what to do next as I folded my dresses back into the suitcase outside Mrs. Vreeland's office, so I asked Kezia. "Take a room at the Gotham Hotel on Fifth Avenue during fashion week. The California fashion companies show there. There will be a traffic flow of buyers around," she told me. "List yourself on the Fashion Calendar and put an announcement in *Women's Wear Daily*." I didn't hesitate. "Can I use your phone?" I asked as I sat at Kezia's desk.

I settled in a room at the Gotham Hotel and spent the first long days waiting for buyers. I had previously done some interviews and those early articles said much more about me being a socialite princess than the clothes I was showing, which, at first, I found frustrating. But that publicity prompted curiosity. Traffic picked up after several early articles in *Women's Wear Daily,* the *New York Post,* and the *New York Times.*

I was so excited to write the first order from a little boutique in New Jersey on my freshly printed custom order forms. Sales really began to gain traction the next season at the Gotham Hotel after my dresses appeared in *Vogue.* I remember large orders from Hutzler's, a department store in Baltimore, and Giorgio's, the fashionable boutique in Beverly Hills. Then Bloomingdale's came in. Their five-person team took over the room, discussing windows and advertising. I was overwhelmed. Not only was my English still a bit shaky; I understood nothing of the rag trade jargon.

Those early years were difficult for many reasons. On one side Ferretti was not easy to deal with. My first orders of a few dozen dresses in a specific style was not what he had expected. "I have a factory, not a sample room," he insisted. Flying to Italy once a month, I would beg for his attention. He would yell. I would cry. "Stick with me," I kept pleading with him. When my orders were finally delivered they were often wrong—wrong color, wrong style, wrong size, wrong everything, yet whatever I shipped to the stores would sell immediately. That is what encouraged me to persevere.

I was totally on my own, with no experience, and the challenges were enormous. I remember Air India's freezing warehouse at Kennedy Airport, where, sitting on the floor sorting out a new shipment from Italy, I had to cross out all the labels written in Italian and rewrite them in English. I can see myself crying from the cold and exhaustion, but now, of course, that experience has become a fond memory. So has the way I stored the folded dresses in our dining room and shipped all the orders myself, while also handling the invoices.

My very first print was the chain link print, a black-and-white geometric design made in a button-down shirtdress that I wore sitting on a cube for the first announcement in *Women's Wear Daily* in 1970. In 2009, Michelle Obama, as the new First Lady, wore that same print I reissued in a slightly larger scale on a wrap dress for the Obamas' first official White House Christmas card. What a lovely surprise! Decades after I introduced the chain link print, it was still relevant, making it truly timeless. At the time I designed it, however, timeless had a different meaning. During those same first two years of my new business, I also had two babies. To say I was busy is a huge understatement.

It was really getting to be too much to do by myself. I could not keep running the business out of my apartment, so I took a tiny two-room office on West Fifty-Fifth Street that became a showroom, a warehouse, and an office all in one. Olivier, my best friend from Geneva who was now a photographer, would come in and help with buyers. I tried to convince some large Seventh Avenue houses to distribute the dresses. One after another turned me down. "These boutiquey little dresses could never sell in large enough volume" became the constant refrain. That door remained closed to me, but another far more important door opened when I met Johnny Pomerantz, the sympathetic son of one of those Seventh Avenue businessmen, who told me all I needed was a showroom on Seventh Avenue and a salesman.

I was twenty-five, in business alone in a new country, and totally inexperienced in the ways of the garment trade. "I don't know any salesmen," I told Johnny. "Call me in a few days," he replied. And so

Dick Conrad, a thirty-nine-year-old salesman with lots of experience who was searching for a new business to run, came into my life. He took a gamble and agreed to join me if I gave him $300 a week and 25 percent of my company. I could find the weekly amount and 25 percent of nothing is nothing, so we struck a deal. I put $750 into our new company, Dick put $250, and I signed a lease for a showroom on Seventh Avenue. We were in business!

I made a few men's shirts for Dick to wear in Ferretti's jersey so that he could experience and understand the uniqueness of the fabric. He did. Dick knew all the best buyers in the specialty stores and better department stores across the country and he called them all. They all came into our new showroom at 530 Seventh Avenue and bought. By the end of 1972, our wholesale revenues were $1.2 million.

Though Ferretti remained very difficult to work with, he generously financed us by allowing a long-term credit of 120 days so we had time to ship and get paid by our customers before paying him. Before we agreed to those terms, at one point we got so far behind I went to a pawnshop across the street from the New York Public Library and pawned the diamond ring Egon and my father had given me when Tatiana was born. (I bought it back four weeks later at enormous interest.)

First there was the simple, perfect T-shirt dress; my favorite, the shirtdress; and a very popular tent dress that came in long and short lengths. Then came a little wrap top, somewhat like the top ballerinas wear to practice, which I designed with a matching skirt. It sold out immediately. The ultimate breakthrough came when I saw Julie Nixon Eisenhower wearing the wrap top and skirt on TV speaking in defense of her father, President Richard Nixon, during the Watergate scandal. "Why not combine the top and the skirt into a dress?" I mused. And the concept for the wrap dress was born.

It wasn't easy to figure it out at first. I wanted to keep the wide belt of the top to keep the waist small, I wanted the skirt to be bias cut, the neckline low enough to be sexy but high enough to be proper, and I wanted a strong collar and cuffs, just like the original top. Bruna and I spent many hours at the factory outside Florence standing around the cutting table playing with paper patterns, figuring out the puzzle. Sue Feinberg, an Italian-trained American designer, worked with us, too. I'd hired her to oversee the production and design at Ferretti's factory. She and I used to spend half of our time naked, wrapping and unwrapping ourselves in dresses as they came off the table to check the fit. Finally, one did.

T/72—that was the number assigned to the first Diane von Furstenberg wrap dress produced in 1974. Forty years later, the dress is still alive. Wrap dresses had existed before, of course. A wrap is a very classical shape: a dress that closes itself without buttons or zippers, like a kimono. But this wrap was different because it was made of jersey. The fabric molded to the body in the most flattering way, and was incredibly soft and comfortable while at the same time tight enough to fit the body like a second skin.

The wrap dress made its debut in 1974 at a fashion show Egon and I, who had separated by this time, shared at the Pierre Hotel. (Egon had left the bank wanting to be a menswear designer and was showing a line of shirts he had designed also out of Ferretti's material.) For the wrap dresses I had chosen two animal prints: snakeskin and leopard. I wanted women to feel sexy, slinky, and feline in the dress and they obviously did. The wrap dresses and the animal prints took off like a stampede, and soon could be seen on the streets of cities all over America. Thanks to the little wrap dress, the business multiplied sevenfold.

Ferretti was very happy, of course; by the end of 1975, production had escalated to over fifteen thousand dresses per week. His factory near Florence was working for us in full capacity. Ferretti had believed in me and I had more than fulfilled his expectations. Over five years, I gave him $35 million in orders.

All of this without a business plan, without any market analysis, without a focus group, without a publicist, without an advertising or branding agency. What I did have was a very good idea, a talented manufacturer who was passionate about his product, and an ambitious salesman who believed in me and sent me all over the country to make personal appearances at different department stores. The stores loved promoting the arrival of a real, live, young princess who was designing easy, sexy dresses that most women could afford. I plunged into the fitting rooms to show the women how to tie the wrap and feel confident about their bodies and themselves.

But it went further. As I was watching women become more confident and beautiful thanks to these new dresses, I was personally becoming more and more confident and, therefore, feeling more beautiful myself. I was projecting what I was selling—ease and confidence. I was becoming one with the dresses and what they stood for. I did not know it then, but I had become a brand.

The pace of growth was dizzying. Suddenly I had close to a hundred people on the payroll, including the staff at the warehouse I'd had to rent on Tenth Avenue to house all the thousands of dresses arriving from Italy. That one little wrap dress had taken the world by storm and I was running behind it as fast as I could. Opportunities were coming in left and right, and as I was young, inexperienced, and not equipped to assess them all, I had very little way to discriminate and decide what offers to choose and for what purpose.

When various entrepreneurs started approaching me as early as 1973 to "license" my name and use my designs to put on their products, I didn't even know what that word meant. They were varied: a mom-and-pop silk scarf company, a Seventh Avenue veteran who wanted to sell shirts made out of Ferretti's fabric, a small luggage company owner who wanted to put my name on a new line of totes, a clever entrepreneur who decided to get into eyewear. I signed contract after contract until my name was on seventeen product categories. By the end of 1976, the licenses were worth more than $100 million in sales. I was twenty-nine.

Everything I touched seemed to turn to gold, including a cosmetics line I started with a friend simply because I loved cosmetics. The idea began to form after I lost all my makeup on one of my trips and went to replace it in an emergency, only to find that makeup lines in department stores looked and smelled old. They were very serious and not fun or relevant to the new, playful fashion mood. "If I dress women so successfully," I said to myself, "why could I not create colorful makeup they could play with that would make them even more beautiful?"

The makeup I was personally using and loved was the professional stage makeup sold at the Make-Up-Center a block from my first office. The little pots of reds, lavenders, turquoises, and purples were irresistible to me and I used to buy all the colors they had. I loved sitting on the big square sink in my bathroom with my feet in the basin to be close to the mirror and play with my face. I had a good face for makeup: lots of eyelid and strong cheekbones. I loved applying the makeup on others, too, and I got good at it.

The idea of turning that passion into a business was solidified in an unexpected way. I was in Los Angeles, staying at the Beverly Wilshire hotel. At the time I was having a mini fling with the movie star Ryan O'Neal. He had come to my room to pick me up for dinner and he teased me about the quantity of makeup I had in my bathroom. "Why do you need all this stuff?" he asked. He may have been a big movie star and I a starstruck young girl, but I could not let his condescension go unanswered. "I don't need it. I just like it," I replied. But when he persisted in patronizing me in that arrogant way, I came up with a boastful reaction. "I'm thinking of buying the company," I said. It was a bluff, of course, but right at that moment I decided to create my own makeup line and go into the beauty business.

It was a ridiculous caper, for sure. As much as I loved cosmetics, I knew nothing about the business. Neither did my friend Sylvie Chantecaille, who had just moved from Paris with her husband, Olivier, and a newborn baby, and was looking for something to do. Sylvie, too, loved cosmetics (she now has a very successful line of her own with her daughter, the grown-up baby Olivia, who I remember learning to walk amongst pots of makeup and creams), so we set out to learn what we needed to do, visiting laboratories and talking to experienced product developers. "You have to create a fragrance," we kept hearing. "That's where the money is."

I had no idea how to do that, so I hired someone who did, Bob Loeb, a beauty business consultant, and the three of us developed my first scent, a light, lovely fragrance named Tatiana after my four-year-old daughter. Tatiana's scent was a wonderful bouquet of white flowers . . . gardenia, honeysuckle, and jasmine. To introduce it, we sent out thousands of free samples by attaching a packet of the scent to the hangtag of the dresses I was shipping all over the country. Tatiana not only quickly became very popular when we officially launched it in

1975, but inspired a generation of new floral fragrances such as Revlon's Charlie, among others.

In the midst of perfecting Tatiana and developing a cosmetics line, I started researching and writing my first book: *Diane von Furstenberg's Book of Beauty: How to Become a More Attractive, Confident and Sensual Woman.* It was bold of me to feel I could dispense that advice at the age of twenty-eight, but wherever I went people wanted to know how I lived, what I ate, what I did for exercise, what makeup I wore. They wanted to know my secrets, so I decided to write the book. I didn't really think I had any secrets, but those questions made me think about the subject of beauty.

I had an ulterior motive as well. I wanted to learn all I could about the business of beauty. Researching for the book, I talked to many experts about nutrition, hair treatment, skin cleansing, exercise, cosmetics—everything to do with beauty. Evelyn Portrait, Bob Loeb's lovely wife, helped me with the research and the book did very well when it was published in 1976.

We officially launched our cosmetics line at the end of 1975 at a small salon I opened on Madison Avenue. I wanted women to have the same fun I did sitting on my bathroom sink and playing with makeup, so in my little store on Madison Avenue (real estate was cheap at the time), I installed four little bars and stools in the front room where women could experiment with testers. The boutique was my version of the Make-Up-Center, and I loved it. So did the women who came in unsure how best to use makeup, and left with lots of products and a personalized chart after a session with Nicholas, our professional makeup artist. Women wore a lot of makeup in the seventies, so our timing was just right.

I was happy with my tiny makeup venture—Sylvie and I did

it on a small budget, using stock packaging and working out of my apartment—and was a bit reticent to grow it beyond my shop on Madison Avenue. I was finally persuaded by the legendary Marvin Traub at Bloomingdale's to open my own cosmetics counter there and to go national. I was very involved with the dresses and my licenses and committing to Bloomingdale's would mean more salespeople, advertising costs, and a lot of my time, of which I had none. But I had fantasized about joining the ranks of such pioneers as Helena Rubinstein, Elizabeth Arden, and Estée Lauder, and did it anyway. It was a blast.

I went on the road with Gigi Williams, a makeup artist and hilarious travel companion, to promote the cosmetics and the dresses, as well as the publication of my beauty book. Gigi was hip and cute, a true downtown little girl with early piercings who was married to artist Ronnie Cutrone, Andy Warhol's favorite assistant. Gigi and I felt like rock stars touring the country, doing interviews at local news stations and visiting all the stores where long lines of women were patiently waiting for makeup applications. We loved doing those makeovers and making women feel more secure with a little eye shadow, a little highlight on the cheekbones, and, equally as important, a little pep talk (and of course a spray of Tatiana perfume).

More and more I was realizing from my conversations with women how many had insecurities. By listening to their insecurities and sharing my own, we all felt stronger. It was an authentic dialogue, a very even give and get. The stronger I became, the stronger I wanted others to be. I realize now that it was at that time, as I was feeling stronger, that my desire to empower women started, a desire that exists to this day, more and more.

Back then, however, my main goal was to be free and independent. I was constantly on the go. I loved being that woman high on her heels walking in and out of places like a tornado, taking planes as if they were buses, feeling pragmatic, engaged, and sexy. I loved the idea of being a young tycooness who smiles at her shadow and winks at herself in the mirror. I loved having a man's life in a woman's body. In a sense I had become the woman I wanted to be, and it was then, at twenty-eight, that I met Barry and we fell in love. He, too, was a young tycoon, barely thirty-three. We both were living an American Dream, separately and together.

My wrap dress had become the "it" dress and I had become a celebrity. I was identified with all my products and was the model for them, all that in no time at all. I had succeeded beyond my wildest dreams.

Even the staid *Wall Street Journal* took notice and on January 28, 1976, ran a feature about my "fashion empire" on the front page. I was beyond proud of myself that morning as I took a very early flight to Cleveland for a personal appearance (having young children, I tried to stay home with them at night and fly early in the morning). There were almost no women on that flight. I sat next to a businessman with my pile of magazines and newspapers on my lap. The *Wall Street Journal* was on top. After a few minutes of staring at me and my legs, huffing and puffing, trying to figure out how to start a conversation, the man asked, "What's a pretty girl like you doing reading the *Wall Street Journal?*"

I looked at him, but said nothing. I could have shown him my front-page story, but it seemed too easy, and to this day, the fact that I did not remains one of the best personal satisfactions I've ever had. I kept my triumph to myself. Though of course I have told that story so many times since that I have more than exploited this poor guy's chauvinist attitude, which was so common at the time.

Exposure attracts exposure and two months later, I was on the cover of *Newsweek*. That was a very big deal in those days before CNN and the Internet. President Gerald Ford had been slated for the cover, having just won the Republican presidential primary, his first since replacing Richard Nixon in the White House, but the editors must have thought I'd make a more appealing sell and decided to put me on the cover instead. When an urgent call came from *Newsweek*, I snatched one of my favorite green-and-white jersey shirtdresses off the rack and raced over to Scavullo's studio, where he squeezed me in for the photo in the midst of a cover shoot for *Cosmopolitan*.

The *Newsweek* cover ended any anonymity I might have had, which, at first, I found intimidating. I'd been invited to the White House just before the cover ran by Luis Estévez, the Cuban-born California designer who made First Lady Betty Ford's clothes. It was my first visit, so you can imagine my amazement to find myself seated at President Ford's table and joking with the president about *Newsweek* choosing me for the cover over him! It all seemed unbelievable, especially when Henry Kissinger introduced himself to me as if I wouldn't recognize him. He subsequently became a good friend and after he and his wife Nancy bought a home near me in Connecticut we often had dinner together.

We all know the value of publicity, but the *Newsweek* cover launched a tsunami. The story spiked sales of the dresses, with more stores fighting for them, and brought me a whole new and very profitable line of work: home design.

There is an energy and an audacity that comes with youth. Older people often find this unchecked spirit uninformed and irritating, and are surprised when that spirit triumphs. And so it was with me and Sears, Roebuck. I'd been approached shortly after the *Newsweek* cover by a bedspread manufacturer who wanted to put my name on the bedspreads he was making for Sears. Bedspreads? I thought. Why stop at bedspreads? At the time, Sears was a very powerful company with many stores and a large catalog on everyone's kitchen counter. They had enormous advertising power and would take out eight- to ten-page magazine ads showing an entire house. Why not give the Sears customers the choice of more interesting home products? Mine.

I put together some sketches and flew to Chicago to see the all-powerful Charles Moran, the head of Sears's huge home furnishing division, which did about $1 billion a year in sales. My mother often reminded me of that day when I left the apartment at six a.m. carrying a huge folder with my presentation. I think even she was impressed by my drive and energy.

I can see myself now in that boardroom with a lot of white, middle-aged midwestern men glancing at my sketches and staring at this strange creature from New York with masses of curly hair, a foreign accent, and a lot of leg trying to sell herself to design home furnishings for Middle America. I can only imagine what they were thinking when, in response to Moran's question of what I wanted in compensation for my work, I said I wouldn't do it for less than half a million dollars. That was an unheard-of amount in those days, but I was young and bold. As weeks passed I became afraid I'd pushed too far, but then I got the call that they had accepted my proposal. What I did not know was that when I signed the contract with Sears I broke a taboo. If you sold to upper-tier stores like Neiman Marcus and Saks you were not supposed to also sell to a mass merchant like Sears. But because my dresses were so hot in department stores, I managed to get away with it.

For the third time I set up a studio in my apartment and hired Marita, a young girl with great taste, to help me design what was in essence a private label line for Sears, The Diane von Furstenberg Style for Living Collection, which quickly grew beyond sheets and towels into curtains, tableware, rugs—eventually even furniture. It was a lot of hard work designing and color-coordinating the different products, then presenting them to the legions of Sears buyers in different categories, and I soon hired an experienced textile designer couple, Peter and Christine d'Ascoli, to manage the Sears collection. It was well worth it. In the seven years I worked with Sears, retail sales of my home furnishings line grew to $100 million a year.

No wonder I call this phase of my business The American Dream. Even I find it hard to believe, as I write this, what I achieved in so little time. In less than five years, I'd gone from a little European girl determined to support herself to achieving success that far exceeded that dream. I was only twenty-seven when I bought Cloudwalk, twenty-nine when I was on the cover of *Newsweek*, barely thirty when I bought a huge apartment on Fifth Avenue as a birthday present to myself.

There was a price for my success, of course. I always felt I had to run faster and faster just to keep up with the business, which filled me with anxiety. The anxiety proved to be justified when the American Dream turned into a nightmare.

I saw it coming, but my partner didn't listen to me. Neither did my lawyer, my accountant, or Ferretti, for that matter. I was the one on the road making personal appearances, noticing the racks and racks of the printed jersey dresses in one department store and the racks and racks of the same dresses in the department store across the street. They, on the other hand, looked at the avalanche of orders after the *Newsweek* cover and supported the decision to up the production at Ferretti's factories, all wrap dresses: blue and white, red and white, green and white! Women all over the country had at least two, five, sometimes ten of those dresses, if not more, already hanging in their closets—and the market for them crashed.

I remember that Sunday in January 1978 when every department store in the city took a full page in the *New York Times* advertising the wrap dress on sale. I was so used to seeing the dress advertised that I wasn't particularly alarmed. I didn't realize the negative impact until the next day, a snowy Monday, when *Women's Wear Daily* announced that the market for my little dresses was "saturated," that the sales marked the "end of a trend." The dresses were still hot with the public, but overnight the market for new sales collapsed in department stores across the country. I was close to panic. Orders plummeted and I faced $4 million of dead inventory. What to do? The only thing I could think of was to immediately stop the twenty-five thousand new wrap dresses Ferretti was making each week. He was furious with me, but I had no choice. My company was on the verge of bankruptcy. I was in shock.

I felt even then, and know now for sure, that we had done it to ourselves. We had behaved like amateurs on a runaway horse. My instincts to diversify the offerings and expand from just making wrap dresses had been ignored when I reported seeing the glut on the market. That little dress was everywhere. I wanted to expand the dress into a collection, a wardrobe, but my associates didn't consider that the demand would ever end. I should have been more forceful in cutting back the orders after the *Newsweek* cover.

I separated with Dick Conrad, paying him $1 million for his 25 percent share of the company, hired a new president, replaced the lawyer and accountant who had ill advised me. I was now chairman, sole owner, and head designer of Diane von Furstenberg, Ltd. So it was I who received the letter from Roy Cohn, the most feared lawyer in America who had been Senator Joseph McCarthy's right hand. Ferretti had hired him to sue me. My heart stopped, but I didn't show my fear. I called Roy Cohn and screamed bluffs: "With all the things I know about Ferretti, I don't think you want to go after me," I threatened. Then I hung up. My bluff worked. I never heard from him again.

But I still had a huge inventory and an even bigger knot in my stomach. Barry was looking at my numbers and looking for a solution. He was incredibly supportive but knew nothing about the fashion business.

The good thing was that success had made me into a household name. The Seventh Avenue companies that had snubbed me a few years before were suddenly all interested in buying my business. It was another flamboyant fashion person who appeared in my life and saved me. I think of Carl Rosen as the "Seventh Avenue Ferretti": passionate and visionary. Carl had just made a deal with Calvin Klein to make a line of jeans. Now he wanted to sign a license with me to make Diane von Furstenberg dresses. Not only would he buy and dispose of my inventory, but he would run the business and pay me a royalty with a guaranteed minimum of $1 million a year. Barry negotiated the deal. Barry is known to be a tough negotiator but so was Carl. They went on for days. Only recently, Barry confessed to me that at one point he had pushed so far he thought he had blown it and that Carl would walk out. But he didn't.

Once again, my mother's credo proved true: What had seemed the worst, turned out to be good. I had managed not only to get rid of a terrible liability but also to work out a profitable arrangement.

My American Dream was still alive and well as I moved forward. Again, I drew on my mother. "If one door closes, another will open," she would say—and it did. My beauty line. It had done very well since I'd launched it in 1975, especially Tatiana, the fragrance, but with the dress business no longer my responsibility, I could now concentrate on taking the beauty line to new heights. Without a moment of nostalgia I got rid of my showroom in the garment district and moved uptown to glamorous offices on Fifty-Seventh Street and Fifth Avenue, in the heart of the cosmetics world. I leased the entire twenty-fourth floor in the old, art deco Squibb building at 745 Fifth Avenue with a view of Central Park and Revlon and Estée Lauder right across the street. I converted what the prior tenant had used as a storeroom into my private, airy, pink office with a terrace. I felt happy and on top of the world!

Since I was chairman and sole owner of the company, it was mine to make or break. I did not think much about funding the beauty business. All my licenses, including the dresses and my home furnishings for Sears, reached $150 million in sales and provided a large income.

My new president was Sheppard Zinovoy, and I hired a professional beauty salesman, Gary Savage, whom I lured from Pierre Cardin fragrance. A ravishing girl, Janet Chin, joined me as a product development person and I even built a state-of-the-art laboratory in the office that was run by an Italian chemist called Gianni Mosca. It all felt very serious when I put on a white coat to enter the lab and test the samples he and his assistant developed, and for me it was a dream come true.

Without the dress business I had the time to play with colors and textures and packaging design. In the seventies we all wore lots of very bright makeup and I had so much fun working with Janet creating and naming the colors and designing the packaging. At Gary's suggestion we named the line "The Color Authority," and indeed it was. I was proud, not annoyed, that other cosmetics companies, from Revlon to Estée Lauder, bought and copied our new colors the instant we released them. To me, anyway, imitation is the sincerest form of flattery. We redesigned the packaging. No more inexpensive stock packaging for us, but a lovely marbleized white plastic compact that looked like mother-of-pearl with my signature in gold. I've always said that makeup is the secret between women and their mirrors, and that makeup is a reflection of our moods. To that end we created compacts that incorporated all the colors you needed, divided into three different moods: Hot Passion Pinks, for a feminine, flirtatious mood; Stop Traffic Red, for strength and authority; and New Wave Metallics, for the browns of more neutral and quiet moods.

As the cosmetics line grew, so did the volume of different bottles, boxes, and caps, which we had to keep stored in a warehouse. It was déjà vu with the inventory of dresses, right down to the multitude of warehouse staff we needed to manage it all. Each product had its own packaging with its own list of ingredients. The many colors we had so much fun creating required their own labels with their own lists of ingredients. On and on. Overseeing and maintaining the line was very expensive.

For all that we loved working on the color line and the attention and success that greeted it, as we had been advised, it was Tatiana, in a new bottle custom designed by sculptor Serge Mansau, that was making the money and we expanded the fragrance into a whole line of bath products.

I also started to conceive of a new perfume. I wanted something very special with a strong scent, a unique bottle, and a passionate message. I called it Volcan d'Amour (Volcano of Love). Since it had been inspired by my Bali days with Paulo, I dedicated it to him.

I went all out with that fragrance, commissioning a magician-turned-designer friend, Dakota Jackson, to create a unique and expensive bottle, and commissioning another friend, Brazilian artist Antonio Peticov, to design the box it came in. Bloomingdale's and

Saks fought for the launch, which was an over-the-top event I staged in my office with pyramids of fresh frangipani I'd shipped from Hawaii to symbolize the offerings to the volcanoes of Bali. From the office we descended Fifth Avenue to Saks, where I dressed the models in blue sarongs I had designed and had had hand-painted with gold volcanoes at the Denpasar market.

What was I thinking? Yes, the company was doing very well. By 1981 we had gross sales of $40 million, but our expenses were enormous. The payroll for over three hundred employees was $1 million a month!

I began to feel tense about meeting that payroll and about the ever-growing inventory of bottles and tops and boxes. The sleepless nights I'd experienced from the panic of failure in 1977 were returning in 1982 because of the speed of our success. As the demand grew, I had to invest more and more money in inventory and a support system of staff and marketing. I was worried we were growing too rapidly again.

I know now, of course, that I should have read the huge, heavy financial reports that Gary Savage and Shep Zinovoy dutifully gave me every week, but I didn't. In my mind, they were in charge of the company's finances. I was the creative end of the operation.

Money, in fact, was the furthest thing from my mind as I explored the islands of Indonesia with Paolo to come up with promotional material for Volcan d'Amour. I trusted the men in New York to manage the money. I had no idea how overextended we were.

The end came as rapidly as that snowy January day when all my dresses suddenly went on sale. This time I was in Paris with Paolo when I got a call from Shep to tell me that I had to come back to sign a personal note of guarantee, and that Chemical Bank was refusing to lend any more money until I did. A personal note? That could mean the loss of Cloudwalk, the loss of my apartment. No way was I going to risk that.

The enormity of the crisis became clear when I got back. Ten million dollars!—that's how much the company owed the bank. I had no idea that we had been borrowing so much money to cover our operating expenses. I'd never read the financial printouts. The only way out was to sell the company. "If you can," the wretched little banker said.

It took months for me to negotiate a deal that could release me from the bank: a sale to Beecham, the big English pharmaceutical company that had started the process of accumulating small cosmetics companies to become a player in the industry. In New York, I felt the bank closing in as I poured my efforts and even more resources into the newly launched fragrance, Volcan d'Amour. But in London, I remember feeling so grown up in my suite at Claridge's hotel, talking with the chairman of Beecham about the future of my business.

To this day, Claridge's is my favorite hotel in the world and I was flattered when they asked me to redecorate a few suites for them in 2010 and make them sexy, luxurious, and glamorous. They were very happy with the result, and the suites have been booked solid ever since. When I see my photo hanging in their lobby, with Winston Churchill and Jackie Kennedy, I am immediately reminded how important I felt staying there, in spite of my panic over the looming debt back home.

The agreement I finally reached with Beecham was a great one. They raised their original offer to $22 million, plus royalties and a large annual consulting fee. I was ecstatic. The nasty banker got his money and I was still $12 million ahead. "Celebration," I wrote in my diary. "I feel free, rich and relieved." But I also felt sad. I'd sold something that really had spirit and was really strong. But I'd had no choice.

And so it was that the first phase of my business life—the American Dream—began to wind down. I'd accomplished more than I could ever have imagined and was extremely proud of the products I'd created. I'd built two companies and sold two companies. I'd more than achieved my goal of financial independence. I could retire, travel the world, and my children would always be secure.

On the one hand, it was liberating. I was thirty-six and for the first time in thirteen years I didn't have the pressure of running a company, and I was excited about that. On the other hand, I felt empty. What I realized later is that I had very little say in the design, quality, and most importantly distribution of the many licensed products. Little by little, the simple dress I'd made had disappeared. In the hands of Carl Rosen, his company Puritan, and the 1980s, the dresses were given shoulder pads and lost their identity as I had lost control. My name was on so many products, but I wasn't designing anymore; I had lost my creative outlet.

I missed that and realized how powerfully I missed it soon after the sale to Beecham when I went to A La Vieille Russie, a wonderful antique store in the Sherry-Netherland hotel, to buy myself a celebratory gift of jewelry. (I often buy jewelry to mark special moments. It signifies a commitment to myself—a ring, for example, when I break up with a man.) This time, while I was buying a beautiful set of aquamarine jewelry, I saw an empty shop for rent across the lobby. I decided to take it and, voilà. Briefly, at least, the American Dream was reignited.

My instincts told me that the elegant Sherry-Netherland on the corner of Fifty-Ninth Street and Fifth Avenue was a perfect location for a very upscale collection I could create for the extravagant eighties. The Carters had left the cloth-coat White House. The Reagans had moved in, complete with Mrs. Reagan's furs and designer clothes.

Millions of people were watching *Dynasty* and *Dallas* on television, and fashion and style changed enormously. The big hairdo and the big shoulder pads were in, as was Donald Trump and a lot of new money. It was not the New York I had fallen in love with, but I thought I could capitalize on the new extravagance and create something new of my own.

I commissioned the well-known architect Michael Graves to design what would be his first retail store. It seems crazy to me now that while he was converting the shop into a beautiful space I didn't even know what clothes I was going to put in it! Once again my impulsiveness had taken over. There wasn't a business plan at all, just a vision of creating couture-like clothes in exquisite fabrics. I thought an expensive, high-end line would strengthen the value of my name, and therefore help the other licensed products over which I had no control.

I hired a talented young Frenchman, Stephan Janson, to help me design this new line and Olivier Gelbsmann to manage the store. I called both the store and the new line by my first name only, Diane, and the first collection was exquisite. We used the most precious and expensive fabrics—silks from Italy, laces from France, cashmere from Scotland—and created elegant ball gowns and other eveningwear. I had lots of money from the Beecham sale, so I didn't need to skimp on anything, including the advertising introducing Diane in 1984. Image is all-important in couture. The clothes have to project high fashion, elegance, and be aspirational, so I hired Helmut Newton, the famous German photographer known for his strong erotic photographs, to shoot the campaign. I had always dreamt of being photographed by him and he loved the idea of using me as a model. We shot in an art deco mansion in the South of France and had a great time. They were beautiful images, which I treasure to this day—me in various Diane ball gowns and in my favorite, a black tuxedo with a veil over my eyes.

The early signs about Diane were very encouraging. An expensive ball gown of pink silk and black lace was bought over the phone and so were the rich tuxedos and evening pajamas. Brooke Shields, Bianca Jagger, and Ivana Trump were among my early enthusiastic customers. It all felt exciting.

The clothes were well made, beautiful, and absolutely right for the time, but looking back, I didn't really like that period in fashion. Nothing felt right. New York of the mideighties was not the same New York that had seduced me in the early seventies, and my personal life was also changing. My children had gone off to boarding schools and, emotionally, I needed something new.

Alain Elkann landed in my life at that very moment—an intelligent, attractive, needy artist in search of his own identity as a writer, as a man, and as a father to his three children. Rather than being excited about building yet another business, I was drawn to being Alain's muse and his partner in life.

I was drawn by the change in Europe, as well. There was the promise of a unified Europe that excited me. I bought lots of blue European Union flags with their twelve stars and displayed them all over my apartment. Newly elected French president François Mitterrand was an intellectual and the whole mood of Paris had become very seductive to me. I packed up, neglecting the fledgling business, and moved to Paris.

A little bit of New York came with me; my assistant, Ellen, who had been with me since she was nineteen, had just married a Frenchman and moved to Paris at the same time. Having each other made us feel a little less homesick.

And homesick I was. I never anticipated the huge identity crisis I would have, both personally and in my own sense of style. I had arrived in Paris with my beautiful newly designed clothes, but Alain didn't like them. That was when he bought me flat shoes and had me order tweed blazers from his tailor in Milan. A woman's style and what she wears reflects a lot of who she is, and I slowly became confused and insecure. I'd had my hair cut very, very short in frustration after the end of my relationship with Paulo, which required frequent visits to the hairdresser, something I'd not done for years. For the first time I began to feel older and started weekly facials. Even though I was in Paris, the epicenter of fashion, I turned my back on fashion and everything I had built. The new line and the Sherry-Netherland store in New York made no sense to me anymore. Soon after my move I closed it all down and sold my Fifth Avenue apartment.

I missed my children and wrote to them daily, while making myself a pleasant life in Paris. I spent my time with writers, and took great pleasure and pride in establishing Salvy, a small publishing company. That was a great plus during this very odd but instructive period in my life. I loved having a literary salon in my apartment and being a publisher, but as a woman I was learning who I didn't want to be.

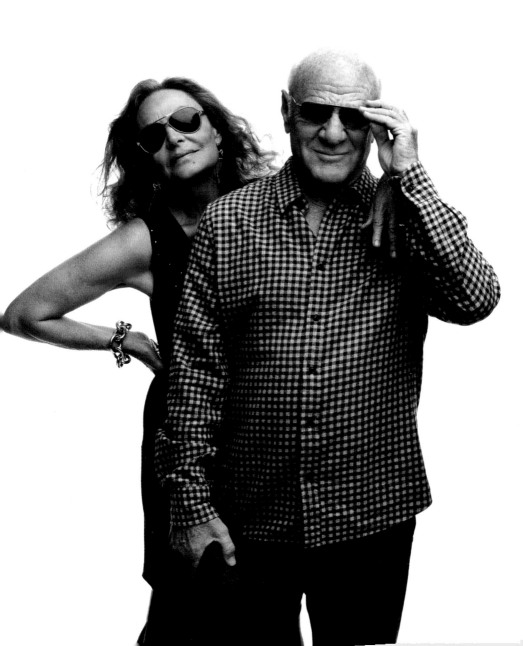

With Barry in Sun Valley, 2013. *(Jonas Fredwall Karlsson)*

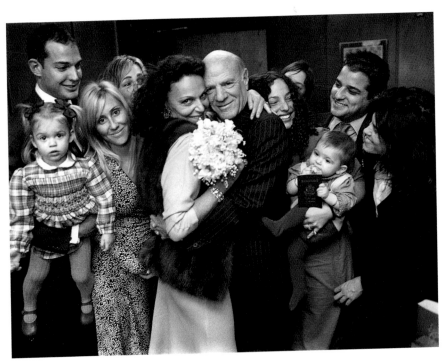

Surrounded by the children, my wedding to Barry, on the day of his birthday, February 2, 2001. *(Annie Leibovitz, courtesy of the artist)*

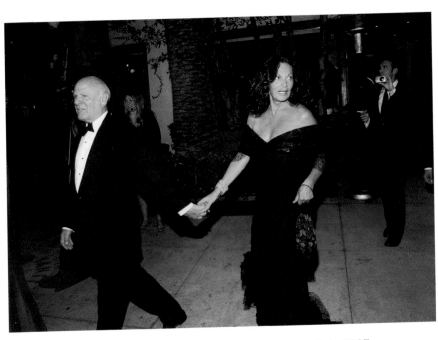

With Barry at the New York Public Library gala in 2007.

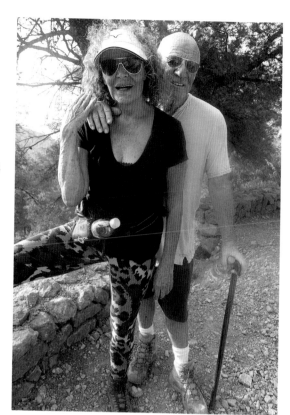

Hiking with Barry.

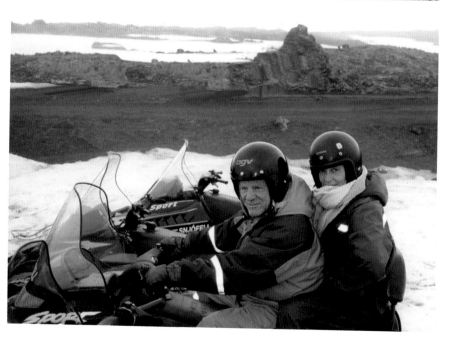

In the glaciers of Iceland with Barry.

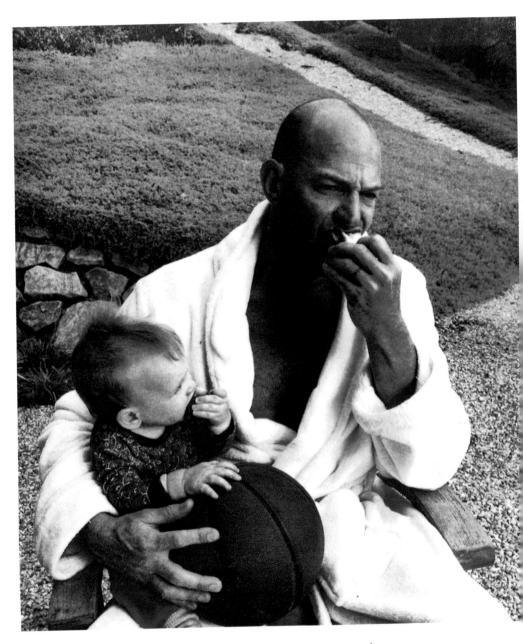

Alexandre with his son Leon, eating peaches.

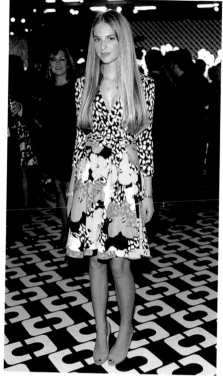

My granddaughter
Talita in a Warhol
wrap at the opening
of *Journey of a Dress*.
(Courtesy of Getty Images)

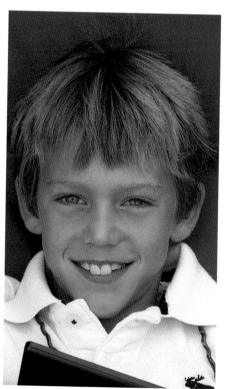

My grandson Tassilo.

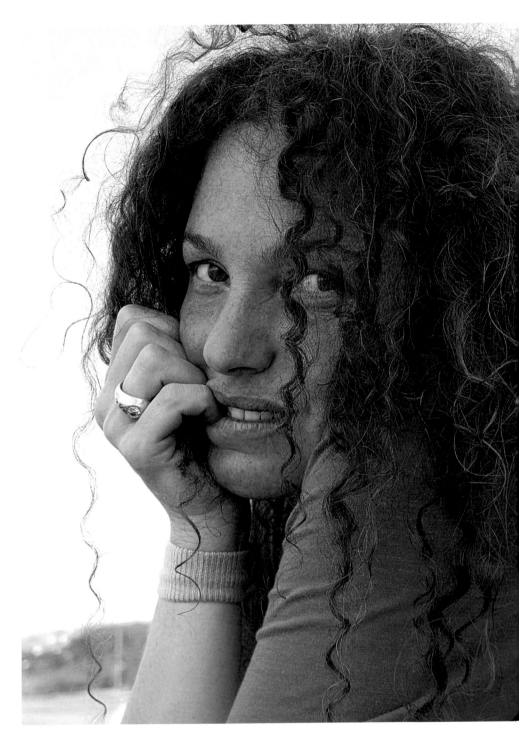

Tatiana in full beauty, captured by me, 2011.

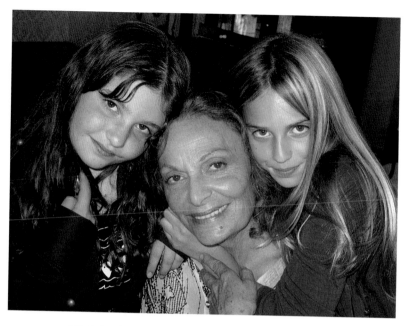

With both my granddaughters, Antonia and Talita.

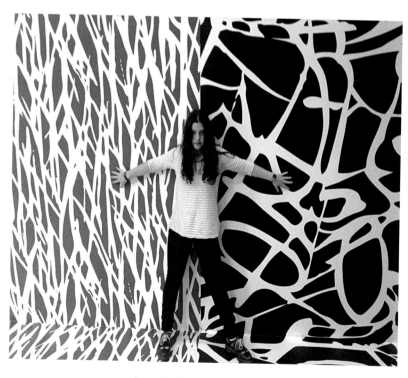

Antonia, Tatiana's daughter.

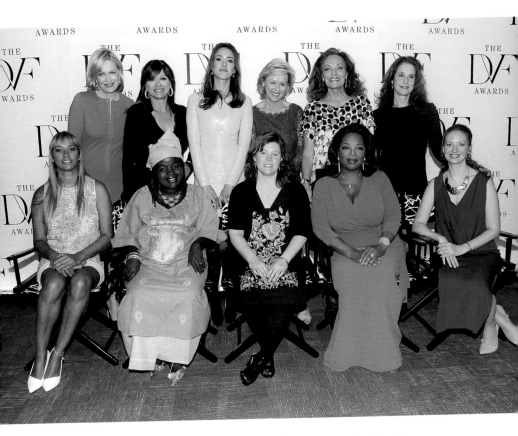

DVF Awards 2012 honorees and presenters. *(BFA Image)*

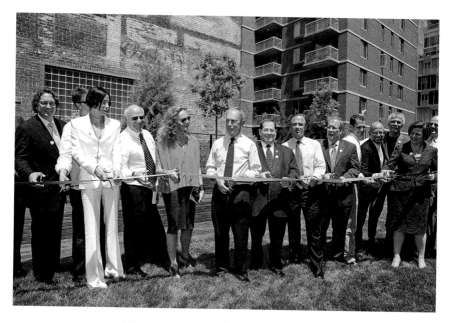

Ribbon-cutting of the second section of
the High Line, 2011. *(Joan Garvin, courtesy of the artist)*

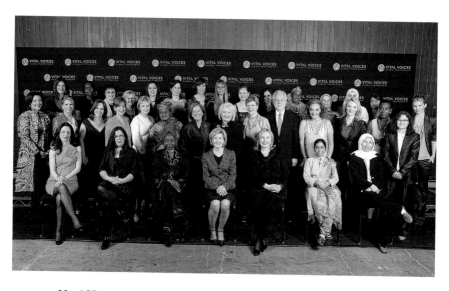

Vital Voices awards ceremony, 2011. *(Joshua Cogan, courtesy of the artist)*

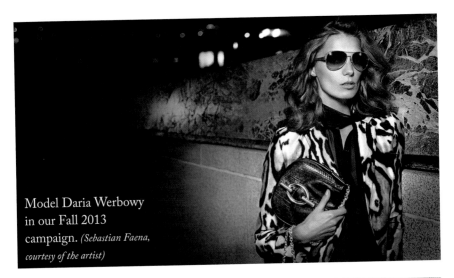

Model Daria Werbowy
in our Fall 2013
campaign. *(Sebastian Faena,
courtesy of the artist)*

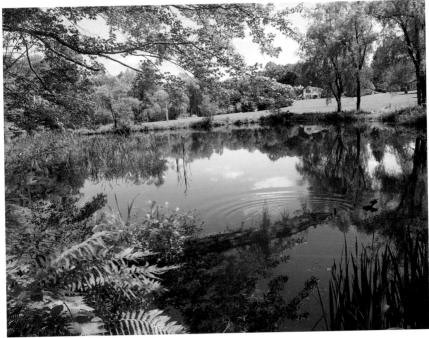

Cloudwalk Farm.

My brother, Philippe, his
wife, Greta, and their two
daughters, Sarah and Kelly.

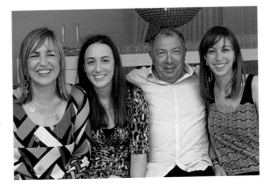

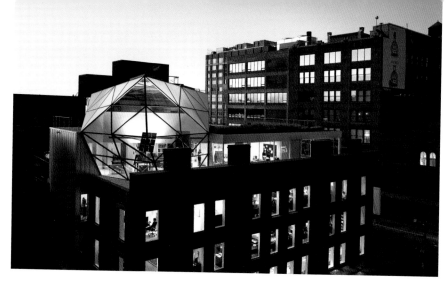

DVF Headquarters. *(Elizabeth Felicella, courtesy of Work AC)*

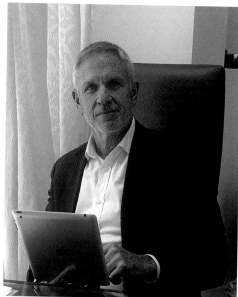

Joel Horowitz,
DVF cochairman.
(Michael Horowitz)

Spectacular Red Ball at Zhang Huan's studio in Shanghai, 2011.

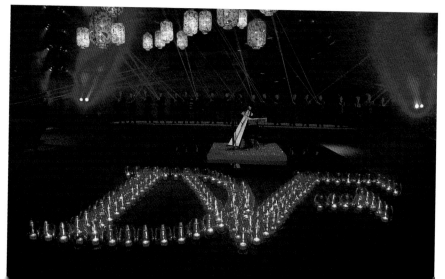

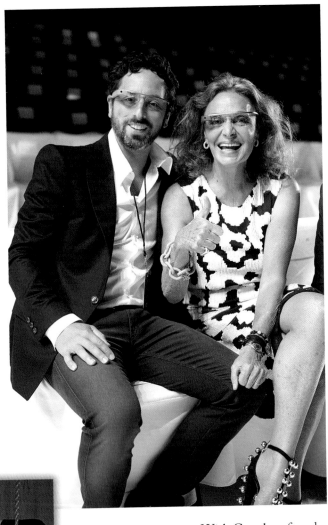

With Google cofounder
Sergey Brin showing Google
Glass for the first time. *(Greg
Kessler, courtesy of Kessler Studio)*

Upside-down doing yoga,
and on the phone.

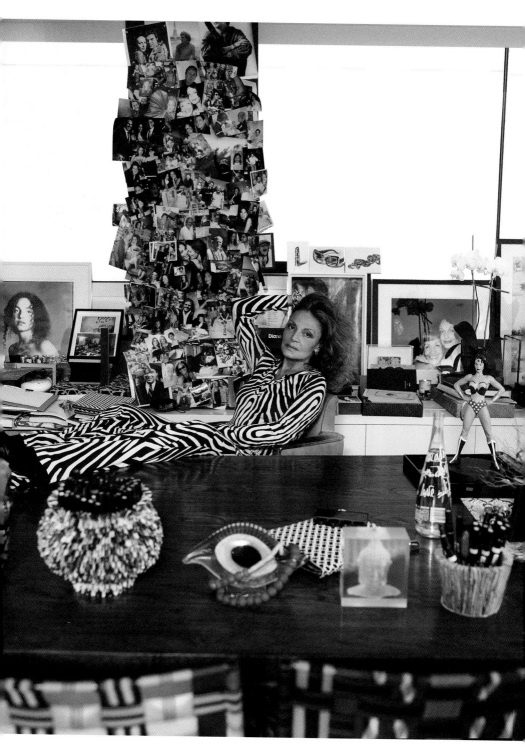

At my desk, surrounded by photos of my loved ones. *(Thomas Whiteside)*

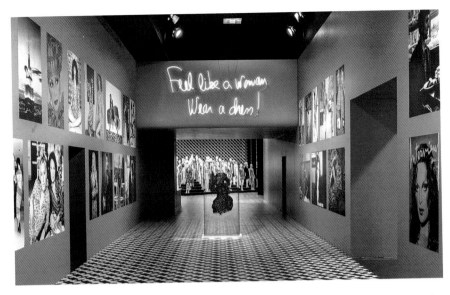

Entrance to *Journey of a Dress*, Los Angeles, 2014. *(Fredrik Nilsen, courtesy of the artist)*

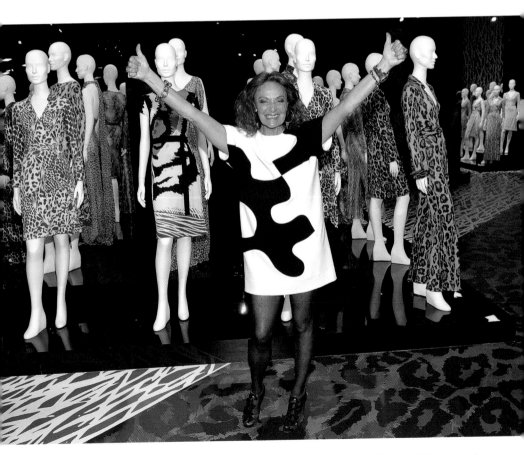

Moment of joy at the press conference for *Journey of a Dress*. *(Courtesy of Getty Images)*

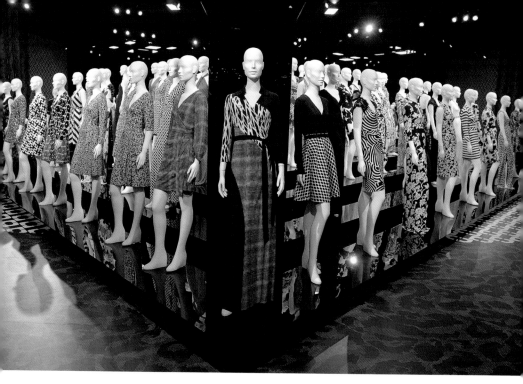

The "army" of wrap dresses at the exhibit. *(Fredrik Nilsen, courtesy of the artist)*

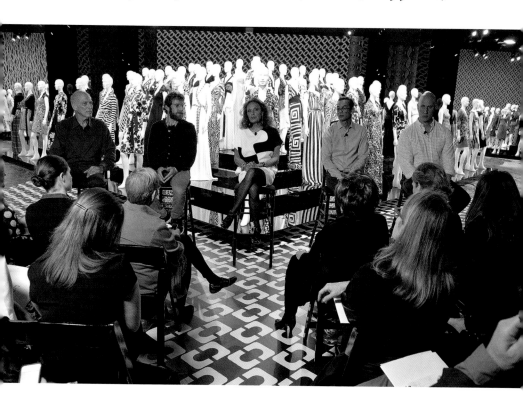

Press conference at the opening of the *Journey of a Dress* exhibit on January 10, 2014. *(Courtesy of Getty Images)*

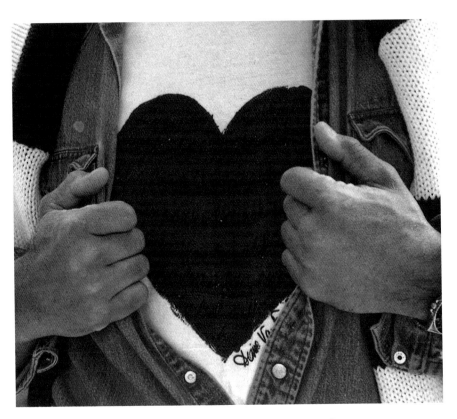

My first "Love is life" on a 1991 postcard.

5

THE COMEBACK
KID

I wish I could say I quickly regained my confident, intuitive self when I left Paris in 1990 for New York, but it isn't true. I was quite lost. My business, what was left of it, was in tatters. The licenses had been sold and resold, and my designs had lost their point of view. My line of cosmetics had vanished in a series of mergers and acquisitions and the only survivor, the light, sexy fragrance I'd named after my daughter, was unrecognizable: Tatiana had been turned purple by its new owner, Revlon, and they had changed the scent.

Not only had I lost my brand, I felt I had lost my identity. I had not realized how much my sense of self had been linked to my work. I did not know who I was anymore. My children were both at Brown University and had blossomed into wonderful young adults. I was very proud of them. I was not proud of me.

What a fool I'd been. By altering my personality, I had now lost myself. By naïvely signing away my name on the licenses without any restrictions and by neglecting my business duties to satisfy my man, the brand had lost its character and much of its value. My income from the royalties had dropped by around 75 percent. When I visited some of the few remaining licensees in their offices, they paid little attention to my design suggestions or to me. In their eyes, I had become irrelevant. I was just someone who'd designed some hot dresses a while back and they couldn't wait for me to leave them alone.

At twenty-five, I was a wunderkind. At forty, I was a has-been. I started straightening my hair again. I hated what the licensees made so I could no longer wear the clothes that bore my name. After the easy jersey dresses, the sarongs of the Bali period, and the tweed jackets of my Paris life, my new personal uniform was couture jackets from YSL with tight Alaïa skirts or narrow Romeo Gigli pants. Trying to feel of the moment, I ordered lavish couture clothes from Christian Lacroix, the talented new French designer: dresses with big pouf skirts and embellished jackets. Those clothes were beautiful and relevant to the time, but not to me. I barely wore them.

I thought my insecurity showed on the outside, but evidently it didn't. Anh Duong, the artist who was modeling for Christian Lacroix at the time and later became a close friend, remembers seeing me for the first time at his haute couture house in Paris. "I was struck by how beautiful you were trying on Christian's clothes," she told me recently. I could not believe she said that. I remember feeling particularly desperate that day and far from beautiful. It proved to me once more that "the woman across the room" may appear perfect, yet does not always feel it. I certainly didn't. Though I spend so much time now telling young women to be their own best friends and that happiness is confidence, I was not practicing what I preached during that lost period of my professional life. I wasn't sure who I was.

I made a few false starts trying to get back to work. I signed yet another unfortunate license deal in 1990 to design a line of dresses, this time with a moderately priced company. The struggling company wanted to upgrade its image and was counting on my name to do it. The chairman had a beautiful smile and blue eyes and he convinced me with his enthusiasm. I went ahead because at least it would get me back into the stores. It did, for a very short time. The company declared bankruptcy the day the DVF division was to launch its second season. By then I had invested a lot of time in developing these new dresses and I quite liked them, so without thinking twice, I told the team I'd been working with at the licensee's office to move the dresses into my office and come work for me. Impulsive for sure, and short-lived. We delivered one more season but I was not equipped nor did I have the desire to rebuild a wholesale business.

"Forget the stores," I said to myself. "Why not go directly to my original, loyal customers who have not forgotten me?" On the wings of that idea, I flew to San Francisco with Barry to visit the powerful catalog house Williams-Sonoma. The catalog industry was booming and I was hoping that Williams-Sonoma would see the value of adding a Diane von Furstenberg catalog to their stable. We had a polite lunch with the chairman but the company was not interested in me, or any designer name. Barry and I left feeling defeated. Now we often laugh and share our fond memories of that day when we felt like two losers with our failed sales pitch.

Still obsessed with direct selling, I had an idea to create a magalog, half magazine, half catalog, and I asked the young graphic artist Fabien Baron to design it for me. He made a beautiful mock-up, but because I did not have the funds or the expertise to make it happen, the ridiculous idea remained on the shelf.

Something just had to happen, and something did, in the summer of 1991 in the Concorde lounge at JFK. I was on my way to join twenty-year-old Tatiana in Venice for a debutante ball given by Count

Giovanni Volpi in his palace. At the airport a man came rushing up to me. "Where have you disappeared to?" he asked me, and introduced himself as Joe Spellman, a marketing executive. "The world of fashion needs you again. You could be a major star of the new century." I looked at him incredulously but I sure enjoyed the recognition. Joe had been a marketing genius at Elizabeth Arden, and later Estée Lauder, and he was also consulting for retired Bloomingdale's chairman Marvin Traub. I met them several times when I returned from Venice. Joe came up with a startling idea: "How about selling on television?" he said.

I had never heard of TV shopping, but why not? Clearly it was a way to reach the customer directly. A few weeks later, on a Saturday morning, we all took the Metroliner train to Philadelphia. Then a car to the suburb of West Chester to visit a company called QVC. I had no idea what to expect when we walked into the live TV studio and saw soap opera star Susan Lucci selling hundreds of bottles of shampoos and hair conditioners in a matter of minutes, sales that raced on the computer up to $600,000! I knew in that moment that we had landed in the future, the world of teleshopping.

As I watched Susan talking directly to her customers through the television screens I became very excited. I envisioned myself reviving my cosmetics line on TV, but the QVC people had something else in mind. They wanted me to design dresses for them. I was hesitant, not really understanding how you could sell dresses on TV and, also, in fairness, a bit concerned about the "tackiness" of their presentation at the time. I told them I would have to think about it.

I reported my QVC visit to Barry. Coincidentally, he knew about the shopping network from discussions he had had with Comcast and Liberty, the cable companies that owned the station. The timing was fortuitous. Barry had left Fox and was also looking for a new direction.

Just as we had been two young, successful tycoons at the same very early age, at that moment we were both "unemployed" and looking for our next opportunities. Little did we know that both our next careers would start from the very same spot: QVC.

Back at my design studio, with the help of the young women I had inherited from the moderate dress company, Kathy and Colleen, we designed not dresses, but a concept we called Diane von Furstenberg Silk Assets. It was a line of washable, coordinated, printed silk separates and scarves. The styles were simple and did not need to be tried on: shirts with a generous cut; easy pants with elastic waists. The colors were bright and cheerful, the prints bold and pretty, and the pieces could mix and match in many combinations. Every mini-collection had an inspiration story. "Giverny" was the print story inspired by the palette of French Impressionist painter Claude Monet. "Pietra Dura" was another collection, inspired by Florentine marble. The stories created a narrative that was easy to discuss on air with enthusiasm.

Here I was, back to my roots, creating color palettes and designing prints. Equally exciting was the financial arrangement I made with QVC for them to buy the clothes directly from the manufacturer in Hong Kong. My responsibility would be to design the line, and make sure it was well made and arrived on time. I would then sell it personally on TV and do all the promotions. For that QVC would pay me 25 percent on top of their cost from the factory. It was a great deal for QVC and for the consumers because there was no intermediate wholesaler. It was an even better deal for me: I had no liability of inventory because the clothes would be shipped directly from the factory to QVC. That arrangement was a huge relief. After all, twice I had had to sell my company because I had not managed inventory properly!

The day I was to have my first Diane von Furstenberg Silk Assets show, in November 1992, I arrived in my hotel room at the Sheraton

Great Valley, next door to the TV studio, and found beautiful flowers with a note: "Welcome home and good luck! I love you, Barry." The "Welcome home" referred to Barry's secret and successful negotiations to take over control of QVC, launching him into the new world of interactive, a move he continued to build on to reach where he is today.

In two hours I sold $1.3 million of Silk Assets while Barry (who surprised me at the show) and the management of QVC watched the galloping sales figures on a computer. They were all cheering! Kate Betts, a young editor at *Vogue,* had come along to witness the first show and documented it with wonderment. "Show and Sell," her article began. "*Vogue* witnesses a fashion phenomenon in the making." Overnight, I went from a has-been to a pioneer once again.

It is not inappropriate to say that Barry and I put the teleshopping industry on the map. Barry's involvement in the new retail phenomenon legitimized it and my participation as a designer glamorized it. A steady stream of people started showing up in West Chester to witness the retail revolution. There were many, many stories about us and QVC in magazines and newspapers.

It just got better and better. Viewers couldn't get enough of Diane von Furstenberg Silk Assets. On one show in 1993, I sold twenty-two hundred pairs of silk pants in less than two minutes!

Success is not only glamorous, it's also a lot of work. Being on live television, often in the middle of the night, was exhausting, and driving back and forth on the New Jersey Turnpike made me feel like Willy Loman in *Death of a Salesman.* But the exhaustion was worth it; in very little time, Silk Assets generated $40 million in sales.

Barry sold his stake in QVC in 1996 and bought controlling interest in the Home Shopping Network. I followed him there with my business and sales continued to grow. The success of Diane von Furstenberg Silk Assets gave me confidence again, but on television

I could not sell the simple, body-hugging, more sophisticated dresses that were my own style. I missed that.

What I desperately wanted was to revitalize my signature brand and return to high-end stores. There were glimmers that it might just be possible. There was a growing nostalgia in the nineties for the fashion of the seventies, spearheaded by Tom Ford, who had revitalized Gucci and put the mood of that legendary decade back into motion.

"You should bring back your dresses," Ralph Lauren told me when I was pitching TV shopping to him, trying to persuade other designers to join me. Karl Lagerfeld and Gianni Versace said the same: "We love your original dresses. You should bring them back." Rose Marie Bravo, then president of Saks Fifth Avenue, agreed, asking me time and again to relaunch the little jersey dresses. Suddenly it occurred to me that I was some kind of icon of the seventies. In the new nostalgia, hip, young designers seemed excited to see me. I remember one day walking past Bar Pitti in the West Village where the edgy new grunge designers Marc Jacobs and Anna Sui were having dinner. They waved enthusiastically. I was surprised, to say the least, and very flattered that such hot young talents would notice me. Another young designer, Todd Oldham, named his fashion show "Homage to Diane von Furstenberg." Again, I was flattered though a little taken aback. "I'm not dead yet," I remember thinking.

The nostalgia for the seventies and my first designs kept growing. In New York, young girls, contemporaries of my cool daughter, Tatiana, were scouring vintage shops and thrift shops in pursuit of original DVF wraps. All the signs were there for a comeback. The question was how. The answer, it seemed at the time, was Federated Department Stores, which, after many mergers and acquisitions, had become one of the largest better retailers in America, owning Bloomingdale's and Macy's, among others. I had breakfast with Allen Questrom, the chairman, whom I had known from the old days, and I proposed designing a private label brand exclusive to his stores. It could start with dresses, and over time expand to an array of products including accessories, intimate apparel, and home furnishings. It was a bit audacious to try and sell myself to Federated considering I hadn't been in the retail world for ten years, but the idea of striking an exclusive agreement with a designer appealed to Allen.

He introduced me to his management and we discussed both the merchandising aspect and the financial side. I wanted to use the same formula as the TV shopping: I would design, and they would buy from the manufacturer and own the liability of the inventory. Since it would require a large commitment and investment on their part, I felt I should show my commitment, too. I would invest in setting up a professional design studio with experienced and talented designers. It sounded like a plan.

Without further ado, I gave up my office at Fifth Avenue and Fifty-Seventh Street, where I had been since 1979. It had shrunk from a full floor to a small corner that was outdated, inadequate, and too expensive for what it was. I needed a larger, new space that would inspire creativity—something that could be both a design studio and a showroom where we would make presentations to buyers and press.

At thirty, I had wanted a very grown-up, glamorous space uptown. Approaching fifty, I wanted something more bohemian and my own. I looked downtown and found an 1858 brick carriage house in the Meatpacking District, way, way west on Twelfth Street, very close to the Hudson River. The fifteen-thousand-square-foot space was both charming and open, with a small pool inside the entrance, exposed beams, and redbrick walls. The building had had many lives—a stable for police horses, a studio for the painter Lowell Nesbitt, and most recently the headquarters of an advertising agency.

I fell in love with it immediately, to the deep concern of Alexandre, who could not understand why I would buy a house in the smelly neighborhood of butchers, meatpackers, and prostitutes. He was so horrified that he called my mother to get her to try and talk me out of it. They failed, though there was some truth to their objections. It was smelly, and in the morning pretty bad to step around the condoms and the trash in the street. Yet I loved it. In a weird way the cobblestone streets reminded me of Belgium, and I paid no attention to the naysayers. I bought myself the carriage house for my fiftieth birthday.

In the West Village there was a lot of energy, diversity, and a sense of community I never felt on Fifty-Seventh Street. I was in a real neighborhood and quickly established relationships with my colorful neighbors. The first was Florent Morellet, the flamboyant son of the famous French painter François Morellet. Florent had a diner nearby on Gansevoort Street that was open twenty-four hours a day where local artists, workers, and drag queens ate. He often dressed in drag himself and was so upfront about being HIV positive that he posted his T-cell count next to the menu over the counter. Florent was really the godfather of the community and determined to preserve the old, low-brick surrounding buildings. Would I help his campaign to turn the neighborhood into a historic district by holding a fund-raiser? "Of course."

The fund-raiser, the first of many I had in the second little building I bought next to my studio, was like a fair, with a lot of local restaurants participating. It was a great success, and in 2003, Florent managed to get local legislation through to declare the neighborhood the Gansevoort Market Historic District. It was a huge accomplishment and saved the wonderful old brick buildings from the wreckers' ball. Florent turned a dream into reality. Alexandre began to appreciate the colorful eclecticism of the neighborhood and soon moved his office there into my space.

Everything seemed new and vital on West Twelfth Street, including my fledgling business. From the moment we moved in, everything seemed to go faster and grow larger—the pressure and stress along with it.

The team was small. Kathy and Colleen handled all of the Silk Assets business I still had with HSN. The design team for my new project with Federated was international: Christian from Holland, Evelyn from Puerto Rico, and Sergio from Colombia. Alexandra, my son's new bride, who had studied fashion at the Parsons School of Design, joined us. Her first role was to go through the prints. Just as I had done decades ago at Ferretti's factory, she came quietly into the studio and began sorting through the archived prints from my early years. Together, we created the first designs during the months we were still negotiating with Federated.

I felt the need to recreate the jersey I had used for my dresses in the seventies. Ferretti had died and his factories were closed, but I had kept swatches of the fabrics. After Ferretti and I parted ways in 1979, a certain Mr. Lam in Hong Kong produced my dresses for Carl Rosen and Puritan Fashions.

I hadn't see Mr. Lam in almost fifteen years when I visited him in Hong Kong to talk to him about re-creating my Italian jersey from the seventies. His factory had been small when I'd last seen him. Now his factories were very large and my business very small, yet he welcomed me with open arms. In return for the investment he would have to make to develop my signature fabric and set up better printing facilities, I moved the production of Silk Assets to his factories. He put his technical people at my disposal and together we developed the perfect jersey fabric, as tight as the original Italian one but this time 100 percent silk and more luxurious. I also shared my knowledge about hand printing, and spent long hours with their technicians. The process took a lot of patience and determination, but it was worth it for sure. The results were astounding.

Working hands-on in Mr. Lam's factories, I felt I had gone back in time, except now I was in China eating noodles with the workers for lunch and not in Italy eating spaghetti. It was exhausting going back and forth from Mr. Lam's office in Hong Kong to the factories in China, accompanied by Patso, his right hand. She worked just as hard, totally committed to what we were trying to do.

Another part of my investment was to write a business memoir to draw a line between the present and future, and introduce myself to new customers. Without hesitation, I went to my friend Linda Bird Francke, who had played such a big part in my life with her articles in *New York* magazine and *Newsweek*, to help me write the book. I would time the publication of *Diane: A Signature Life* to coincide with the launch of my first collection for Federated. The plan was to do personal appearances in their stores across the country, promoting the book and the clothes. I was close to finishing the book in the summer of 1996 when the crushing news came in: the deal with Federated had fallen through.

I got the call in my car on a Friday afternoon, while driving to the country. Allen Questrom, the chairman, had left the company. The collaboration no longer seemed right for them. They were sorry. I'm sure there were other reasons, too, but if they ever told me, I've forgotten them. I was in total shock. I was devastated. I had counted so much on this arrangement. What was I going to do?

That weekend Barry was with me in Cloudwalk. As usual, he reassured me and encouraged me to move on. By Monday morning, I had a new plan. An obvious plan. One that had been under my nose the whole time. The wrap dress. My quintessential symbol of the seventies. I would relaunch the wrap and once again I would do it on my own.

There were many positive signs. The success of QVC had made my name extremely well known again; I was surprised to see how high I ranked in a poll of brand-name recognition published in *Women's Wear Daily* that year. So there I was, with name recognition, a demand for the dress, and the perfect fabric at my disposal.

I called Rose Marie Bravo and my mother's adage proved right once again. One door closed. Another door opened. "How exciting," Rose Marie said. "We would be proud to launch your wrap dresses at Saks."

I had retired at thirty-six, and here I was beginning again, at fifty. I was nervous but it was unbelievably exciting. Reintroducing my brand successfully in a high-end department store like Saks would prove to the world, and to myself, that the first time hadn't been an accident. But first I had to make it happen.

I decided to call the new line "Diane," the same name I had used, with a label in my handwriting, for my short-lived couture line. That label also became the first new print I designed: an allover "Diane" signature print. The idea had come to me while I was talking on the phone, looking at the label and doodling on a piece of paper. All those intertwined "Dianes" looked very much like the original prints and felt right. That led me to rework the original twig print by adding more colors. I reissued the original wood print and added a few new ones, all geometric and bold in the style of the seventies.

The announcement of my exclusive arrangement with Saks set off an enormous buzz about the return of the wrap, and me! Newspapers and magazines revisited my marriage to Egon, the children, and the phenomenon of the wrap. The *International Herald Tribune* described the dress as "The Image of an Era," over the subhead, "The Charmed Lives and Free Spirit of Diane von Furstenberg." The *New York Times Magazine* saw me as a fairy tale—"Once upon a time, there was a princess with an idea. The idea was a dress"—and *Women's Wear Daily* really got it right: "Diane's Wild Ride."

Beginning again made me feel young and fearless, but, looking back, my diary of that year also reveals many fears. As usual, I did not show my insecurities. I sounded full of confidence in all the interviews I gave, but it was a complicated time for me. On the one hand, I felt excited and rejuvenated, restarting the adventure of the wrap dress, flattered by the reaction of young girls and the excitement of Rose Marie Bravo. On the other hand, I was scared and constantly questioning myself. I did not feel secure. I was going ahead but I was afraid to fail. My rejection by Federated had left me off-balance in my business life and I was also living a major rejection in my private life: Mark Peploe had left me for another woman and I was hurting. What a strange time it was. Part of me felt old and for the first time ever, on a trip to LA, I consulted a few cosmetic surgeons. Those visits made me feel even more scared, insecure, and confused, although I did know that cosmetic surgery was not the solution. I did, however, get my teeth fixed; I'd had problems since a bad fall when I was ten years old, and seven weeks of radiation made the situation much worse.

Alexandra introduced me to her dentist, Dr. Irwin Smigel, and after months of work he left me with two gifts: a beautiful smile for the first time in my life, and the phone number for Tracie Martyn.

The launch at Saks was set for September 1997, and during the summer countdown there were a few unexpected and very welcome confidence boosters. I went to an elegant wedding of friends of my children, in Virginia, where all the young girls were wearing the "it" Tocca dresses: simple, colorful shifts by the then very popular Dutch designer Marie-Anne Oudejans. However the young hip Marie-Anne herself had asked to borrow a sample of a new DVF wrap in the beige-and-white signature print, and to my delight, she wore it to the wedding. I was extremely flattered. It meant a lot.

I got another boost in July at the Dior couture show in Paris. I'd brought a new wrap dress with me and wore it, a choice that was equally daring and nerve-racking. Here I was in the most sophisticated circumstances, a Dior couture show in an elegant greenhouse, wearing a dress that was basically the same as I would have worn twenty years before. But amazingly, it was that little dress that created a buzz in Paris and caught the attention of Amy Spindler, the talented young fashion editor at the *New York Times*.

"She slipped one on for John Galliano's Christian Dior couture show in July in Paris, over a bathing suit," Amy wrote for the Sunday *New York Times Magazine*. "By the time the sun began blazing through the roof, everyone near her was envying her wrap: She pulled the skirt aside to reveal leg, pushed up the sleeves to reveal arms, and was left with a dress the size of the bathing suit beneath. Actresses Rita Wilson and Kate Capshaw, seated across from her, raved about her look. So did the models backstage. And that was when she knew." I did know it was happening but it was still unbelievable. "Oh, I'd like a dress like that," one model after another said to me as they stood in their beautiful ball gowns when I was taken backstage to see John Galliano. There was such enthusiasm for the dress in Paris that I called my office in New York to arrange for more samples to be brought over by a friend so I could wear another wrap to the Chanel couture show. I wore a different print every day.

Amy was just as enthusiastic back in New York at the first, unconventional fashion show I gave on West Twelfth Street in September. It was only wrap dresses and a few beaded printed shirts over white pants. The models came down the carriage house's steep, narrow spiral staircase onto a carpet I'd designed for the little runway that was printed with the black-and-white "Diane" signature print. Looking back, I cannot believe that at age fifty I was once again a little do-it-yourself start-up. It was not so different from my first show at the Gotham Hotel. I was following my instinct, determined to make it work. The press loved it, including Amy.

"Yes, yes, yes, Diane Von Furstenberg's bold bias-cut wrap dress is back," she wrote in the *Times*. "Redesigned for the 90's, it is sleek and sexy, but still a dress with a sassy mom quality." I cannot calculate how much I owe to Amy. The influential fashion reporter, who wore the dresses herself, was such an editorial supporter that she became as important to the new line as Diana Vreeland had been to the original wrap. (Sadly, Amy died of cancer in 2004. She was only forty.)

I needed to find the right image, with the right spirit, for the first ad campaign for Saks. I went to my friend, French photographer Bettina Rheims, who is a master at photographing women, and we chose Danielle Zinaich to be our girl. Danielle was in her late twenties, had great legs and perfect body language. Her brown hair was shoulder length and her face quite long and distinctive, but what we loved most about her was her personality and her huge laugh that revealed her prominent gums shamelessly. Danielle and I flew to Paris and we shot the relaunch of the wrap dress in my Left Bank apartment. Most of the shoot was in vivid color, except for one dress that we photographed in black-and-white. I had no idea how fortuitous that would be.

The problem arose when I proudly called Rose Marie Bravo to my studio to see the edgy photos that Bettina and I had done in Paris. She and I were accomplices in this venture, relaunching the wrap, but she didn't like the pictures at all. She found them too hard, too decadent, too reminiscent of a recent controversy: "heroin-chic" images of pale, ill-looking models. I was devastated. All those beautiful photos in vivid colors rejected. Rose Marie must have felt sorry for me because on her way out, she pointed at the black-and-white photos of Danielle, one serious and one laughing, showing her exaggerated gums and declared, "Use these. She looks happy!"

I stared at those two black-and-white pictures for hours after Rose Marie left. I didn't know what to do after spending so much time and money with Bettina shooting hundreds of images for the beautiful color ads, but I had to do something. And then it came to me. "I'll make them speak," I said to myself, "and give them a reason to be." I put them next to each other and under the serious shot of Danielle, I wrote "He stared at me all night" and under the laughing one, I wrote "And then he said, 'Something about you reminds me of my mother.'"

The copy was funny but also risky, leading people at my office to call it ridiculous. "Nobody wants to look like their mother," they said. But I thought it was provocative and I liked it, and more to the point, so did Rose Marie, who agreed to endorse the campaign, which turned out to be very successful.

We launched at Saks in New York on September 9 with great fanfare. Television cameras and print photographers crowded around the women standing in line in the dress department, many with their daughters, to buy the new dresses. The demand was so great the dresses quickly sold out and the women who had to go home without one put their names on waiting lists for the next shipment. "It feels like déjà vu," I kept telling the hordes of press. They saw explosive success that looked familiar, but I meant it also as a cautionary tale.

Once again I was on a runaway train without a business plan or a strategy. I didn't even have a president to manage the new company. There'd been no time. Our new West Twelfth Street studio was still in disarray. I hadn't finished renovating it, there weren't enough phone lines, and the computers kept crashing. I remember feeling distracted and exhausted during the launch at Saks, a state exacerbated by my return to the fitting rooms with the customers and seeing my face twenty years older looking back at me in the mirrors. Still, the return of the wrap was a dream come true.

Alexandra and I toured the country, making personal appearances at the Saks stores from coast to coast selling the dresses with lots of hype. We got a lot of press—a beautiful new von Furstenberg princess in one wrap, her mother-in-law in another—illustrating the agelessness of the dress. The dresses sold well when we were in the stores, but the excitement, and sales, didn't hold after we left. The reintroduction of the wrap started like a big soufflé, and the soufflé fell flat. I didn't know what to do. "Business hard, losing money, no plan," I wrote in my journal.

I had been out of the stores for so long that I didn't know the new reality: Young girls in the nineties rarely shopped in the dress department, and that is where we were placed at Saks. The older generation still shopped there, but Alexandra and her friends bought their clothes at smaller boutiques. And that's where the wrap dress, newly and more sleekly designed, was truly reborn.

Scoop. What would we have done without Scoop? Owned by a friend of Alexandra's, Scoop was a very hip, new little shop on Broadway, way downtown in SoHo, where just about everything they sold was black, including the combat boots. But Scoop's owner, Stefani Greenfield, loved the colorful new wraps and simply hung them on hangers in her window. They sold out in half an hour. She couldn't keep them in stock with the huge demand from the downtown girls—and soon from the uptown girls when Scoop opened another shop on Third Avenue in the seventies. Where young people shopped, the dresses sold at meteoric speed, but it was just not the case in the old-fashioned dress departments we were also counting on.

At the beginning of 1998, I hired Susan Falk, the former president of Henri Bendel, to be my president. We also hired a well-known consulting company to advise us on what distribution channel we should pursue. Susan introduced me to Catherine Malandrino, a talented young French designer with whom she had worked previously. Catherine came to see me at the Carlyle, where I was living at the time. We talked about her journey as a designer and I showed her my newest wrap in a dark-green camouflage leopard print. She loved it and agreed to join us.

We introduced new wraps, and some simple solid-color dresses with soft drape, to the buyers by staging a presentation that was inspired by the old Paris couture houses. I transformed the studio into a living room, decorating it with the sofa, some paintings, a huge mirror, and a piano from my old Fifth Avenue apartment. Every fifteen minutes or so, models would appear in different designs and strike motionless poses by the piano or around the indoor pool as the pianist played Gershwin or Joplin.

Catherine brought a lot of value to the fledgling company. I wore one of her designs myself the following year when I sat for my portrait by Francesco Clemente on the day Talita was born. I remember joking about being a sexy grandmother as I posed for Francesco that day. The painting hangs now in the lobby of my studio on Fourteenth Street and will be forever in my memory as the day I become a grandmother for the first time. That dress was called Angelina and was cleverly draped and very flattering with all kinds of details from old-fashioned dressmaking. Angelina proved to be very successful.

Alexandra was getting more and more involved and was a wonderful image for the company. Though she liked the new draped dresses well enough, she was still concerned about our lack of direction. She had a point. Between the wraps and the new drape dresses we clearly had a viable collection but we didn't have a clear path of how to distribute it and move the business forward. The consultants we had hired advised us to go into the moderate market, but it didn't match the sophistication of the designs. I was confused and stressed.

That summer as I was driving to Teterboro Airport in New Jersey to meet Barry and fly to Alaska, I took a very bad turn. Having passed the airport turnoff, I swerved, bumped into something, and was spun back onto the highway where I hit an eighteen-wheeler. I had a big, huge pain in my chest and I remember asking the ambulance crew, "Can you live if you have a hole in your heart?" It turned out that in addition to the eighteen stitches I needed in my head, I had broken five or six ribs and punctured a lung. (I also totaled Barry's BMW.)

I spent the next two painful but peaceful weeks in a small hospital in Hackensack, New Jersey, with great doctors and such tight security that I was convinced there was a mob boss on my floor. Barry and the children wanted desperately for me to be transferred to a hospital in New York, but I refused. I loved that little hospital and I loved the time alone, as Hackensack was far enough from Manhattan to discourage visitors. I needed a break. I knew I was exhausted and confused, and so did Alexandre. "You had the accident because you don't know what you're doing," he said, not as a reproach but out of concern. That was perhaps a harsh comment, but I think he was totally right. Just as a few years before I'd thought my tongue cancer symbolized my inability to express myself, I saw the accident as a symptom of my lack of a road map for my business.

The nights were long and painful in the hospital, despite my wonderful nurse with whom I became friends. I have few memories of those two weeks in a no-man's-land, as I never wrote about it in my diaries. All I know is that I had a tube in my lung, did not read or watch television, and waited motionless for my body to heal. It did. Slowly and steadily I sweated out all the bad.

I knew I had to make a change and the catalyst presented itself the moment I arrived back at my apartment in the Carlyle—and discovered water pouring into the bedroom from a leak in the ceiling. "That's it," I said to myself. "I'm moving downtown."

And another new life began.

I created a wonderful living space next to my private office on the top floor of the West Twelfth Street studio carriage house. I decorated the living area with Balinese artifacts and put an iron canopy bed against the exposed brick wall. I made a large dressing room that was also a yoga studio. I loved the décor of my new bohemian lifestyle, so different from the Carlyle. In the morning I would make a cup of coffee and cross the highway practically in my pajamas to walk along the river. I had a small guest room where my mother stayed when she visited me. She was never really comfortable there; years later it occurred to me that the exposed brick may have reminded her of the camps.

On the other hand, Christian Louboutin loved staying in that guest room and practically lived there as he showed his early collections of shoes on my dining room table. At the time he had just begun selling his sexy, red-soled heels to Barneys, Jeffrey, and Neiman Marcus. As I watched him develop new, spectacular shoes every season, selling only a few styles at a time, I suggested he build a core line he could offer every season, and was proud that I was able to help him build his talent into a huge global brand. We became the best of friends, going on to share personal appearances across the country, and began taking lots of holidays together. We've walked and driven the dusty Silk Road in Uzbekistan all the way from Tashkent to Samarkand, Bukhara, Khiva, and Fergana, to end up on the border of Afghanistan. Christian and I are both Capricorns, and like two little goats we love to climb. We've hiked up and down the hills of Egypt and the steep mountains of Bhutan.

What I loved most of all about my West Twelfth Street carriage house was the feeling that I belonged there. My personal style and designs were one and the same again—simple, happy, sexy—and everything in my life was beginning to feel coherent for the first time in years. All of this, including the creative characters in my vibrant neighborhood, made me feel like a young new me. Once again I was giving lots of fun parties, including one for the publication of *Signature Life*. Tatiana asked a friend of a friend to organize the music, and that is when we all met Russell Steinberg, who soon after became father of my second grandchild, Antonia.

The business was still limping along, but little by little we were gaining traction and I was certainly happier than I'd been in a while.

I was very touched and proud when the CFDA asked me to join its board of directors in 1999. It was very reassuring to be recognized by my colleagues. For the first time in many years, I no longer felt like an outsider. I was back in the world of fashion.

What I didn't anticipate was a run-in I had with Alexandre in what has become known as the "family intervention." The whole family was gathered in Barry's office in New York where we were discussing the creation of the Diller–von Furstenberg Family Foundation for charitable donations. After that discussion, Alexandre, who manages our family money, confronted me. "You've got to refocus your energies on making a plan for what you want to do with the company and stop hemorrhaging money," he said. "Or else pull the plug."

I was very angry at being confronted like that—or being confronted at all, for that matter. It was my money after all, and there was progress. I did understand Alex's concern, but in my mind, this time it was less about money and more about me. When I'd first started out in business, my goal had been financial independence and I had achieved it. This time my goal was to prove to myself and the world that the first time around hadn't been a fluke. My pride was more important than the cost of achieving that goal. It was also about the wrap dress, the style that was mine and had a place in women's closets again. Pull the plug? Now?

I slammed my fist down hard on the table. "Give me six months!" I said. "I'll turn it around. You'll see." Alex backed off and we all agreed to the six months.

He was right, of course. I couldn't just keep spending money without a plan. But I felt I might be on my way with the enthusiasm of young women for my dresses again, and that's what I wanted to work on. I did, however, need professional sales help.

And that's when Paula Sutter came into my life.

Stefani from Scoop introduced me to Paula, her young friend and former colleague, over lunch at Balthazar, the French downtown bistro. Paula, who was then greatly pregnant, had been the vice president of sales and marketing for DKNY. She and Stefani had both been part of Donna Karan's dream team that was so successful in the eighties launching DKNY. Many of the women on that team went on to have spectacular careers. "You should hire her," Stefani said. It was I who had to do the convincing when Paula visited me in my office. She didn't want to commit to a full-time job because of her impending motherhood, but I managed to persuade her to come on as a part-time consultant. That was 1998. When Susan Falk, who wanted to return to corporate life, left the following year, Paula became president of Diane von Furstenberg Studio. She remained the company's invaluable president for fourteen years.

It was a struggle for her at first, accentuated when Alexandre came to see Paula to reissue his now familiar ultimatum. "You've got six months to turn a profit or close it down," he told her. Not a great welcome. Paula, however, was on my side.

With her credentials she could have gone to bigger, more successful names at the time, but she saw that our company had really good DNA and really good bones but needed "Windexing," as she put it, to get rid of the messiness. She was as excited as I was about the possibilities that lay in the young, not in the middle-aged dress department. The demographic model had been wrong from the start, so we changed course.

The retail experience was trending toward a new, more modern approach. Department stores were beginning to establish contemporary or "affordable luxury" divisions and that's where Paula thought we belonged. It would be a great opportunity for us to go after the younger consumer and pretty much retell our story in a new and modern way, but to get there, we first we had to reposition the brand as universally cool.

Paula was enthusiastic and determined. She had such energy talking to the luxury stores like Bergdorf Goodman, but it was difficult. My name was "polluted" they claimed because we were still selling on television, and some buyers still thought of me as an old brand even though by that time we had an enviable track record with contemporary girls. The signature label, Diane, was also problematic. They thought it old-fashioned. Luckily an old boyfriend, Craig Brown, the graphic designer who made the Rolling Stone logo of Mick Jagger's tongue, reappeared in my life at that moment and he redesigned the label as a typeface "Diane von Furstenberg."

We took other steps as well. "Diane von Furstenberg Silk Assets" became "Silk Assets." I eased myself out of the HSN broadcasts and Alicia, a young woman from the office, replaced me.

Paula established monthly deliveries to create an ongoing fresh flow of merchandise in the stores. For our next press day I had the idea of creating evocative *tableaux vivants* around the studio's pool illustrating the themes of those monthly deliveries: the plants, the flowers, the sea. The models were ravishing in the small, focused collection of featherweight chiffon and jersey dresses in trademark prints and matching colors. The buyers and press walked into a living painting. It was colorful, sexy, edgy, and different from what anyone else was doing at the time.

We continued our show-and-tell in Paris. We packed up and took a booth at Tranoï, an international fashion trade fair for young designers at the Carrousel du Louvre during French Market Week. The best specialty stores from around the world go there. These shops set the taste for everyone else. We were hoping to be a presence in those stores and it happened when Colette, one of the coolest shops, ordered our sexy, printed dresses for its store in Paris. It was at that time that Betsee Isenberg, the hot showroom rep in LA, also took the line on to sell on the West Coast.

Alexandre was still skeptical. We weren't really making any money, but there was definitely traction. Paula did some projections and a small business plan when we came back to New York. She showed them to Barry and Alexandre. "I understand," Barry laughed when she finished her presentation. "You want to try and give the business a blood transfusion." We adopted those words because that was exactly what we were trying to do—and six months later, it was back to Paris with the next collection.

I remember those days with tremendous affection. Five or six of us from the New York studio would pile into my apartment on the rue de Seine along with all the clothes, essentially camping there for the duration of the fair. We were a skeletal crew—Paula, of course, and Astrid, the best salesperson ever, speaking every language and trying every dress on herself. There was Maureen from marketing and Luisella, the smart Italian girl who at the time was my assistant. We laughed a lot and were very successful at getting orders in the very best international shops.

I felt young again, propelled by the girls around me, and I shared their excitement and enthusiasm. I felt their age. There were no big business meetings, no big marketing plans. None of that. The second time started just as organically as the first. It was, after all, a small business. It was really like incubating a new, young brand and we did it on a shoestring, living off my profit from HSN.

Soon we were selling, selling, selling to specialty stores in England, France, Italy, Spain—all over Europe—as well as shops in the US. Scoop was, of course, our mainstay in New York, and in LA it was Fred Segal, the brilliant retailer who had been the first, in the sixties, to open a denim-only store. Both stores were big fans of the brand and getting the word out through their very loyal client base. Relaunching amid the nostalgia for the seventies turned out to be perfect. Colette loved paying glamour homage to the seventies and Studio 54, all of which I had thoroughly lived. That I was an original player of the time gave authenticity to my clothes, interviews, and personal appearances. There we were in our booth at the fair, right beside the cool, young designers, and it was all encouraging, but the income was still small.

I looked for a shortcut. On a flight from London to New York I sat next to Tom Ford, and he expressed great interest in what I was doing. I had a flash: Why not sell a piece of the company to Gucci to raise some money so we could go on smoothly? A few months later I flew to London with Barry and Alexandre and Paula met us there. It was the summer of 1999 and Barry was involved in a huge deal trying to buy up Universal, but he took the time to come with us to Gucci. Our meeting didn't get off to a great start. Tom and his partner Domenico De Sole were late, and Barry was upset. Nonetheless, we went ahead with our presentation and they seemed interested. We had several meetings with their people in New York over the next few months, but somehow shortcuts don't work for me. In the end, they were not interested and invested in Stella McCartney instead. I was disappointed.

In the midst of all this, Catherine Malandrino left us to develop her own line and open her own shop. In came Nathan Jenden in 2001. He stayed with me for almost ten years.

Nathan was English, thirty I think at the time, and had worked with John Galliano and Tommy Hilfiger so he understood both high fashion and Main Street, and he had a little funky side. I liked him from the beginning when I'd asked him to make a presentation (which he promptly lost but found again) and he came back with a sketch of a girl wearing a crossword puzzle print dress that he titled The Rebel Princess. When he came into my office he was impressed by the numbers of books I had around me, and I was impressed that he'd noticed them.

Nathan brought a lot of feng shui and a little rock 'n' roll to the clothes and we had a great run together. Nathan was incredibly talented and he was able to create magic during fittings with his aggressive scissors. The first show we did together happened two days before 9/11, which left us all in a state of shock and disarray. His work was so sharp, it managed to keep our numbers up as the city's economy took a huge hit. That year he came we also opened our first shop in New York next door to the carriage house. It was a tiny boutique you could barely find. Calvin Klein came to the opening of my hidden-away shop and looked at the little dresses. "What a wonderful concept," he said. Coming from Calvin, who doesn't like color or print, that was a huge compliment. I was really beginning to feel on a high, even though Gucci had rejected me.

The high continued in Los Angeles at the Academy Awards. Barry and I have always given a Saturday picnic lunch for our friend Graydon Carter, the editor of *Vanity Fair* and host of its longtime Oscar party. A lot of beautiful stars come to our lunch and more and more started arriving in DVF. Now we were definitely gaining ground!

From just a few little dresses, we expanded into a full collection. Twice a year we held formal runway shows at our studio. The names—Working Girl, Under the Volcano, Rebel Princess—reflected the easy, sexy, independent, on-the-go, slightly mischievous woman we designed for. After the successful Dolce Diva fashion show, a light fell and hurt two editors. I felt terribly guilty. I visited Hilary Alexander, the highly respected editor of the *Daily Telegraph* in the hospital and she was an incredible sport. In spite of her injury, she gave us a great review, but the time had come to join the big leagues and show in the official New York Fashion Week tents.

By 2002 we were in virtually every quality department store, including the grande dame of them all, Bergdorf Goodman. I let my hair go curly again. The Comeback Kid had arrived! In three amazing years, I had gone from losing money, and being advised by my concerned family to shut down, to being very profitable. No one in the industry could believe it. No one expected us to do what we did, and a lot of people were surprised by how we were able to reinvent the brand. Paula and I positioned the business in a very modern way, and here we were—a 1970s business that had successfully transitioned into the twenty-first century with the original centerpiece dress surrounded by new, multigenerational global designs.

We grew as opportunities arose, without a master plan. We opened a shop in Miami in 2003, and the next year in London in a little boutique in Notting Hill, where we were hot, hot, hot. Paris followed the next year, with a spectacular launch. Madonna happened to be in Paris so I sent her an email. She came to the opening with her daughter and a retinue of paparazzi and bought a wrap that she wore at a press conference she gave in Israel. You can't ask for a better friend or better publicity than that!

Madonna came through again a few years later in Los Angeles at the 2008 Oscar after-party she cohosted with Demi Moore. They surprised me by wearing the same gold wrap dress the stylist Rachel Zoe had ordered for them from my spring fashion show! I really felt that as a designer, I had arrived. I was exhilarated that same night by the commercial American Express ran twice during the Oscars broadcast. They had commissioned Bennett Miller, the Academy Award–nominated director, to do it, and we shot at Cloudwalk and at the studio. Bennett refused to have me read a script; he interviewed me instead, and used that for the voice-over. That night millions of people heard me say: *I didn't really know what I wanted to do, but I knew the woman I wanted to become.* Even though I must have said that sentence many times before, hearing it on TV made me realize its power. That desire is the spirit of my brand.

Over the next few years we opened shops in Tokyo, Jakarta, St. Tropez, Brussels, Shanghai, Hong Kong, Moscow, Madrid, second and third shops in Paris, São Paulo, Beijing. Opening the shop in Antwerp, run by my sister-in-law, was particularly rewarding because it was my first store in Belgium. Axel Vervoordt, the renowned architect and interior designer, gave a big, beautiful dinner for me in his castle; for the first time ever, I felt recognized as a designer in my native country.

Moscow presented another wonderful opportunity. Our collection in 2005 was Russian-inspired and was carried by a shop called Garderobe that invited me to Moscow. They held a little fashion show and dinner for me at Tolstoy's house on the Ulitsa Lva Tolstogo! After the show, sitting in Tolstoy's garden under the lilac trees, drinking champagne and giving interviews made me think how thrilled my Russian father would have been.

Another great memory is the visit to Cloudwalk by Roberto Stern, the Brazilian jewelry designer who co-owns and runs the jewelry company H. Stern. I had always wanted to design fine jewelry and had approached his father, Hans, thirty years earlier to collaborate. I loved the quality of their jewelry, but Hans had turned me down.

I had tried again with the son in 2001, but again not much happened. Roberto, I found out later, had been a little bit intimidated by me at our first meetings, but intimidation turned to inspiration during his visit to Cloudwalk, and we entered into a wonderful collaboration. He did a phenomenal job of interpreting my vision and was not afraid to make the really bold jewelry I love—huge, crystal rings and the heavy, 18-karat yellow-gold Sutra link bracelet that I wear every day, each link engraved with one of my favorite sutras: Harmony, Integrity, Peace, Abundance, Love, Knowledge, Laughter, and Creativity.

The business was growing so rapidly the carriage house on West Twelfth Street filled, then overflowed with staff. The DVF family had outgrown our home and we needed more room.

I bought two historic buildings on the corner of Washington and Fourteenth Street, still in the Meatpacking District. Part of the buildings had been used by John Jacob Astor as housing for his workers. It took three years to build a new six-story headquarters and studio because we were in a historic district, which I'd helped create via the first benefit I'd held on West Twelfth Street six years before. Instead of tearing the buildings down to create my new headquarters, I had to go to the land-marks commission and present a wildly expensive plan to preserve the two brick façades, gut the interior, and build from within. I even created a bedroom, however eccentric it might seem to sleep in a glass tree house on the roof. West Twelfth Street turned out to have been a wise invest-ment, despite all the resistance I'd faced. I'd bought the two carriage houses for $5 million in 1997. I sold them in 2003 for $20 million.

All this growth was boosting my confidence, which is vital to how you view opportunities. My self-assurance was reinforced in 2005 when I received the CFDA's Lifetime Achievement Award, then again when the next year I was elected president of the CFDA. Recognition by peers is the most valid recognition, and without it I doubt I would have undertaken the most audacious challenge of all, China.

"I want to be "known in China." These words topped my New Year's Resolutions on the eve of 2010, and I take resolutions seriously since New Year's Eve is also my birthday. It was a huge goal, of course, but it was a goal to make happen.

I have always been fascinated with China. I had been there many times, starting in 1989 when there were barely any cars in the streets. I had made friends in Beijing and Shanghai over the years: artists, writers, businesspeople. Suddenly everybody was looking at China as a great business opportunity, but I didn't want to be just another opportunistic brand. I wanted to understand their culture as well as explain my own. By being the face of my brand from the beginning, I'd always had a relationship with my customers, an understanding, and I wanted to do the same in China.

I had a way: the exhibit of my work, life, and art that I'd already mounted in Moscow and São Paulo to introduce myself to the markets there. Bill Katz, who designs exhibitions and interiors and is a longtime friend, suggested an extraordinary venue: Pace Beijing, the largest privately owned art gallery in the world. Arne Glimcher, the gallery's owner, enthusiastically agreed to host the show.

I was so excited. Others were not. Paula was against my China campaign; by this time Nathan had left and Yvan Mispelaere had joined as creative director. There was a lot to do, and he needed to be fully briefed and integrated into the company. Furthermore, she argued—legitimately—that it was premature to do an exhibition in China. Our presence in mainland China was limited to two stores in Beijing and one in Shanghai, and from a business perspective, mounting the exhibit wouldn't justify the huge commitment of money, time, and effort from the company. "Wait a few years until we're better established in China," Paula said. But my instinct told me the timing was right and I insisted on pressing ahead. The opening for the six-week exhibition was set for April 4, 2011.

I explained the Beijing exhibition to friends at a dinner given for me in Shanghai by Pearl Lam, the flamboyant art dealer. "What about Shanghai?" they asked. They were eager for me to do something in their city. "Give a ball," suggested Wendi Deng Murdoch, then the wife of media mogul Rupert Murdoch. "No one in China gives a ball." My Chinese friends loved the idea and so did I. "We'll call it the Red Ball," I decided.

The next day I visited the celebrated artist Zhang Huan in his cavernous pipe-factory-turned-studio in an industrial suburb of Shanghai. From the first moment, I knew it would be the perfect venue for a ball—much more interesting than any grand hotel. Zhang loved the idea, which in turn delighted the Shanghainese, who have an informal rivalry with their counterparts in Beijing. The Red Ball would be March 31, four days before the opening of the retrospective.

We expected seven hundred guests at the ball but more than a thousand came. It was a who's who of Chinese talent, including the Academy Award–winning composer Tan Dun (*Crouching Tiger, Hidden Dragon*), the multi-award-winning actress Zhang Ziyi (*Crouching Tiger, 2046*), China's beautiful top international model Du Juan, and many, many others. I wore a sequined gown with the Chinese character for love on the bodice, and I really did love that spectacular evening. So did the hordes of Chinese press. My Chinese partners, David and Linda Ting and Michael and Jess Wang, were ecstatic.

People in China are still talking about the DVF Red Ball, I am told by my friend Hung Huang, the highly influential author, blogger, the founder of the magazine *iLook* and the first Chinese designer store, BNC. Scores of masked men dressed in black manipulating red laser beams around the thirty-foot-high studio, Zhang Huan's Ming dynasty temple floating on red mist, Jin Xing's modern dance troupe snapping giant red fans in the temple and performing to kettle drums, the after-dinner disco amid spinning lights and a red glitter floor—all brilliantly designed by my friend Alex de Betak, the magician who designs the sets of my fashion shows.

I was so proud that night, especially because my entire family was with me: children and grandchildren, cousins, and Philippe who came from Belgium with his family. "What do you like best about your job, Didi?" Tatiana's daughter, Antonia, had asked me the day before the Red Ball. "What I like best about my job is the fact that I can dream of something and make it happen," I replied. That trip was even more special because Tatiana shot the DVF ad campaign and a spectacular film, both titled "Rendezvous," at Zhang Huan's studio in Shanghai.

Four days after the ball, a thousand people came to the opening at Pace Beijing. Chinese people were fascinated by my journey in New York in the seventies and the Andy Warhol portraits, such a contrast to where China was in the 1970s. I also commissioned four new portraits by leading Chinese artists, Arne Glimcher's idea.

Each time I walk into my office and see the ash painting Zhang Huan did of me, or into my library at Cloudwalk, where there's a portrait by Li Songsong, I'm glad I followed my instinct; they are masterpieces. I also achieved my New Year's Resolution. We have twenty-one stores in China and plans to open fourteen more in the next four years. And I am certainly "known." When I started working on the China project, I had no followers on Sina Weibo, China's version of Twitter. After the Red Ball and the exhibition, the numbers grew to three hundred thousand. As I write this, my followers have grown to over two million!

We were all on a high when we left China. We had succeeded beyond our wildest dreams, and the DVF team had performed magnificently. Little did I know that within three years, we'd be mounting the exhibition yet again, this time in Los Angeles. It would be different though. I'd pushed alone against my team's resistance to make the China campaign happen. When we returned to New York, I realized making those solo decisions was a bad habit. So many things had to change. It was time for the business to enter a third phase, a phase I would call The New Era. The change was not easy for any of us.

6

THE NEW ERA

The realization had begun before the trip to China. Change, both exciting and painful, was in the air. Paula and I had been like Thelma and Louise, hurtling cross-country beautifully for ten years. We were the pretty girls on the block. The brand was young again, a shining star in fifty-five countries. We had opened fifty of our own shops. We had brought the business from nothing to $200 million in sales. Now what?

My goals had shifted. No longer was I striving to be financially independent. I was. I didn't need to prove that the first time around wasn't an accident. I had. What I wanted now was to turn a good company into a great company, to leave a legacy, something that would live beyond me. I had reached the age where you begin to think about what you leave your grandchildren and their children.

I was already building a legacy outside the business. Having empowered myself, it was my duty to empower other women. That is why I got involved with Vital Voices and established the DVF Awards. It was also my turn to support the fashion and New York communities that had given me so much. In fashion, the opportunity came from the CFDA. I can't overstate how honored I was to be elected its president in 2006. *Women's Wear Daily* put my election on the front cover: "Von Furstenberg Elected: Brings Power Contacts, Jet-Set Savvy to CFDA." Steven Kolb, the new executive director, and I became a team. My first goal was to turn the organization into a family, bring in fresh blood, and make sure the more established designers helped and mentored the newer ones. Together we would have more power, more leverage than on our own. The first month I was elected, Steven and I flew to Washington, DC, to lobby Congress for copyright protection against design piracy. When we arrived that morning, our lobbyist, Liz Robbins, told us it was a bad day. Everyone was busy and we would probably spend hours waiting and meet no one. To her surprise and our delight, it turned out we had more clout than she had thought. We met with Senators Hillary Clinton, John McCain, Olympia Snow, Charles Schumer, Dianne Feinstein, and Representative Nancy Pelosi, the future Speaker. We explained the urgent need to protect our designs, posed for photos, and left excited. We have yet to pass the law, but we certainly raised the profile of design and showed mass merchants the value of hiring designers instead of simply copying them.

After the disaster of 9/11 and its effect on the New York economy, my friend Anna Wintour, the powerful editor of *Vogue*, had the idea of creating a fund to identify and promote young American designers. The CFDA/Vogue Fashion Fund was created and being part of it is one of my biggest sources of pride. Some of today's brightest talents and most successful businesses have emerged from the fund. Alexander Wang, Proenza Schouler, Rodarte, Rag and Bone, Prabal Gurung, Joseph Altuzarra, Jennifer Meyer—to name just a few—all came up through it.

CFDA is committed to promoting diversity and protecting the health and well-being of models. It supports Made in NY, an initiative spearheaded by Andrew Rosen (son of Carl who saved my business in 1979) to reenergize the local garment industry. CFDA helps develop American design talent with many scholarship programs. It also rallies in times of need. We raised over one million dollars for Haiti's earthquake relief and support the Born Free campaign to eliminate the transmission of HIV from mothers to babies.

Steven and I will never forget the day we went to City Hall to meet with the newly elected mayor Michael Bloomberg. "What can the city do for fashion?" he asked. "We need a place for our fashion shows, we need a fashion center. I would love to get one of the piers along the Hudson River," I told him presumptuously.

We never got a pier, but the mayor's deputy, Dan Doctoroff, did not forget my request. We will get a home for Fashion Week at Culture Shed, a new two-hundred-thousand-square-foot, highly flexible cultural institution, which will be a crossroads for the full range of creative industries. I joined the board of Culture Shed, which will stand at the northern end of the High Line, the immensely popular park that is the pride and joy of my family.

The High Line was the dream of Josh David and Robert Hammond, young neighbors from Chelsea and the West Village, who had the audacious idea of reversing one of Mayor Giuliani's last acts, signed a few days before he left office: a demolition order for the old elevated railroad that runs from Gansevoort Street to Thirty-Fourth Street. They wanted to recycle it into a park. My family joined in their dream and we succeeded, with the help of so many. The old railway was transformed by the amazing design work of James Corner Field Operations, Diller Scofido + Renfro, and Piet Oudolf, and opened in 2009. Millions of visitors and New Yorkers enjoy strolling along the beautiful, long green ribbon of wild flowers, shrubs, and grasses above the urban streets. I am one of them.

For all of this, Forbes named me one of the twenty most powerful businesswomen in the world! Yet my own business was moving along an uncharted path from one opportunity to another without a clear set of goals or much discipline. While we had been lulled by our remarkable growth, companies that had started only a few years before, but had a clear road map and were driven by smart marketing, were suddenly worth much more.

Our new creative director Yvan Mispelaere had just started, coming in with big credentials from Gucci, where he was head designer for women's wear. Gucci's designs and ours are very much in the same sexy seventies style so it seemed a perfect fit. He came to New York in 2010 to meet Paula and me and we hired him on the spot.

It started well, with a first "inspiration" walk through the streets of Paris. I took him to see an exhibition on Isadora Duncan at the Musée Bourdelle in the 15th Arrondissement, and decided to base our next spring collection on that. We called it "Goddess." It was modern but timeless, and very sexy. The prints were bold, the colors luminous, and I loved it. Our collaboration was well received and it seemed like a match made in heaven. After that first collection that we did together, I relinquished all of my design authority. I had China to take care of, and many projects that needed my time and energy.

As I spent more time working outside the studio, Yvan was left to run the design department. A perfectionist, he took his role very seriously. Everyone was intimidated by this European designer who came from Gucci and was changing everything. Yvan's idea was to divide the collection into a vintage group called "DVF 1974," add accessories to it, and create another, elevated, more designed line to exist by its side.

It sounded great in principle, but the problem was that every one of his many ideas was produced, resulting in too many products and eventually a lack of focus. I started to sense this when I went to Honolulu just before Thanksgiving in 2011 for the grand opening of my first store in Hawaii. The manager, Marilee, and my old friend Princess Dialta di Montereale had organized a fantastic party with the who's who of Honolulu. It was a glamorous evening, we sold a lot of clothes, and everyone was happy. But I felt something was wrong . . . the assortment of products was overwhelming, and though it looked good and was colorful, I wondered whether that kind of output could be sustained long term.

Furthermore, when I returned to New York, I found a lot of confusion. Design had taken over so completely in less than a year that it was affecting merchandising and production. Calendars and deadlines had started to lag, making everyone nervous. I was fond of Yvan, respected his talent, and knew how hard he worked. So I would come in and out, not digging into the problems but spending my time pacifying everyone and ceding more and more authority to him. More importantly, I also ignored Paula when she said the clothes were going off brand, confusing our buyers, and our customers.

Though I hadn't yet realized the full importance of DNA and staying on brand, we started taking an inventory of the brand's assets, and our first project was to reexamine the DVF monogram. Over the years, those three letters had become so familiar that even my family calls me DVF now! Our new, brilliant graphic designer, Diego Marini, played with the *V* and the *F*, opening it up and creating a flow the monogram had never had. He placed it between a scattering of lips on our shopping bag and stationery. I loved this bold, elegant new image that represents all I endorse: strength, love, and freedom.

I remember taking an early-morning helicopter from Cloudwalk to a windy runway at a deserted airport on Long Island in the summer of 2012. As we approached, I looked down to see our new monogram, gleaming, fifteen feet tall, surrounded by the huge team of Trey Laird, the advertising guru I had hired to shoot our next ad campaign. Designed to look metallic, and as tall as a house with nothing but sky above it and space beyond it, the logo was made almost surreal by the water we kept hosing across the ground. I loved that huge logo, and the images of our model for the season, Arizona Muse, posing in and around it. After the shoot I collapsed laughing into the juncture of the *V* and someone took a snapshot. I love that photo and fought to put it on the cover of this book!

It was a fun day. What wasn't fun was the disciplined process of creating a "brand book," a task Paula and Trey were insisting on. The goal of a brand book is to clarify what a brand stands for, to define one vision everyone can follow. At first I found this project an annoying and unnecessary exercise. But I soon realized how wrong I was when I had to struggle with the questions being posed. What is the brand? What does it stand for? What message does the brand project? Is the message consistent? What is the core design? What are the core colors? Who is the customer? Describe her. The answer to the last question should boil down to a few words, Trey said. A few words? How could forty years in fashion and millions of customers be encapsulated in a few words? Marketing genius Lapo Elkann, Alain's son, refers to my brand as the ultimate Love Brand. How could we explain that? The whole company was going through therapy and I was very stressed.

Trey was excited though. "The brand is you, it is your story. The European princess who comes to America with a few jersey dresses and turns them into an American Dream. Who else can claim that story? And your huge archive of prints, that also needs to be part of the brand book, it is unique." I decided to let him work it out.

The problems ran deeper than just improving branding and marketing. I wasn't a great manager and never will be. This became clear when Alexandre started to do a detailed audit and overview of the company. I was shocked to learn that he had trouble tracking the numbers. He was shocked by the casual and inefficient structure of the company, which was run as one entity without each division, wholesale and retail, having accountability and transparency. We'd grown fast and profitably yet we hadn't invested in the infrastructure. We didn't even have a proper CFO.

Alexandre's list of grievances was very long, yet he held some back because he didn't want to upset me. He kept on talking about transparency and accountability. I resented hearing those words but I knew he was right.

In all of my years in business I had never stuck to a business plan. I always followed my impulses and grew them into businesses. Some were huge successes, some were poorly executed and failed. That kind of energy gives authenticity and a human factor to a company, but it creates a lot of chaos, and chaos it was! Paula and I knew that if we were going to move into the big leagues, we would have to completely rework the structure, invest in experienced division heads and give them authority, add financing, and expand our family board with at least one member with a strong business and retail background.

Once I realized we desperately needed help on all levels of

management, I was shameless in seeking it. I had lunch with the chairman of Coach, the chairman of Calvin Klein, and Mickey Drexler, the retail superstar at J.Crew, among other professionals. They all said the same thing: Your name and your brand are so much bigger than your business. The growth potential is enormous. It was both frustrating and instructive—frustrating because they thought I was much bigger than I was, instructive because even though I had achieved a remarkable level of success and recognition, I was still acting like someone who was just starting.

"Build accessories," they told me. "It is critical to your growth and profitability." As it was, accessories were 10 percent of our sales, and ready-to-wear 90 percent, which had made our success to date even more astonishing. Still, to move into the next world we would have to close that gap.

Meeting these retail experts for lunch wasn't enough. I needed one on my team and on my board. We already had one board member from outside the family, Hamilton South, former president and CMO of Polo Ralph Lauren who now runs his own marketing and communications firm, HL Group. Besides being a loyal friend for over twenty years, Hamilton has an excellent strategic mind. I needed to find that trusted expertise in business as well.

During my hunt, I realized I knew the king of them all, Silas Chou. Silas is the wealthy superstar apparel investor based in Hong Kong who had bought Tommy Hilfiger some years before when the company was in trouble, then helped build it up successfully before taking it public. More recently, Silas had bought Michael Kors and done another IPO in 2011 for billions of dollars.

I knew Silas socially, and as I set out for my events in China, he had offered to give me a party at his home in Beijing to introduce me to everyone. It was a memorable dinner at his penthouse replica of a courtyard house, with a dramatic view of the Bird's Nest stadium and all across Beijing. He'd filled the apartment with celebrities and brought in dancers for the occasion. Silas also came to the Red Ball in Shanghai. He came to the exhibition in Beijing, and, back in New York, he came to lunch at my studio.

I was in awe of Silas's success in business, but he was too busy to join my board. Still, he was very enthusiastic. "You don't understand how valuable DVF is," he told me. "In order for you really to grow, Diane, you need a machine behind you. You could be so big."

"I have an idea," Tommy Hilfiger told me at yet another lunch. "Joel Horowitz. He was my partner and I owe him everything. You should meet him."

What I didn't know about Joel when he walked into my office a few weeks later in February 2012 was that he'd turned down one business idea after another that Tommy had proposed to him. He had worked hard with great success all his life, retired, and now he loved playing golf and living a pressure-free life in the Florida sun.

What I did know was that I liked him immediately, so immediately that the first thing I did was to hug him. I'd never met the man but there was something about the openness of his smile and his blue eyes.

Like the other industry professionals, he was shocked when I told him our numbers. He found them "unimaginably low" for a "lifestyle" designer, as he called me, with such recognition. "It should be a $2 billion business," he said.

Soon afterward I emailed him to ask if he could be on my board. "Yes," he replied, "I could." I immediately sent him the date of the next board meeting, and was taken aback when I got his reply: "I said I could, I didn't say I would." His loss, I thought and wrote him off.

It was Silas who got the relationship back on track when he invited Barry and me to dinner at his home in New York. Barry and I were leaving for India that night and I told Silas we couldn't stay for dinner but we'd drop in on our way to the plane. Silas took us into a side room. "I know you met with Joel Horowitz," he said. "He's your guy. You should have him on your board and make him a partner." "Really?" I said. Silas nodded. "Really," he said. "I'm going to see him next weekend and tell him." And that's how wonderful Joel joined the board and the company.

My son started to negotiate the contract with Joel over the phone in July of 2012 when we were at Herb Allen's annual conference in Sun Valley, Idaho. He didn't know I was sitting on the floor outside his door listening, my heart swelling with pride and gratitude that I had such a loving, smart son to represent the company and protect me. It turned out that Joel's hesitation was my invitation to be only a board member. "I don't do boards," he explained. "I'm not interested in giving general advice four times a year. I'd need to be an active partner." In the end, we agreed that Joel would invest for a small share of the company, my family would increase our investment, and Joel and I would cochair the board.

I was thrilled, and so was Alexandre, though for different reasons. I was excited about Joel's business expertise and Alexandre was excited that he would be an authority figure with the stature and respect to hold me in check. DVF was still reeling from the very expensive blunder I'd made the year before when I launched a new fragrance called Diane with a company too small and too inexperienced to market and distribute it properly. It was costing us a lot of money to terminate the contract. I'm sure I wouldn't have been allowed to sign with that company had Joel been there.

What was there when Joel arrived at DVF in August of 2012 was mayhem. Even thinking about it now is painful, and I blame myself. Myself only. Everyone was running around feeling my panic and the lack of direction. All along I had been trying to find solutions but there was never any time to stop and think; the bullet train just kept going.

It was during those terrible days just before the Spring 2013 collection that I finally had to confront another major problem: Our product had lost its identity. On one side the design department was making complicated fashion, while on the other side, to counterbalance it, merchandising was making banal commercial pieces. Everyone was working hard and doing what they thought was right, but truly none of it was on brand, and I didn't like any of it. My own history and the brand's heritage, the iconic dress, the archive of fifteen thousand prints—why weren't we focusing on those assets? What we had lost along the way was everything we had put in the "DVF 1974" capsule collection, which we then abandoned to address overproduction. I realized much, much later that that little capsule collection was truly the essence of the brand.

I remember those days as the worst time ever. I was going back and forth from my office to the design staging area as we prepared the fashion show, and getting more upset by the minute. Looking at racks and racks full of clothes that I knew were useless was wrenching. I couldn't sleep. I even cried. I couldn't quietly doubt anymore. It was so clear that the product was wrong. Only the beautiful colors—Yvan is a genius with colors—felt on brand but that was not enough. Still the show had to go on.

The unexpected gift that turned out to save that show was the debut of the wearable computer: Google Glass. Two months before, at the Sun Valley conference, the cofounder of Google, Sergey Brin, had called to me from where he was hiding behind a tree. He didn't want to be seen as he was wearing his new, very secret technology: glasses that were capable of taking pictures and videos and displaying email. There was a minicomputer on his brow! We continued to chat, and when I learned he had never been to a fashion show, I invited him and his wife to mine the following September.

As fashion week approached, Sergey called me with an intriguing offer: "What if you introduced Google Glass on the runway?" I almost fell out of my chair. I would be launching Google Glass? I thought it was a fantastic idea. My design and PR teams did not. "It's going to distract from the clothes and ruin the show," they claimed. "Wait a minute," I interrupted. "What is the main purpose of a show? To get beautiful photographs, right? Not only will we introduce this incredible technology that has never been seen, but we will be making a film that has never been made before: from the point of view of the models on the catwalk!" I also saw it as my secret weapon to turn around a show I was not feeling great about.

Indeed, it became a historic moment, especially when I grabbed Sergey from the audience to take the victory walk. The show was on every evening news broadcast around the world and the film, *DVF [through Google Glass]* was seen by millions on YouTube. Google Glass saved the day.

Yvan and I parted soon afterward. What we had to do to get the brand back on track would compromise his creativity. Joel insisted that I step back in to be the creative director and lead the designs back to our DNA. "What better person to do DVF than DVF?" he argued. Easier said than done. It took me more than a year to regain my confidence, find clarity, and slowly and painfully bring us back on brand.

One morning, my friend François-Marie Banier called me from Paris. He must have felt that I was insecure, and said something enlightening to me: "*assume-toi*," a French expression that means own yourself. What he was telling me was "Trust your own talent, learn to respect it." He was absolutely right. Though I always tell others "Dare to be you," I wasn't applying it to myself. "Make me a drawing of it, to remind me," I told him, laughing. That drawing now hangs on the wall next to my desk.

As I got much more involved in the creative process, Joel reorganized the company into divisions, with a unified team between design, merchandising, and sales, and a clear, nine-month time frame for design development. He hired a president of retail, a division head of accessories, a chief operating officer, our first chief marketing officer, and several others.

Joel also took it upon himself to ask each executive to define the DVF woman in one sentence. To his mounting frustration, he got a different answer each time, so he organized a focus session with Trey.

The goal of the daylong brainstorm was to come up with three words that exemplified DVF. Three words to identify our brand, our customer, and our designs. I was skeptical. We formed different groups and broke down words and sentences. Joel locked us in a room with coffee and pizzas so we wouldn't lose our momentum. By the end of the day I was surprised to see how many of the different groups came up with the same words: effortless, sexy, and on-the-go. Everyone applauded.

When the fog lifts, all of a sudden you see the light and everything becomes easier. Those three words brought us clarity. If it isn't effortless, if it isn't sexy, if you cannot put it in a little suitcase, it's not DVF. By the next day Joel was inundated with suggestions about what we had to do next, how to relate this definition to every facet of the business. Design and merchandising went back to edit the next collection with a new lens.

Joel's son found some old Ron Galella paparazzi pictures of me in a blur of motion, and Joel declared that's what DVF's image should be: on-the-go and caught in the moment. "She's glamorous, she's crossing the street, her hair is flying and she looks like somebody you want to be," he said. We needed to find the right model who was sophisticated and had confident body language—a girl who resembled, in a sense, the woman that I'd always wanted to become.

I turned to Edward Enninful, the talented fashion director of *W* magazine, whom I love and respect so much. "Who do you think should be in my ads?" I emailed him. Within the hour he responded with photographs of me as a young woman he'd pulled from the Internet alongside pictures of Daria Werbowy.

And there she was: a thirty-one-year-old Canadian woman of Ukrainian descent, extraordinarily beautiful and interesting-looking with long legs and wide-set blue eyes. Although she appears on the covers of *Vogue* worldwide, Daria is not your average supermodel. You never see her at parties, she is a world traveler, a hiker. She is the epitome of cool.

Daria's first DVF campaign was evocative and gritty. Night in New York. A beautiful young woman alone, confident, knowing where she is going, glancing behind her. "The images channel seventies-era paparazzi shots," wrote *Women's Wear Daily*, "with a spotlight on DVF's iconic wrap dresses." I knew we were on the right track.

As insurance that we didn't stray again, Paula brought in Stefani Greenfield, the friend who had originally brought Paula to me. Stefani, who sold Scoop in 2008 and now has her own consulting firm, understands the brand perfectly. Furthermore, she personally has a huge collection of DVF products and I was delighted to have her by our side.

Through all these transitions, many drawing from the strengths of the past and streamlining them for the future, was the unbelievable reality that in 2014 the wrap dress was turning forty! Joel called a meeting to discuss ideas for its birthday. Focusing on the wrap dress seemed a déjà vu for Paula and me. We needed to be convinced, but the young girls in marketing, and Stefani, were excited. Ideas were brought to the table: an exhibition, some collaborations.

As I started to think more and more about the dress I had created decades ago, and that was still selling, I realized I had always taken it for granted. Sometimes I even resented it when people talked about it as if it were the only thing I had ever done. Slowly but surely I began to look at it with fresh eyes and appreciated not only what it had done for me but also the value of the design itself. Effortless, sexy, and on-the-go, that little dress was very much the spirit of the brand! I decided to design a new one as an anniversary present to the original that had paid all my bills and had become part of fashion history.

In our line, we had a fit-and-flare dress that was very popular with young women, the Jeannie, named for our superstar head of production. Sleeveless, fitted stretch knit top, a flared skirt. It is simple and comfortable, sexy and effortless, easy to dress up or dress down. It quickly became a bestseller. When Victoria Beckham came to lunch at my office one day, she noticed it on a girl in the elevator and, after touching the easy stretch fabric, ordered one for herself on the spot.

If that flared skirt is so popular, I thought, I should turn it into a wrap dress. So I went to the sample room and called in Emily, the talented young woman I had discovered at the Savannah College of Art and Design when I spoke there at graduation years ago. I had noticed the simple but clever long jersey dress she had designed to wear for the occasion and offered her an internship. Emily has been working with us ever since. I told her that we would do this new wrap dress together. I explained that the top had to feel like a ballerina cover-up: tight jersey to flatter the bust and pinch the waist. For the circle skirt we chose a woven fabric that holds its shape well, but is still light.

We set to work building it and we fit it until it was perfect, just as I'd done with the first wrap dress in the factory outside Florence forty years before. I wanted to name the dress Emily, but along the way it became Amelia instead. We reissued the original snake print, the one that had danced down the runway at the Cotillion Room of the Pierre Hotel, and used it to make the new Amelia wrap. At first, our sales department did not even notice the dress; it had come so late that they barely showed it to buyers. In spite of my insecurity at the time, I forced our retail stores to buy it. I was right, Amelia was a hit, got a full page in *Vogue,* and became a bestseller! Reliving the magic with the birth of a new wrap, I became convinced. We would celebrate her fortieth birthday with pride. I was totally on board and excited when we all met again.

It was more or less at that time, as I started to regain my confidence and excitement, that Paula came to me and hinted that she wanted to leave. She was tired and felt it was time for her to look for a new horizon and new challenges. At first I refused to believe it; I always thought we were joined at the hip, that she was my partner in crime. We had built the new company. We were the Comeback Kids. "I can't imagine you not being here," I said. As she continued to discuss our separation with Joel, I slowly started to accept that she would leave.

Plans for the anniversary were accelerating. We decided to mount an exhibition and this time it would really earn its name: Journey of a Dress. It would be only about wraps: vintage wraps from the archives, current wraps, and we would create some anniversary wraps. A collaboration with Andy Warhol immediately came to my mind. What would be more DVF, more seventies yet modern than a Warhol wrap dress?

The first big decision was where to mount the exhibition. Los Angeles was my choice . . . not only is it a city I love and where both my children live, but it has the right mixture of edginess, style, and pop culture. I love the light in LA, that very light that attracted the movie industry in the 1930s, a light that reinforces colors and boldness.

I made an appointment to see Michael Govan, the dynamic leader of the Los Angeles County Museum of Art (LACMA) and husband of the equally dynamic Katharine Ross, the superstar of fashion communications—art, fashion, and culture in one couple. In the museum parking lot, I got cold feet. "What am I going to tell him? Let's cancel," I told Grace Cha, my trusted VP of global communications. "We're already here," she said, incredulous. "Let's go in." And so in we went.

Of course as soon I began talking to Michael my adrenaline started racing. I relived the success of the exhibition in Beijing and how I had commissioned Chinese artists for it. I could feel his excitement and, with nothing to lose, I asked him, "How can I make this happen within your world? Do you know of any space near LACMA that I could use?" "Maybe," he said smiling.

The old May Company department store building sits on the LACMA campus and they had been using it for storage. They had begun clearing it out as it was going to be rebuilt by mega architect Renzo Piano into the spectacular Academy Museum of Motion Pictures. "You should meet with the Academy people and ask them," Michael suggested. "The timing may very well work for you."

An old famous department store on the LACMA campus that will become the museum of the film Academy? Was I dreaming? It sounded perfect!

When I entered the movie poster–lined hallways of the Academy to meet Dawn Hudson, the CEO, and Bill Kramer, director of development for their future museum, I was determined to seduce them. I guess Dawn felt the same way. She was wearing a DVF top, which I considered a good omen. She suggested we see the space, and if we liked it, she would ask the board.

The big, gloomy storage building was divided into endless large rooms packed with crates of art. It wasn't a pretty sight but I knew my friend interior designer Bill Katz could turn this gloom into glamour. It was full speed ahead.

What I did not know is that the Warhol Museum in Pittsburgh, where I'd never been, was also planning an anniversary, its twentieth. When Eric Shiner, the director, called to invite me to participate, he mentioned that there were lots of photos of me in their archives, and it tickled my curiosity. The next night, I ran into my good friend Bob Colacello, who had been *Interview* magazine's editor in the Warhol years, and as close to Andy as anyone could be. Stars were lining up and I decided to organize a field trip to Pittsburgh with Bill Katz, his assistant Kol, and Bob so that ideas for the exhibition would start to gel. But before that, I wanted Bob to take me on a day trip to Brooklyn to visit some young local artists. He planned the day guided by Vito Schnabel, Julian Schnabel's son, who is a successful independent art curator. As we visited the Bruce High Quality Foundation and Rashid Johnson's studio, I explained Journey of a Dress, and how I wanted to incorporate young artists in it. I invited Vito to come to Pittsburgh, too.

We took off early in the morning to fit in a visit to Fallingwater, Frank Lloyd Wright's beautiful nature-intensive house that I had always wanted to see, have a picnic on the way, and end up at Andy Warhol's museum in downtown Pittsburgh. We toured the museum, marveled at the paintings, watched the movies, and ended up in the private archive rooms where Eric had pulled out all of the photos

Andy had taken of me over the years. Bob and I felt as if we were back at Warhol's Factory.

For a few weeks I continued to visit artists' studios with Vito. I commissioned Dustin Yellin to make me a sculpture the minute I entered his studio in Red Hook, Brooklyn. He had never heard of the wrap dress, so I gave him a wrap for his girlfriend. Apparently he wore it around his studio instead, seeking inspiration from my early motto: "Feel like a woman, wear a dress!" I guess it worked, because he created a stunning 3D collage of the wrap frozen midmotion without a body inside. The "dress" is made up of hundreds, probably thousands of tiny, scanned black-and-white paper images of prints and newspaper articles cut into the shape of my first link print and laminated on multiple layers of glass inside a glass case. The dress floated in what looked like an aquarium to me and was the perfect blend of art and the wrap. Finding similar concepts with other artists, however, was getting very cerebral and confusing.

"Don't make it too complicated," Bill scolded me. "This exhibition has to be about the dress and about you. The art should only be from artists who have known you, painted you, worked with you . . . it is your journey and the journey of the dress. That is what this show has to be about. Use your bold prints, honor them, paste them on the walls, on the floors! Don't be shy!" Bill is the most visually secure person I know . . . no wonder Jasper Johns, Anselm Kiefer, and Francesco Clemente don't hang a painting without his advice. I was convinced. I kissed him.

Next, we met with Stefan Beckman, who designs the magnificent sets for Marc Jacobs's runway shows, and that was when the exhibit started to find its shape: we would have a time line, an art room, and one big room with an army of mannequins. I had always said I wanted an army of wraps, like the terra-cotta army of warriors I had seen in

Xi'an, China; a huge army of mannequins wearing the wraps. We'd started that idea with a group of thirty-six in Beijing, but I wanted many more for LA. I took Stefan to the mannequin manufacturer Ralph Pucci, whose in-house sculptor proceeded to design a mannequin by studying old photos of my face. He brought them to life with high cheekbones and, at my request, strong noses. I also wanted the mannequins to have a powerful pose, and so they did, inspired by the contrapposto of Michelangelo's *David*. I went many times to check on how those mannequins were evolving, and when I was satisfied that they looked strong and fearless, I ordered 225 of them.

Stefan designed the display of the mannequins, which would be divided into five diamond-shaped pyramids: a large one in the middle and four smaller ones around it. On the floor around the diamonds would be wide stripes of six "hero" prints chosen from the archives that we now call the six sisters: the nature-inspired Twigs, the geometric Cubes and Chain Link, the Leopard and Python, and the graphic print of my Signature. They would be greatly enlarged, printed on vinyl, and run across the floor and up the walls, making the whole thing look like a flag. I was thrilled. I had always wanted us to have a flag!

Now that Bill and Kol were designing the rooms, Stefan the sets, and Pucci the mannequins, Franca Dantes, our valuable archivist, was pulling images for the time line: Diana Vreeland's 1970 letter of encouragement, early advertisements, and memorable photos of women in wraps—everyone from Madonna to Ingrid Betancourt to Michelle Obama to Cybill Shepherd in *Taxi Driver*, Penélope Cruz in *Broken Embraces*, and Amy Adams in *American Hustle*. For the art room we would send all the works by Warhol, Francesco Clemente, Anh Duong, a new work by Barbara Kruger, photos by Helmut Newton, Chuck Close, Mario Testino, Horst, Annie Leibovitz, and the contemporary works we had commissioned for China. Luisella, once my assistant and now our VP of global events and philanthropy, was working on the logistics with Jeffrey Hatfield, our production person who had done Moscow, São Paulo, and Beijing. We were almost set except I did not have the most important link: Who was going to curate the dresses? Who was going to look at our huge archives, make sense of it all, and put it in a clear presentation? I certainly could not do that nor could anyone at DVF. For us they were just a bunch of old dresses!

Serendipity presented the answer. In June 2013 I went to England with my granddaughter Antonia to her boarding school orientation day, and to celebrate the eightieth birthday of Bob Miller, the founder of Duty Free shops and my cograndparent of Talita and Tassilo. When I go to London, I often take the opportunity to meet designers, to evaluate the pool of talent available. One of them was Michael Herz, creative director for Bally Switzerland.

We had met many years before when he was still a student and had a conversation sitting outside the Victoria & Albert Museum. This time, we had tea and a pleasant chat at Claridge's. He confessed that I always appeared on his inspiration boards. I liked his humorous take on things and I loved his description of women. There was poetry in everything he said and I was intrigued. He told me he was finishing his contract and would be taking time off. "It would be fun to do a project together," I said, having no idea what the project could be.

The moment I landed back in New York, I called Michael. "I may have a project for you," I said, and I invited him to Cloudwalk for the following weekend. Maybe he could curate the exhibition.

When Michael walked into my archive room and started putting the dresses on himself, I smiled. I left him to work alone for two days, to absorb it all. His first selection was very interesting. He had pulled out dresses I hadn't seen in years. He had spent hours in the old press books, taking photos, making notes, and sketching. By the end of his stay, I knew he should curate the show. "You have three months, three months to divide the dresses into groups and make sense of it all. I want you to mix them, old ones, new ones, and show the timelessness and the relevancy of the dress. You are allowed to reissue old prints, play with scales, and design new dresses ... but it has to be seamless and effortless." He worked for one month alone and then we took two long days to go over it together.

Michael showed me the groups he wanted to do. The huge central diamond would be black-and-white dresses. "Black-and-white is perfect, but only if you mix it with colors. Black-and-white mixed with bright color, that is very DVF," I insisted. The other groups' themes were Nature, Animal, Geometric, and Pop. We rearranged them many times and he showed me sketches and the fabrics he wanted to reissue. I loved his choices. He disappeared into the sample rooms and factories for weeks. I let him do his thing, thinking I always had time to edit later.

The opening was planned for Friday, January 10, 2014, two days before the Golden Globe Awards. Eran Cohen, our new, much-needed CMO, and his team were in full planning now: construction, marketing, PR, and, last but not least, party planning.

When I went to check on the progress in early December, we met with the party planner but I was frustrated. I refused to have the party in a tent outside. I wanted the party to be inside, yet not in the exhibition. That is when I spotted an extra space adjacent to the large mannequin room and decided to convert its thirty-seven-hundred-square feet into my own Studio 54 with banquettes, mirrored columns, and disco balls!

Everything was in motion, no turning back.

Jeff and his team had started the construction after Thanksgiving and were going nonstop through all the holidays. The art was on the road, the new dresses were being made, and the old ones assembled. Franca was getting rights for the photos for the time line. Luisella, the grand conductor of it all, wanted to be on site. So she took Lensa, her adorable four-year-old daughter who is also my goddaughter, to LA to spend the holidays.

During the holiday while with my family on the boat, I kept pestering Jeffrey to send me photos. I was terrified that plastering the prints on the walls and floors would be too much. I flew back on January 2 and went straight from the plane to the museum. The space was magnificent and there was excitement in the air. The prints were on the floors and, although very bold, it looked almost neutral. I loved it.

We were still debating about the time-line gallery: pink walls? white walls? white floor? chain link floor? When Bill arrived the next day, everything crystallized. There was no more doubt. Pink walls. Chain link floor. Black and white and pink, the core colors of DVF. He started to hang the art, placed the Dustin Yellin in the middle of the time-line gallery and the original picture I had signed on the white cube in the entrance hall under the quote: "Fashion is a mysterious energy, a visual moment—impossible to predict where it goes."

Franca was sorting out the photos Bill wanted posted in the gallery. Michael was in the side rooms with dozens of interns, dressing the army of mannequins. Looking at the gallery that was shaping up, I decided that I wanted "Feel like a woman, wear a dress!" in neon right above the entrance. Jeffrey made it happen. We needed benches. He made that happen, too. As I walked through the dressed mannequins, I was in awe. I changed almost nothing of Michael's curation—except for the very central dress, at the front of the first big pyramid. I had a revelation: "We need the original black-and-white leopard!" I remembered that on my last trip to Miami, at the opening of the new Coral Gables store, a woman had walked in wearing it. I had looked at the label and confirmed that it was an original: 1974. She was very proud. "Call Adis, the Miami manager, and see if she can track that lady down. See if she will agree to lend it." She did.

Everything was ready.

Friday, January 10, 2014

I woke up early. Barry was asleep next to me, calm and reassuring. There we were, in the same bedroom where I landed thirty-nine years before. So much had happened and nothing had changed.

Before getting up, I lay still, imagining the day. A press conference was scheduled for 9:00 a.m. followed by a series of one-to-one interviews in different languages that would take most of the day. I had lined up different outfits in order to not look the same in all the photos. For the night, I had chosen a long black gown called the Geisha Wrap, a glamorous dress with dramatic sleeves and an obi sash lined in chartreuse silk.

I got up and, as I ate a bowl of pomegranate seeds, saw my face in the mirror. My eyes were puffy. Not a good start. I put on a mask and got into the steam shower. As usual, I did my own hair and waited for Sarah, the makeup artist, to arrive, though the last thing I wanted was to put on makeup. Sarah's touch was light and slowly I started to feel better.

I put on my python jacquard pants, my camouflage leopard shirt, my leather jacket, and my booties, and kissed Barry goodbye. I took the clothes I had prepared and everything I would need to survive the press day and threw it all in the car.

Off I went in my little rental Mercedes. As I drove down Sunset Boulevard, turning on Fairfax, I checked myself in the mirror and winked. As I arrived at Wilshire, I saw the huge building with large banners of my face by Warhol all around it. "Dianette," I told myself in French, "Your whole life is in that box!" I smiled.

Walking into the long time-line gallery, my clothes over my arm, I felt like the Diane who used to love walking into Studio 54 alone, feeling like a pioneer in a saloon, confident, with the desire to conquer . . . a man's life in a woman's body.

I went into the back office where, in the chaos of the last-minute preparations, I changed into a little black-and-white dress, nude fishnet stockings, and high-heeled sandals . . . feel like a woman, wear a dress!

Inside my shoe, for good luck, I scotch-taped one of my father's gold coins, the ones he smuggled into Switzerland in 1942. For a moment, I closed my eyes and I felt thankful.

Thankful to God for having saved my mother,

To my mother for giving me life,

To my children for being who they are,

To Barry for always being there for me.

I was then ready for the day, ready to honor the little dress that started it all.

Everyone came to the party. Like a cast at the end of a movie, all the actors of my life showed up.

My modern family first: Barry; my children, Alexandre and Tatiana, with their significant others; Ali Kay; Russell Steinberg; Francesca Gregorini; Alexandra and her companion, Dax. My granddaughter Antonia was unfortunately at boarding school and Leon was too small to show up, but Tassilo was there with Talita and her friends, who represented the new generation of wrap girls in their DVF/Andy Warhol dresses. My brother, Philippe, his wife, Greta, and his daughters Sarah and Kelly flew in from Belgium; Martin Muller from San Francisco; Ginevra Elkann from Rome; Olivier Gelbsmann and Hamilton South from New York; Konstantine Kakanias and Nona Summers.

TV host extraordinaire Andy Cohen and model Coco Rocha welcomed all the guests on the red carpet, and we live-streamed their arrival. California governor Jerry Brown and his wife, Anne, followed by my fashion friends Anna Wintour, André Leon Talley, and Hamish Bowles. Then came my actor friends, Gwyneth Paltrow; Raquel Welch; Demi Moore; Rooney Mara; Robin Wright and her daughter, Shauna; Tobey Maguire and his designer wife, Jennifer Meyer; Julie Delpy; Ed Norton; Seth Meyers; Allison Williams; and the Hilton sisters. Hollywood aristocracy was represented by David Geffen, Bryan Lourd, Sandy Gallin, and many more. My American friends Anderson Cooper, restaurateur Bruce Bozzi, Amazon's Jeff Bezos and his wife; CFDA's Steven Kolb; Alyse Nelson from Vital Voices; Vito Schnabel; Dustin Yellin and Bob Colacello; Linda Bird Francke. Joel Horowitz led the DVF contingent with Stefani Greenfield and many DVF executives, as well as Ellen, my loyal assistant who came back to my side as my chief of staff. My first boss, Albert Koski, and his wife,

Danièle Thompson, flew in from Paris, as did Christian Louboutin, François-Marie Banier, Martin d'Orgeval, and Johnny Pigozzi.

The exhibit was a huge success and lasted for four months. Almost 100,000 visitors, tens of thousands of posts on social media, rave reviews from all over the world. Even the most critical fashion experts loved it and acknowledged the undeniable timelessness of the dress and its infinite versatility. It was no longer just about the past, but also about the future.

It had a great impact on the business and created a demand for the wraps for yet another generation. But for all the effects it had on others, the most surprising and exciting is the effect it had on me. Seeing the body of my work in that show made me so proud and, for the first time ever, I felt totally legitimate. It propelled me into what I call the new era, the next chapter of my company that will last after me.

Like my life, my work has been a wonderful adventure. It allowed me to become the woman I wanted to be as I helped other women to feel the same. I went into it looking for confidence and spread confidence along the way.

I don't know if I have reached wisdom, but hopefully my experiences, told with all the honesty and candor I could find in my heart and in my memory, will inspire others to take their lives in their hands, be their best friends, and go for it fearlessly.

About the Author

DIANE VON FURSTENBERG first entered the fashion world in 1972 with a suitcase full of jersey dresses. Two years later, she created the wrap dress, which came to symbolize power and independence for an entire generation of women. By 1976, she had sold more than a million of the dresses and was featured on the cover of *Newsweek*. After a hiatus from fashion, Diane relaunched the iconic dress that started it all in 1997, reestablishing her company as the global luxury lifestyle brand that it is today. DVF is now sold in over fifty-five countries. In 2005, Diane received the Lifetime Achievement Award from the Council of Fashion Designers of America (CFDA) for her impact on fashion, and one year later was elected the CFDA's president, an office she continues to hold. In 2012, Diane was named the most powerful woman in fashion by *Forbes* magazine.